DICTIONARY OF

ORTHOPEDIC TERMINOLOGY

DICTIONARY OF

ORTHOPEDIC

TERMINOLOGY

Julio Gonzalez, M.D.
Saul Bernstein, M.D.
Deborah Collins

TRIAD PUBLISHING COMPANY   GAINESVILLE, FLORIDA

Library of Congress Cataloging-in-Publication Data

Gonzalez, Julio, 1964-
    Dictionary of orthopedic terminology / Julio Gonzalez, Saul Bernstein, Deborah Collins. -- 1st ed
            p. ; cm.
    ISBN: 978-0-937404-69-0
    1. Orthopedics--Dictionaries.
    I. Bernstein, Saul, 1935- II. Collins, Deborah, 1951- III. Title.
    [DNLM: 1. Orthopedics--Dictionary--English. WE 13 G643d 2008]
    RD723.G66 2008
    616.7003--dc22
                        2008011959

Published and distributed by
Triad Publishing Company
Post Office Box 13355
Gainesville, Florida 32604

*Additional copies of the Dictionary of Orthopedic Terminology
(1st ed.) are availble from the publisher by sending $29.95 per copy,
plus shipping and handling ($8 1st book, $1 each addl.) plus
Florida sales tax, if applicable. Foreign orders are payable
in U.S. funds; contact Triad for shipping charges.*

Illustration "Musculoskeletal System" reprinted with permission from The Merck Manual of Medical Information - Second Home Edition, pp. 336-337, edited by Mark H. Beers. Copyright 2003 by Merck & Co., Inc. Available at: http://www.merck.com/mmhe. Accessed Oct. 2007.

CONTENTS

Illustration: Musculoskeletal System, 6–7

Guide to the Dictionary, 8

Pronunciation Key, 9

Symbols, 9

Numbering of Digits and Joints, 9

Abbreviations & Acronyms, 11

Dictionary of Orthopedic Terminology, 17

MUSCULOSKELETAL SYSTEM

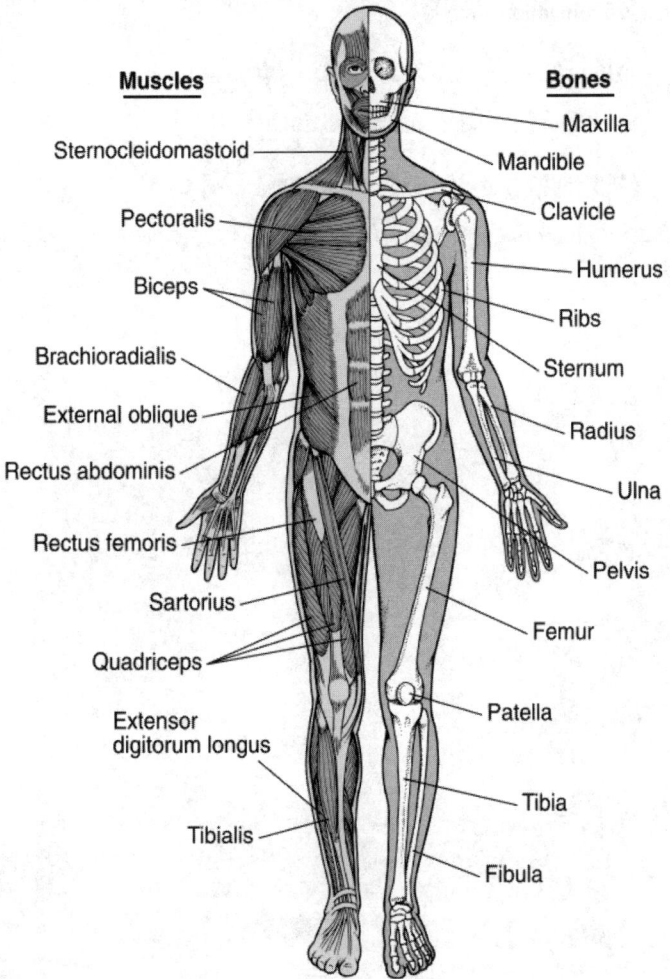

Muscles

Sternocleidomastoid

Pectoralis

Biceps

Brachioradialis

External oblique

Rectus abdominis

Rectus femoris

Sartorius

Quadriceps

Extensor
digitorum longus

Tibialis

Bones

Maxilla

Mandible

Clavicle

Humerus

Ribs

Sternum

Radius

Ulna

Pelvis

Femur

Patella

Tibia

Fibula

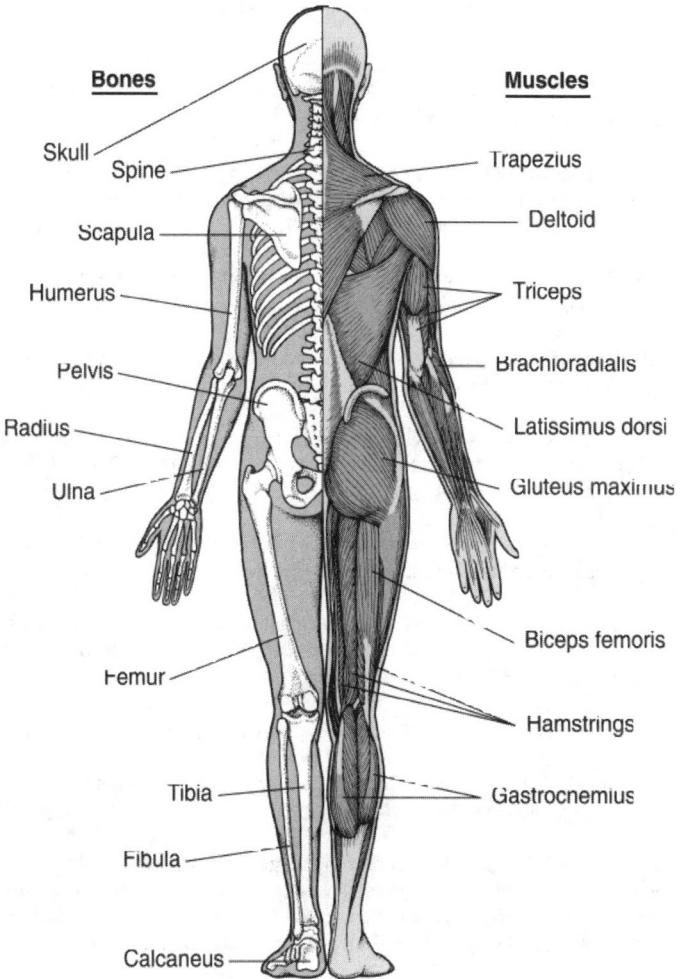

Bones

Skull

Spine

Scapula

Humerus

Pelvis

Radius

Ulna

Femur

Tibia

Fibula

Calcaneus

Muscles

Trapezius

Deltoid

Triceps

Brachioradialis

Latissimus dorsi

Gluteus maximus

Biceps femoris

Hamstrings

Gastrocnemius

GUIDE TO THE DICTIONARY

The *Dictionary of Orthopedic Terminology* is written so that a science background is not necessary for understanding the terms or their definitions. Lay language has been used wherever possible, and throughout the dictionary short clarifications are included (in parentheses) within the definitions. Sometimes, for clarity, this is reversed, with the lay word used in the definition and its clarification in parentheses.

MAIN ENTRIES, the word or phrase being defined, are printed in **bold** type and set out to the left of the margin.

SYNONYMS and words having the same application as the entry (though not necessarily the identical meaning) are printed in **bold** type alongside the entry. Most of these also have their own listings.

SUBGROUPS are listed in **bold** type and indented below main entries; subgroups apply only to main entries and not to the synonyms.

CAPITALIZATION: upper case letters are used only when the word is normally capitalized, such as for a proper name.

An ABBREVIATION for an entry follows it (in parentheses). If the abbreviation or acronym is in common usage, it may also be a main entry. A complete listing of abbreviations and acronyms precedes the dictionary listings.

CATEGORY: most listings are followed by a word or phrase printed in *italics* *(pathologic condition, surgical procedure)* that will instantly categorize it.

COMMONLY MISSPELLED WORDS are alphabetized as main entries, printed in italics: *"Incorrect spelling of (correct spelling)."* This makes it easy to find a term without knowing its spelling.

CROSS REFERENCES are minimized by providing, whenever possible, sufficient information to understand a definition within that definition. "See also" is used to indicate related information. References to other terms in the dictionary are printed in SMALL CAPITAL LETTERS.

PRONUNCIATION: phonetic spelling follows (in parentheses) entries whose pronunciation is not readily apparent. No attempt has been made to indicate fine gradations of sound by diacritical marks. The pronunciation given may not be the only correct way; there is wide variation in pronouncing medical terms.

PRONUNCIATION KEY

Accented (stressed) syllables are indicated by CAPITAL LETTERS.

Vowel sounds are pronounced as follows:

A	as in day	ay
	as in map	a + consonant (at end of syllable: aa)
	as in father	ah
E	as in see	ee
	as in net	e + consonant (at end of syllable: eh)
	as in term	ur
I	as in eye, site	i (or i + consonant + e)
	as in tin	i + consonant (at end of syllable: ih)
O	as in go	o, oh
	as in mother	uh
	as in dot	ah
	as in fog	aw
	as in do	u, oo
U	as in blue	u, oo
	as in cute	yu, yoo
	as in cut	uh
Y	as in family	ee
	as in myth	ih

SYMBOLS

♂	male
♀	female
△	change
◡	combined with
∞	infinity
>	greater than
<	less than
↑	increased
↓	decreased
1°	primary
2°	secondary

NUMBERING OF DIGITS AND JOINTS

Finger and toe joints (DIP, DP, MCP, MP, MTP, PIP, PP) are numbered as follows, with the number specifying the digit following the abbreviation for the joint (e.g., PIP IV):

Thumb = I	Great toe = 1
Index finger = II	2nd toe = 2
Long finger = III	3rd toe = 3
Ring finger = IV	4th toe = 4
Small finger = V	Pinky toe = 5

*If any word you need is not in the
Dictionary, we'd like to know, so it
can be included in the next edition.
List words as well as any comments
you'd like to make and email to
dictionary@triadpublishing.com.*

ABBREVIATIONS & ACRONYMS

The use of shortcuts in medical notation has evolved over many years. So far, there is no universally accepted list, nor is there any consistency as to the use of periods and capitalized letters. The following list has been collected from many sources and are all in common usage.

A

a	before
@	at
AA	ankle arthroplasty
AAOS	Amer. Acad. of Orthopaedic Surgeons
AARF	atlanto-axial rotary fixation
AAS	ankle arthroscopy
Ab	antibodies
ABC	aneurysmal bone cyst
AbDM	abductor digiti minimi
AbDQ	abductor digiti quinti
AbH	abductor hallucis
AbPB	abductor pollicis brevis
AbPL	abductor pollicis longus
a.c.	before meals *(ante cibum)*
ACL	anterior cruciate ligament
ACLS	advanced cardiac life support
AD	ankle disarticulation
	autosomal dominant
ad. lib.	as desired *(ad libitum)*
AFO	ankle foot orthosis
AFP	alpha-fetoprotein
AI	auto-immune
AIDS	acquired immunodeficiency syndrome
AIIS	anterior inferior iliac spine
aka	also known as
ALL	anterior longitudinal ligament
	acute lymphocytic leukemia
ALS	amyotrophic lateral sclerosis
AML	acute myelogenous leukemia
ANA	antinuclear antibodies test
ANCA	anti-neutrophil cytoplasmic antibodies
ANS	autonomic nervous system
AODM	adult onset diabetes mellitus
AP view	anterior to posterior view x-ray
AR	AIDS-related complex
	ankle replacement
	autosomal recessive
ARDS	adult respiratory distress syndrome
AS	arthroscopy
ASA	aspirin (acetylsalicylic acid)
ASAP	as soon as possible
ASC	ambulatory surgical center
ASCVD	atherosclerotic cardiovascular disease
ASIS	anterior superior iliac spine

ASSF	Assn. for Study of Internal Fixation
AV	arteriovenous
AVM	arteriovenous malformation
AVN	avascular necrosis

B

B, B/L	bilateral
BBB	blood brain barrier
	bundle branch (heart) block
BBFA	both bones forearm
BCC	basal cell carcinoma
BEA	below elbow amputation
BF	black female
b.i.d.	twice a day *(bis in die)*
BKA	below knee amputation
BL, B/L	bilateral
BM	black male; bowel movement
BMD	bone mineral density
BMP	bone morphogenic proteins
BMR	basal metabolic rate
BP	blood pressure
BR	brachioradialis
BUN	blood urea nitrogen level
Bx	biopsy

C

c	with *(cum)*
C	centigrade; cranial nerve
C	cervical vertebra (used with specific number, e.g., C1)
C1	1st cervical vertebra, the atlas
C2	2nd cervical vertebra, the axis
Ca	calcium
CA	carcinoma, cancer
CAD	coronary artery disease
caps	capsule
CAT	computeried axial tomography
CBC	complete blood count
cc	cubic centimeter
CC	chief complaint
CCU	coronary care unit
CD	Cotrel-Dubousset instrumentation
CDH	congenital dysplasia/dislocation of the hip
CEA	carcinoembryonic antigen
CE	center edge angle of Wiberg

CHF	congestive heart failure
CICU	cardiac intensive care unit
CJD	Creutzfeld-Jakob disease
CLL	chronic lymphocytic leukemia
cm	centimeter
CMC	carpometacarpal joint
CME	continuing medical education
CML	chronic myelogenous leukemia
CMT	Charcot-Marie-Tooth disease
CMV	cytomegalovirus
CN	cranial nerve
CNS	central nervous system
c/o	complains of
CO2	carbon dioxide
CP	cerebral palsy
CPK	creatinine phosphokinase
CPM	continuous passive motion
CPR	cardio-pulmonary resuscitation
CPT	current procedural terminology
CR	closed reduction
CrCl	creatinine clearance
CRPP	closed reduction and percutaneous pin fixation
C & S	culture and sensitivity
CSF	cerebrospinal fluid
CT	computerized tomography
CTD	connective tissue disease
CTR	carpal tunnel release
CTS	carpal tunnel syndrome
CTX	chemotherapy
CVA	cerebrovascular accident; stroke
CVD	cardiovascular disease
CVICU	cardiovascular intensive care unit
CW, C/W	consistent with
CXR	chest x-ray

D

D & I	debridement and irrigation
DC	discontinue
DC, D/C	discharge (from hospital/clinic/care)
DCE	distal clavicular excision
DCP	dynamic compression plate
DCR	distal clavicular resection
DDD	degenerative disc disease
DDH	developmental dysplasia of the hip
DEXA	dual x-ray absorptiometry
diam	diameter
DIP	distal interphalangeal
DJD	degenerative joint disease
dl	deciliter (100 cc)
DM	diabetes mellitus
DMD	Duchenne muscular dystrophy
DNA	deoxyribonucleic acid

DNR	do not resuscitate
DO, D/O	disociation, disorder
DOA	dead on arrival
DOB	date of birth
DP	distal phalanx (numbered 1-5)
DR	distal radius
DTR	deep tendon reflex
DTs	delirium tremens
DTR	deep tendon reflexes
DU	distal ulna
DVT	deep venous (or vein) thrombosis
DW, D/W	discussed with
Dx	diagnosis
Dz	disease

E

EBV	Epstein-Barr virus
ECG	electrocardiogram
ECRB	extensor carpi radialis brevis
ECRL	extensor carpi radialis longus
ECU	extensor carpi ulnaris
ED	emergency department
EDB	extensor digitorum brevis
EDC	extensor digitorum communis
EDL	extensor digitorum longus
EDM	extensor digiti minimi
EEG	electroencephalogram
EHB	extensor hallucis brevis
EHL	extensor hallucis longus
EHRS	electronic health record system
EI	extensor indicis
EKG	electrocardiogram
ELISA	enzyme-linked immunoabsorbent assay
EMG	electromyogram
EMR	electronic medical record
EPB	extensor pollicis brevis
EPI	epinephrine
EPL	extensor pollicis longus
ER	emergency room
ERF, ESRF	endstage renal failure
ErYAG	erbium-yttrium-aluminum-garnet laser
ESR	erythrocyte sedimentation rate
ESRD	endstage renal disease
ESRF	endstage renal failure
et	and
ETOH	ethanol alcohol
EUA	examination under anesthesia

F

FA, F/A	forearm
Fam Hx	family history
FB	foreign body

FBS	fasting blood sugar	HMSN	hereditary motor sensory neuropathy
FCR	flexor carpi radialis		
FCU	flexor carpi ulnaris	HNP	herniated nucleus pulposus
FDL	flexor digitorum longus	h/o	history of
FDP	flexor digitorum profundus	H & P	history and physical
FDS	flexor digitorum sublimus	HPI	history of present illness
	flexor digitorum superficialis	h̄r	hour
FG	fiberglass	HR	heart rate
FH	family history	HS	hip spica
FNA	fine needle aspiration	h.s.	at bedtime (hora somni)
FPL	flexor pollicis longus	HS	herpes simplex
FSH	follicle-stimulating hormone	HSV	herpes simplex virus
FT	full-time	HTN	hypertension
FTA-ABS	fluorescent treponemal antibody absorption (test for syphilis)	Hx	history
		Hz	hertz
FTSG	full thickness skin graft	HZ	herpes zoster
FTT	failure to thrive		
f/u	follow-up		
FUO	fever of unknown origin		
FWB	full weight bearing		
Fx	fracture		

I

I/A	infusion- (or irrigation-) aspiration
ICD	International Codes of Diseases
ICP	intracranial pressure
ICU	intensive care unit
I & D	incision and drainage
IDDM	insulin-dependent diabetes mellitus
IDDM I	IDDM type 1
IDDM II	IDDM type 2
IDET	intradiscal electrothermal therapy
IgA	immunoglobulin A
IgD	immunoglobulin D
IgE	immunoglobulin E
IgG	immunoglobulin G
IgM	immunoglobulin M
IHD	ischemic heart disease
IL	interleukin (+ specific no.)
IM	intramedullary; intramuscular
IO	intraosseous
IP	interphalangeal
IR	infrared
ITT	internal tibial torsion
IV	intravenous

G

GC	gonococcus
GCA	giant cell arteritis
GFR	glomerular filtration rate
GSW	gun shot wound
GTT	glucose tolerance test
Gy	Gray

J

JRA	juvenile rheumatoid arthritis
JXG	juvenile xanthogranuloma

H

h, h°	hour
HA	headache; heart attack hemiarthroplasty hydroxyapatite
HAS	hip arthroscopy
HATTS	hemoagglutination treponema (test for syphilis)
Hb	hemoglobin
HBP	high blood pressure
HCFA	Health Care Financing Administration
Hct	hematocrit
HCVD	hypertensive cardiovascular disease
HD	hip disarticulation
HDL	high-density lipoprotein
Hgb	hemoglobin
HHC	home health care
HID	herniated intervertebral disc
HIPAA	Health Insurance Portability and Accountability Act
HIV	human immunodeficiency virus
HKAFO	hip-knee-ankle foot orthosis
HKO	hinged knee orthosis hip-knee orthosis
HLA	human leukocyte antigen

K

K	potassium; degrees Kelvin
KAFO	knee-ankle-foot orthosis
KAS	knee arthroscopy
KD	knee disarticulation
KI	knee immobilizer; knee injection
KOH	potassium hydroxide
KUB	kidney-ureter-bladder x-ray
K-wire	Kirschner wire

L

L	left
	lumbar vertebra (+ specific number, e.g., L1)
LAC	long arm cast
LASER	light amplification by stimulated emission of radiation
LB	leg brace
LC	leg cast
LCDCP	low-contact dynamic compression plate
LCH	Langerhans' cell histiocytosis
LCL	lateral collateral ligament
LDL	low-density lipoprotein
LFT	liver function test
LGV	lymphogranuloma venereum
LH	luteinizing hormone
LLC	long leg cast
LLD	leg (or limb) length discrepancy
LLE	left lower extremity
LLL	left lower limb
LLQ	left lower quadrant
LLS	long leg splint
LLWC	long leg walking cast
LOC	loss of consciousness
LP	lumbar puncture
LR	lactated ringers
LS	lumbar spine, lumbosacral
L-spine	lumbar spine
LUE	left upper extremity
LUL	left upper limb
LUQ	left upper quadrant
LVH	left ventricular hypertrophy

M

Max	maximum
MC	metacarpal bone (numbered MC1-5)
MCA	middle cerebral artery
MCC	motorcycle crash
MCL	medial collateral ligament
MCP	metacarpophalangeal joint
MD	muscular dystrophy
MFH	malignant fibrosis histiocytosis
MG	myasthenia gravis
MHA-TP	microhemagglutination assay (for *Treponema pallidum*)
MI	myocardial infarction; heart attack
MICU	medical intensive care unit
MIH	mini-incision hip replacement
MIS	mini-incision surgery
MIK	mini-incision knee replacement
MMI	maximum medical improvement
mm Hg	millimeters of mercury

M/O, MØ	macrophage
MP	metacarpophalangeal joint (no. 1-5)
	metatarsophalangeal joint (no. 1-5)
	middle phalanx (numbered 1-5)
MRA	magnetic resonanance angiography
MRI	magnetic resonance imaging
MRSA	methicillin-resistant staph aureus
MS	multiple sclerosis
	muscle strength
MT	metatarsal bone (numbered 1-5)
MTP	metatarsophalangeal joint (numbered 1-5)
MVA	motor vehicle accident
MVC	motor vehicle crash

N

N/A	not applicable
Na	sodium
NaCl	sodium chloride; saline
NB	neck brace
NCV	nerve conduction velocity
NdYAG	neodymium yittrium-aluminum-garnet laser
NF	neurofibromatosis
NFI	neurofibromatosis type I
NFII	neurofibromatosis type II
NICU	neonatal intensive care unit
NIDDM	non-insulin-dependent diabetes mellitus
NKA	no known allergies
NKDA	no known drug allergies
nl	normal
nm	nanometer
nml	normal
NMR	nuclear magnetic resonance
non rep	do not repeat *(non repetatur)*
n.p.o.	nothing by mouth *(nil per os)*
NR	non-reactive
NS	normal saline
NSAID	nonsteroidal anti-inflammatory drug
NWB	non-weightbearing
N & V	nausea and vomiting
NV, N/V	nausea and vomiting

O

Ø	no; none
OA	osteoarthritis
O2	oxygen
OCRL	oculocerebrorenal dystrophy
OD	overdose
OJT	on-the-job training
OM	osteomyelitis
OR	operating room

ORIF	open reduction and internal fixation
OS	osteonecrosis
OSHA	Occupational Safety & Health Adm.
OT	occupational therapy
ØWB	no weightbearing

P

p	after (post)
p	post prandial
p.c.	after meals (post cibum)
P.A. view	posterior to anterior view x-ray
PAN	polyarteritis nodosa
PCL	posterior cruciate ligament
PCN	penicillin
PCR	polymerase chain reaction
PDR	Physicians Desk Reference
PE	physical exam; pulmonary embolus
PEMF	pulse electromagnetic field
PFFD	proximal focal femoral deficiency
PFT	pulmonary function test
pH	acidity/alkalinity of a solution
PH	past history
PHN	post herpetic neuralgia
PI	present illness
PICU	pediatric intensive care unit
PIP	proximal interphalangeal joint
PKU	phenylketonuria
PMH	past medical history
PMNs	polymorphonuclear leukocytes
PN	polyarteritis nodosa
PNS	peripheral nervous system
p.o.	by mouth (per os)
po, p/o, p-op	post-operative
polys	polymorphonuclear leukocytes
p.p.	after eating (post prandial)
PP	proximal phalanx (numbered 1-5)
PPD	purified protein derivative (tuberculin skin test)
PPDs	packs per day (tobacco use)
PPM	parts per million
PPN	peripheral parenteral nutrition
prn	as needed (pro re nata)
pt	patient
PT	physical therapy, physiotherapy prothrombin time
PTA	prior to admission
PDB	patellar tendon bearing
PTT	partial thromboplastin time posterior tibial tendon
PTTD	posterior tibial tendon dysfunction
PVC	premature ventricular contraction
PVNS	pigmented villonodular synovitis

PWB	partial weightbearing
Px	prognosis; prophylaxis

Q

q.	each, every (quaque)
q2h	every 2 hours (quaque 2 hora)
q.a.m.	every day before noon (quaque ante meridiem)
q.d.	every day (quaque die)
q.h.	every hour (quaque hora)
q.h.s.	every bedtime (quaque hora somni)
q.i.d.	4 times a day (quater in die)
q.l.	as much as desired (quantum non satis)
q.n.	every night (quaque nocte)
q.n.s.	quantity not sufficient (quantum non sufficiat)
q.p.m.	every day after noon (quaque postmeridiem)
q.s.	sufficient quantity (quantum sufficiat)

R

RA	rheumatoid arthritis
RAST	radioallergosorbent test
RBBB	right bundle branch block
RBC	red blood cell, RBC count
RCR	rotator cuff repair
RCT	rotator cuff tear
RF	rheumatoid factor; renal failure
RICE	rest, ice, compression, elevation
RLE	right lower extremity
RLL	right lower limb, right lower leg
RLQ	right lower quadrant
RNA	ribonucleic acid
r/o	rule out
ROM	range of motion
ROS	review of systems
RSD	reflex sympathetic dystrophy
RT	radiation therapy
RTC	return to clinic
RTO	return to office
RUE	right upper extremity
RUL	right upper limb
RUQ	right upper quadrant
RVA	rib vertical angle
RVAD	rib vertical angle difference
RVU	relative value unit
Rx	prescription: medicine, etc.

S

s	without (sine)
SA	septic arthritis
SAC	short arm cast
SAD	subacromial decompression

SAI	subacromial injection	TEA	total elbow arthroplasty
SAS	shoulder arthroscopy	TENS	transcutaneous electrical nerve stimulation
SB	spina bifida		
sc	subcutaneous	TER	total elbow replacement
SCC, SCCA	squamous cell carcinoma	TFCC	triangular fibrocartilage complex
SCDs	sequential compression devices	TFL	tensor fascia lata
SCF	supracondylar femur	TFT	thyroid function test
SCFE	slipped capital femoral epiphysis	THA	total hip arthroplasty
SCH	supracondylar humerus	THR	total hip replacement
SD	shoulder disarticulation	TIA	transient ischemic attack
	standard deviation	t.i.d.	three times a day *(ter in die)*
SEP	sensory evoked potentials	TKA	total knee arthroplasty
SICU	surgical intensive care unit	TKR	total knee replacement
SI joint	sacroiliac joint	TLSO	thoracolumbosacral orthosis
sig	instructions *(signetur)*	TMT	tarsometatarsal
SJS	Stevens-Johnson syndrome	TNF	tumor necrosis factor
SL	scapholunate	TNTC	too numerous to count
SLAP	scapholunate advanced collapse	TPN	total parenteral nutrition
SLC	short leg cast	TS	thumb spica
SLDO	scapholunate dissociation	TTWB	toe-touch weightbearing
SLE	systemic lupus erythematosus	TW2	Tanner-Whitehouse system
SLL	scapholunate ligament	tx	treatment; therapy; traction
SLN	solution	txn	traction
SLR	straight leg raising		

U

SL splint	short leg splint	UA	urinalysis
SLWC	short leg walking cast	UBC	unicameral bone cyst
SOB	shortness of breath	UCBL	U. of Calif. Berkeley Lab. (orthosis)
SOJRA	systemic onset juvenile rheumatoid arthritis	UKA	unicondylar knee arthroplasty
		UKR	unicondylar knee replacement
soln	solution	URTI	upper respiratory tract infection
s/p	condition after *(status post)*	URI	upper respiratory tract infection
SQ	subcutaneous	US	ultrasound
SS	shoulder spica, shoulder splint spinal stenosis	UTI	urinary tract infection
		UV	ultraviolet
stat	immediately *(statim)*		

V

STD	sexually transmitted disease	VAC	vacuum assisted closure
STS	serologic test for syphylis	VDRL	Venereal Disease Research Lab
STSG	split thickness skin graft	VZV	varicella-zoster virus
subcut.	subcutaneous (under the skin)		

WYX

sub q	subcutaneous (under the skin)	w	with
SVT	superficial vein thrombosis	WB	weightbearing
Sx	surgery; symptoms; syndrome	WBAT	weightbear as tolerated
		WBC	white blood cell (count)

T

T	thoracic vertebra (used with specific number, e.g., T1)	w/o	without
		WSS	wrong-site surgery
tab	tablet	XRT	radiation therapy
TAL	tendoachilles lengthening	YAG	yittrium-aluminum-garnet laser
TAR	thrombocytopenia with absent radius	y/o, y.o.	years old
TB	tuberculosis		

abduct (ab-DUKT). *Function.* To move away from the midline of the body. See also ADDUCT.

abduction (ab-DUK-shun). *Function.* Movement away from the midline of the body. See also ADDUCTION.

abduction bar /or/ **bar splint, Denis Browne bar** /or/ **brace** /or/ **splint, Fillauer bar, Tarso abduction bar**. *Orthopedic appliance.* Metal bar that holds a pair of shoes together, to position the feet. Used to control leg rotation in infants.

abduction boot. *Orthopedic appliance.* Cast that extends from the upper thighs to the feet, with a bar between the legs to keep the hips and legs immobilized and the hips in abduction.

abductor (ab-DUK-tor). *Anatomy.* Muscle that pulls a part of the body away from the midline. Opposite: adductor.

   a. digiti minimi (AbDM) (DIJ-uh-tee MIN-ih-mee), **a. digiti quinti**: 1. Muscle in the hand that abducts the little finger. 2. Muscle in the foot that abducts the little toe.

   a. digiti quinti (AbDQ) (DIJ-uh-tee KWIN-tee): same as A. DIGITI MINIMI.

   a. hallucis (AbH) (HAL-uh-sus): muscle in foot that abducts the big toe.

   a. pollicis brevis (AbPB) (PAHL-uh-sus BREH-vus): muscle in the hand and wrist that abducts the thumb.

   a. pollicis longus (AbPL) (PAHL-uh-sus LONG-us): long muscle in the forearm that abducts the thumb.

ablate (ab-LAYT). *Function.* To remove or take away, as by radiation, chemotherapy or surgery.

ablation (ab-LAY-shun). *Process.* Removal or destruction of tissue, as by radiation, chemotherapy or surgery.

abrachia (uh-BRAY-kee-uh). *Congenital anomaly.* Absence of arms.

abrade (uh-BRAYD). *Pathologic process, treatment.* To wear away; to scrape off.

abrasion (uh-BRAY-zjuhn). *Pathologic condition.* Loss of the epidermis (top layer of skin) by mechanical action, such as by rubbing against a rough surface. See also ATTRITION, EROSION, PLANING.

abscess (AB-sess). *Pathologic condition.* Collection of pus within a localized area, surrounded by inflamed tissue.

absorptiometry (ab-sorb-she-AHM-uh-tree). *Radiologic test.* Measurement of the amount of x-ray absorption by a bone, to gain an idea of its density.

   dual x-ray a.: compares absorption to a control substance of known density. Test of choice for the diagnosis and evaluation of osteoporosis.

accessory communicating tendons. *Anatomy.* Two connective tissue bands (tendons) that are joined so that when one moves, the other also moves. Usually found between the extensor tendons of the hands and feet.

acetabular (ass-uh-TAB-yu-lur). *Anatomic description.* Refers to the acetabulum (hip joint socket).

   a. anteversion: the degree to which the opening of the acetabulum is angled toward the front of the body; generally about 15° to 25°.

   a. dysplasia (dis-PLAY-zjuh), **congenital** /or/ **developmental dysplasia of the hip**. *Pathologic condition.* Incomplete formation of the acetabulum (hip joint socket), leaving head of the femur (thighbone) partially uncovered, with less-than-normal or no cartilage contact between the femoral head and the acetabulum.

a. fossa. *See* ACETABULUM.

a. angle. Same as ACETABULAR INDEX (below).

a. index */or/* **angle, CE angle, center edge (angle of Wiberg), Wiberg angle**. *Radiologic measurement.* On a front view of the pelvis, the angle formed between a vertical line passing through the center of the femoral head and a second line from the center of the femoral head to the outer edge of the acetabulum. An angle greater than 25° is normal; less than 20° is suggestive of dysplasia.

a. retroversion. *Anatomic abnormality.* The degree to which the opening of the acetabulum is angled toward the back of the body. Usually seen in hip replacement in which the cup was placed in a less-than-ideal position (retroverted); leads to subsequent hip dislocations.

a. roof. *Anatomy.* Upper part of the acetabulum; partly covers the head of the femur (thighbone) and provides stability to the hip joint.

acetabuloplasty (ass-uh-TAB-yu-loh-plas-tee). *Surgical procedure.* Remodeling of the bony hip socket; refers to deepening the acetabulum (hip joint socket) to improve the seating of the head of the femur (thighbone), usually performed in hopes of prolonging the useful function of patient's natural hip.

acetabulum (ass-uh-TAB-yu-lum), **acetabular fossa**. *Anatomy.* Cup-shaped socket on the hipbone surface that holds the head of the femur (thighbone).

acetylsalicylic acid (aspirin). *Drug.* NSAID for treating pain and inflammation. Trade name: Aspirin (Bayer).

acheiria (uh-KI-ree-uh). 1. *Congenital anomaly.* Absence of one or both hands. 2. *Pathologic condition.* Absence of sensation in the hands; associated with hysteria.

Achilles tendon (uh-KIL-eez), **tendoachilles, heel cord**. *Anatomy.* Strong connective tissue band that joins triceps surae (calf muscles) to the calcaneus (heelbone); comprised of the tendons of the gastrocnemius and soleus muscles.

achondrodysplasia (ay-kahn-droh-dis-PLAY-zjuh). See ACHONDROPLASIA.

achondrodystrophy (ay-kahn-droh-DIS-troh-fee). See ACHONDROPLASIA.

achondroplasia (ay-kahn-droh-PLAY-zjuh), **achondrodysplasia, achondrodystrophy, chondrodystrophia fetalis, chondrodystrophy, osteosclerosis congenita, Parrot's disease**. *Congenital abnormality.* Abnormality of the growth cartilage of the extremities, resulting in a short-limbed dwarf, generally accompanied by an apparent enlargement of the front of the skull. Trunk length is normal. Hereditary.

aclasia (uh-KLAY-zee-uh), **aclasis**. *Pathologic condition.* Abnormal tissue arising from and continuous with a normal structure; example: achondroplasia.

   diaphyseal a.: imperfect formation of cancellous bone in the cartilage between the diaphysis and epiphysis.

acrocephalosyndactylia (ak-roh-sef-lo-sin-DAK-tuh-lee-uh). See ACROCEPHALOSYNDACTYLY.

acrocephalosyndactyly (ak-ro-sef-lo-sin-dak-TIL-ee-uh), **acrocephalosyndactylia, Apert's syndrome**. *Congenital abnormality.* Syndrome characterized by skull malformation, flat forehead, wide spaced eyes, depressed nose, and fusion of the fingers and toes; the jaw and eyes may protrude.

acromegaly (AK-ro-meg-uh-lee). *Pathologic condition.* Disorder marked by progressive bone enlargement in the head, face, hands and feet, due to abnormal secretion of growth hormones in the pituitary gland.

acromium (uh-KRO-mee-un), **acromium process**. *Anatomy.* Finger-like projection from the shoulderblade (scapula); forms the roof (bony ceiling) of the shoulder.

acromionectomy (uh-kroh-mee-uh-NEK-tuh-mee). *Surgical procedure.* Full or partial removal of the acromium (outer end of shoulderblade), usually for chronic irritation against the head of the humerus (upper armbone).

Actron. *Drug.* A trade name of ketoprofen, NSAID for treating pain and inflammation.

acute. *Description.* Of sudden or recent onset. See also CHRONIC.

acute idiopathic polyneuritis, Guillain-Barre syndrome. *Pathologic condition.* Viral syndrome that affects the central nervous system; rapid onset, results in progressive paralysis.

adactyly (uh-DAK-tuh-lee). *Congenital anomaly.* Absence of fingers or toes.

adamantinoma (ad-uh-man-tuh-NOH-muh), **ameloblastoma.** *Pathologic condition.* Rare, slow-growing bone tumor, usually in the tibia (shinbone) or jaw bone. Generally benign, but may metastasize.

adaptive equipment, assisting device. *Orthopedic device.* Any device (e.g., wheelchair) used to help an individual attain highest functioning capability.

adduct (ad-DUKT). *Function.* To move toward the midline of the body. Opposite: abduct.

adduction (ad-DUK-shun). *Function.* Movement toward the midline of the body. Opposite: abduction.

adductor (ad-DUK-tor). *Anatomy.* Muscle that pulls a part of the body toward the midline. Opposite: abductor.
  a. brevus: muscle in the thigh that adducts, flexes and rotates the thigh.
  a. hallucis: muscle in the foot that moves big toe toward midline of foot.
  a. longus: muscle in thigh that adducts, flexes and rotates the hip joint.
  a. magnus: muscle in thigh that adducts, rotates and extends the thigh.
  a. pectineus: muscle in the thigh that adducts and flexes the thigh.
  a. pollicis: muscle in the hand that adducts the thumb.

adhesion (ad-HEE-zjun). *Pathologic condition.* 1. Sticking together of two surfaces; may be united by growth or the formation of fibrous tissue resulting from an inflammatory process or injury. 2. The newly formed uniting tissue; the union of wound edges.

adhesive capsulitis, frozen shoulder. *Pathologic condition.* A shoulder that is stiff and painful to move. The patient refuses to move the arm, leading to fibrosis (scar tissue) and markedly reduced motion that is difficult to regain.

adiposogenital dystrophy, dystrophia adiposogenitalis, Frölich's syndrome, Launois-Cleret syndrome. *Pathologic condition.* Obesity and delayed secondary sexual characteristics, sometimes seen with a pituitary tumor; occasionally associated with slipped capital femoral epiphysis.

advancement flap, Atasoy. *Surgical technique.* Triangular flap of skin moved from an adjacent area to cover an amputated fingertip.

Advil. *Drug.* A trade name of ibuprofen, NSAID for treating pain and inflammation.

Albers-Schönberg disease, chalk bones, ivory bones, marble bones, osteopetrosis, osteosclerosis fragilis. *Pathologic condition.* Rare disorder characterized by extreme density and fragility of the bones, and obliteration of the marrow spaces. Symptoms include pathologic fractures, osteomyelitis of the mandible, cranial nerve palsy, enlargement of spleen and liver, severe anemia, and possible deafness and blindness. Hereditary.

Albright's disease /or/ syndrome, Albright-McCune /or/ McCune-Albright disease /or/ syndrome, polyostotic fibrous dysplasia. *Congenital disorder.* Syndrome characterized by multiple skin lesions (cafe-au-lait spots), endocrine abnormalities (especially precocious puberty) and multiple fibrous dysplasia lesions.

**Albright's hereditary osteodystrophy, pseudohypoparathyroidism, Sea-
bright Bantam syndrome**. *Pathologic condition*. Syndrome characterized by resistance to the effects of parathyroid hormone; includes small
stature, obesity, mental deficiency, delayed teeth formation, short
metacarpals with a relatively long index finger, and tendency to develop
cataracts. Calcification of the basal ganglia of the brain, hypocalcemia,
and hyperphosphatemia may occur. May be hereditary.

Aleve. *Drug*. A trade name of naproxen, NSAID for treating pain and inflammation.

-algia. *Suffix*. Pain (arthralgia: pain in a joint).

Allis sign. *Clinical sign*. Seen in fractures of the neck of the femur (thighbone).
A finger pressed forcibly between the trochanter of the femur and the iliac
crest will sink deeper into the muscle on a fractured hip than it will on a
normal hip.

Allis test, Galeazzi sign. *Clinical test/sign*. For determining hip dislocation or
limb length discrepancy in an infant. Patient lies on back, both knees
bent and feet on the table; knee is noticeably lower on the side with a dislocation or shortening.

    reverse: used to evaluate leg length discrepancy and help determine
whether the femur (thighbone) or tibia (shinbone) is responsible for the
shortening. After Allis test is done, the patient is moved onto prone position (face down), with knees and ankles bent 90°. If one knee sits farther
down the table than the other, it indicates that the discrepancy stems
from the femur, and if one ankle sits higher than the other, it indicates the
discrepancy stems from the tibia.

Allman classification. *Fracture classification*. Groups pediatric clavicle fractures into three major types.

allograft (AL-oh-graft), **homograft**. *Surgical implant*. Tissue transferred to a
member of the same species, e.g., human to human. May be from anoth-
er individual or a cadaver. See also AUTOGENOUS GRAFT.

alpha-fetoprotein (AFP) (fee-toh-PROH-teen). *Blood test*. Protein found in
blood and amniotic fluid; elevated concentrations can be found in multiple conditions identifiable while still in utero, including spinal bifida, open
neural tube defects, Down syndrome or certain cancers.

ALS. Abbreviation for AMYOTROPHIC LATERAL SCLEROSIS.

ambulation. *Function*. Walking or moving about freely.

    classification scheme: grading system for documenting a patient's
ability to walk; mostly used in reference to lower extremity amputations. K-
0, nonambulatory; K-1, household ambulation; K-2, limited community
ambulation; K-3, unlimited community ambulation; K-4, ambulate without
significant limitation.

amelia. *Congenital abnormality*. Congenital absence of the extremities.

ameloblastoma (am-uh-loh-blas-TOH-muh). See ADAMANTINOMA.

amniotic band /or/ **groove, annular band, ring constriction**.*Congenital
abnormality*. Constricting ring produced by thin band of amniotic membrane that may encircle an arm, leg or digit in utero; may be so deep as to
sever blood vessels and nerves. See also STREETER'S DYSPLASIA.

amphiarthrosis (am-fee-ahr-THROH-sus). See AMPHIARTHROTIC JOINT.

amphiarthrotic joint (am-fee-ahr-THRAH-tik), **amphiarthrosis, juncturae
cartilaginae, slightly moveable articulations**. *Anatomy*. Type of synarthrosis (nonmobile joint). Called a symphysis if the bones are connected
by flattened disks of fibrocartilage (e.g., the symphysis pubis connecting the
two pubic bones at the front of the pelvis), or a syndesmosis (if connected
by an interosseous ligament).

amputation. *Surgical procedure*. Removal of a part of the body. See also DIS-
ARTICULATION.

Chopart a.: removal of the foot at the midtarsal joint.

cineplastic a. (sin-uh-PLAS-tik): amputation with preparation of the
stump for suspending and activating a prosthesis with straps; most frequently in the arm. Alternate spelling: kineplastic.

closed a.: the amputation site is covered by skin.

forequarter a.: removal of arm through the shoulder.

guillotine a. (GEE-yoh-teen): removal of an extremity, cutting the
muscle, skin, and bone at the same level; the wound is left open.

interscapulothoracic a.: same as FOREQUARTER AMPUTATION (above).

Lisfranc a.: removal of the foot through the tarsometatarsal joint.

Littlewood technique: same as FOREQUARTER (above).

open a.: amputation site is left open to allow for drainage, with a
dressing covering the soft tissues and bone.

amyloid (AM-ih-loyd). *Biologic substance*. Protein polysaccharide deposited
in organ tissues in certain pathologic conditions.

amyloidosis (am-ih-loy-DOH-sus). *Pathologic condition*. Condition characterized by accumulation of deposits of amyloid (protein-like material) in organ
tissues, e.g., skin, lungs, tongue, intestinal tract, kidneys. Associated with
chronic diseases such as multiple myeloma.

amyoplasia congenita (uh-mi-oh-PLAY-zjuh kuhn-JEN-ih-tuh), **arthrogryposis multiplex congenita**. *Congenital abnormality*. Most often recognized
of the congenital contracture syndromes (arthropryposis); characterized by
featureless, tubular joints with significant stiffness. Etiology unknown.

amyotonia (uh-mi-oh-TOH-nee-uh). *Abnormal condition*. Deficiency or lack
of muscle tone.

a. congenita (kun-JEN-uh-tuh), **benign myotonia congenita,
Oppenheim's syndrome**: rare disorder affecting newborns; characterized
by muscle weakness and decreased muscle tone. Normal lab data and
imaging studies; apparent normal alertness. Usually improves spontaneously. See also FLOPPY BABY SYNDROME.

amyotrophic lateral sclerosis (ALS) (uh-mi-oh-TROH-fik), **Charcot's disease,
Lou Gehrig disease, motor neuron disease**. *Pathologic condition*. Progressive degenerative disease of the spinal cord nerves that control motor
function (muscles); leads to gait and motor abnormalities and eventually death.

amyotrophy. *Pathologic condition*. Muscle atrophy or wasting.

a. neuralgica: muscle atrophy or wasting resulting from nerve injury.

analgesia (an-ul-JEE-zee-uh). *Treatment*. Reduced sensitivity to pain while
conscious.

analgesic, analgetic (an-ul-JEE-sik, an-ul-JEH-tik). *Drug*. Medication that reduces pain, e.g., aspirin.

Anapron. *Drug*. A trade name of naproxen, NSAID for treating pain and inflammation.

anastomosis (an-ass-tuh-MOH-sus). *Surgical procedure*. 1. The connecting
of two tubular structures such as blood vessels or intestines. 2. The result
of the procedure.

anatomic ankle ligamentous construction, Bröstrom procedure. *Surgical
procedure*. Technique for repair of ankle ligaments after sprain or injury.
Involves supplementing the repair with a rotational flap from the extensor
retinaculum.

anatomic position. *Anatomic description*. Convention for anatomic reference:
body is erect, facing forward, with arms at the sides, palms facing forward.

Anderson classification. *Fracture classification*. Describes osteochondral lesions of the talar dome (rounded part of the talus).

anencephaly (an-en-SEF-uh-lee). *Congenital anomaly*. Severe failure of brain development with associated skull malformation.

anesthesia. *Treatment*. Loss of sensation, usually from disease or from anesthetic drugs that decrease sensitivity to pain.

anesthetic. *Drug*. Medication that temporarily removes sensation, including pain.

    general: affects entire body, with loss of consciousness.

    local: affects a part of the body without loss of consciousness; may be regional or topical.

    regional: affects an area of the body.

    topical: applied directly to the surface of an area; affects only that area.

aneurysmal bone cyst (ABC) (an-yur-IZ-mul). *Pathologic condition*. Benign bone tumor containing abnormal anastamosing (communicating) hollow spaces filled with blood. Thin bony walls result in a balloon-like appearance.

angiogram (AN-jee-oh-gram). *Radiologic test*. X-ray study of the blood vessels after injection of a radiopaque dye. See also ARTERIOGRAM.

angiography (an-jee-AH-gruh-fee). *Radiologic test*. X-ray study of the blood vessels after injection of a radiopaque dye.

angiolipoma (an-jee-oh-li-POH-muh). *Pathologic condition*. Benign tumor of fat and blood vessels seen as a nodule below the skin.

angioma (an-jee-OH-muh). *Pathologic condition*. Benign tumor composed of tiny blood vessels or lymph channels. Frequently visible on the skin.

angiomatosis of bone (an-gee-oh-muh-TOH-sus). *Pathologic condition*. Multiple angiomas (benign tumors) within a bone.

angiomyolipoma (AN-jee-oh-MI-oh-li-POH-muh). *Pathologic condition*. Benign tumor of fatty tissue containing muscle cells and tiny blood vessels.

angiosarcoma (an-jee-oh-sahr-KOH-muh), **hemangiosarcoma**. *Pathologic condition*. Rare, malignant tumor arising from the cells of the inner wall of blood vessels; occurs most often in skin, soft tissue, breast or liver.

angle of Wiberg, **acetabular angle** /or/ **index**, **CE angle, center edge** /or/ **Wiberg angle**. *Radiologic measurement*. On a front view of the pelvis, angle formed between a vertical line connecting the center of the femoral head to the outside bony tip of the acetabulum (hip joint socket) and a line connecting the center of the femoral head with outer edge of the acetabulum. An angle greater than 25° is normal; less than 20° is suggestive of dysplasia.

angulated fracture. *Pathologic condition*. Broken bone bent at point of fracture.

angulation deformity. *Pathologic condition*. An abnormal bend in a structure; generally refers to a long bone having a change from normal alignment.

anisomelia (an-i-soh-MEEL-yuh). *Congenital abnormality*. Inequality of limb lengths, e.g., right leg longer than left leg.

ankle (ANG-kuhl). *Anatomy*. Joint between the foot and the leg; area where the leg and the foot articulate (loosely connect).

ankylosing spondylitis (an-kil-OH-sing spahn-dih-LI-tus), **Bechterew's disease**, **Marie-Strumpell disease**, **rheumatoid spondylitis**. *Pathologic condition*. Autoimmune connective tissue disorder resulting in the gradual fusion of the joints between vertebrae; causes severe limitation of spinal motion, with back and hip pain.

ankylosis (an-kil-OH-sus). *Pathologic condition*. Fusion or stiffening of a joint, by disease or surgery. May also be congenital.

    artificial: surgical fusion of a joint by removing the cartilage and compressing the joint surfaces allowing the bones on either side of the joint to heal together into one bone; eliminates motion.

bony: abnormal bone growth that crosses a joint, preventing motion.

annular (AN-yu-lur). *Anatomic description.* Circular, ring-shaped.

> **a. band**. See AMNIOTIC BAND.

> **a. groove**. See AMNIOTIC BAND.

> **a. ligament**. *Anatomy.* 1. One of many connective tissue bands that surround the wrist, elbow or ankle joint, or the flexor tendons of the fingers. 2. At the elbow joint, the ring-shaped cartilage that surrounds the radial head (bone on thumb side of forearm), helping to keep it from dislocating.

annulus (AN-yu-lus). *Anatomy.* A ring-shaped or circular structure. Pl. -li, -luses.

> **a. fibrosis** (fi-BRO-sus): ring of fibrous tissue that encloses a vertebral disc.

> > **rupture**. *Pathologic condition.* Tear in the annulus fibrosis; may result in a herniated disc (disc extruding through the tear and causing pressure on the nerve root).

anomalous (uh-NAHM-uh-lus). *Anatomic description.* Deviating from normal, as of a body part or function.

anomaly (uh-NAHM-uh-lee). *Pathologic condition.* Any body part or condition that is different from normal in appearance or function. Example: absence of a hand.

Ansaid. *Drug.* A trade name of flurbiprofen, NSAID for treating pain and inflammation.

antalgic gait (an-TAL-jik). *Pathologic condition.* Characteristic limp that occurs when an individual shortens the duration of weightbearing on the involved leg because of pain.

antebrachial cutaneous nerves (an-tee-BRAY-kee-ul kyu-TAY-nee-us). *Anatomy.* Superficial nerves supplying sensation to inner surface of the arm and hand.

antebrachium (an-tee-BRAY-kee-um), **forearm**. *Anatomy.* The part of the arm between the elbow and wrist; comprised of two bones, radius and ulna.

antecubital (an-tee-KYU-bih-tul). *Anatomy.* Pertaining to the front of the elbow.

> **a. fossa** (FAH-suh): front part of elbow where the crease forms. Contains biceps tendon, median nerve, brachial artery, and other structures.

antecubitus (an-tee-KYU-bih-tuss). *Anatomy.* Inner or front surface of the forearm.

anterior, ventral. *Anatomic location.* The front of the body or body part in the anatomic position; the anterior surface of the hand is the palm. Opposite: posterior, dorsal.

anterior cord syndrome. *Pathologic condition.* Paralysis from trauma to the spinal cord; sensation remains intact.

anterior cruciate ligament (ACL) (KRU-shee-ut). *Anatomy.* Connective tissue band connecting the femur (thighbone) to the top of the tibia (shinbone) across the knee joint; prevents the tibia from slipping forward on the femur.

> **rupture/tear**. *Pathologic conditon.* A tearing of the ACL.

> **sprain**. *Pathologic conditon.* Stretching of the ACL without actual rupture.

anterior drawer sign/test. *Clinical test.* For determining whether the anterior cruciate ligament is torn. With the knee flexed 90°, the tibia (shinbone) pulled forward. Excessive motion indicates that the ligament is torn.

anterior horn cell, motor neuron. *Anatomy.* Cell located in the front side of the spinal cord; innervates muscles.

> **disease**. *Pathologic condition.* Viral disease involving the anterior horn cells; leads to paralysis of muscles supplied by those cells. Example: polio.

anterior inferior iliac spine (AIIS). *Anatomy.* Front, lower edge of the iliac wing of the pelvis. See also ANTERIOR SUPERIOR ILIAC SPINE.

anterior longitudinal ligament (ALL). *Anatomy.* Tight connective tissue band within the front surfaces of vertebral bodies, securing them to each other.

anterior scalene (skay-LEEN), **scalenus anticus** /or/ **anterior**. *Anatomy.* Muscle that elevates the clavicle (collarbone) and bends the neck. Attaches from the transverse processes of the cervical vertebrae to the clavicle.

anterior spinal artery syndrome, Beck's syndrome. *Pathologic condition.* Occlusion (blocking) of the anterior spinal artery of the spinal cord, leading to motor abnormalities without sensory impairment.

anterior spinal cord. *Anatomy.* The front portion of the spinal cord, through which traverse the motor nerves to the extremities.

anterior superior iliac spine (ASIS). *Anatomy.* Front, upper edge of the iliac wing of the pelvis. See also ANTERIOR INFERIOR ILIAC SPINE.

anterior tibial artery. *Anatomy.* Continuation of the popliteal artery to supply the front of the lower leg and the knee joint. Continues to become the dorsalis pedis artery.

anterior tibial nerve, deep peroneal nerve. *Anatomy.* Branch of the common peroneal nerve that travels around the back of the fibula (smaller lower leg bone) and innervates muscles at the front of the leg and the area between the first and second toes and the skin at the dorsum of the foot.

anterolateral. *Anatomic location.* In front of and to the outer side.

anteromedial. *Anatomic location.* In front of and toward the center.

anteversion (an-tee-VUR-zjun). *Anatomic description.* Forward rotation of a structure relative to the rest of the body. Most commonly refers to the acetabulum (hip socket) or neck of the femur (thighbone).

> **femoral a.:** arterior rotation of the neck of the femur about its long axis.

antibiotic. *Drug.* Medication designed to act against a bacterial organism that is causing or may cause an infection. Generally derived from a mold or bacteria.

antibody. *Biologic chemical.* Immunoglobulin (immune system protein) produced by the body in response to a specific foreign antigen, which is then available to neutralize, inhibit or destroy that antigen. Part of the body's immune system.

anticoagulant (an-ti-koh-AG-yu-lunt). *Drug.* Substance that slows or prevents blood clotting. Example: heparin, warfarin.

antigen (AN-tuh-jun). *Biologic chemical.* Any substance (usually a bacteria or virus from outside the body) that the body recognizes as foreign; stimulates production of antibodies.

anti-inflammatory agent. *Drug.* Reduces redness, swelling and pain associated with inflammation without eliminating the causative agent. Example: aspirin.

antinuclear antibody (an-ti-NU-klee-ur). *Biologic chemical.* Immune system protein that has an affinity for or reacts with the cell nucleus.

antisepsis. *Germicidal process.* Counteracting or preventing infection.

antiseptic. *Chemical.* Substance that can prevent or ward off infection by halting the growth of or killing the infecting organism.

anular. Incorrect spelling of ANNULAR.

anulus. Incorrect spelling of ANNULUS.

AO (Arbeitsgemeinschaft für Osteosynthesefragen). *Organization.* Foundation established by a group of Swiss orthopaedic surgeons in 1958. Known in English-speaking countries as ASIF (Assn. for Study of Internal Fixation).

AO Müller classification. *Fracture classification.* Codes fractures according to anatomic location and degree of comminution (fragmentation).

AO technique. *Surgical technique*. Use of special patented screws and plates for fixation of bone.

Apert's syndrome (uh-PEHRZ), **acrocephalosyndactyly, acrocephalo-syndactylia**. *Congenital abnormality*. Syndrome characterized by skull malformation, flat forehead, wide spaced eyes, depressed nose, and fusion of the fingers and toes; the jaw and eyes may protrude.

aphalangia (ay-ful-AN-jee-uh). *Congenital anomaly*. Absence of one or more long bones of a finger or toe.

apical stitch (AY-pih-kul, AP-uh-kul). *Surgical technique*. Suture placed at the apex of a triangular skin flap or fascial flap.

aplasia (uh-PLAY-zjuh). *Congenital abnormality*. Incomplete development or absence of an organ or tissue.
> **a. of the odontoid** (oh-DAHN-toyd): partial or complete absence of the odontoid process of the axis (2nd cervical vertebra).

Apley's grind test, grinding test. *Clinical test*. Test for a meniscal tear; with patient lying face down, the knee is flexed 90° and a downward, twisting force is exerted on the leg, compressing the knee cartilage. Pain in the knee indicates tearing of the meniscus in the knee joint.

apodia (uh-POH-dee-uh). *Congenital anomaly*. Absence of one or both feet.

aponeurosis (ap-ohn-yu-ROH-sus). *Anatomy*. Wide band of connective tissue spanning between bones or attaching muscle fibers to a bone.

aponeurotic fibroma (ap-ohn-yu-RAH-tik fi-BROH-muh). *Pathologic condition*. Benign calcifying tumor within an aponeurosis in a child or adolescent; most frequently seen in hands and feet as a slow-growing and painless nodule.

apophyseal (uh-pah-fuh-SEE-ul). *Anatomic description*. Refers to an apophysis.
> **a. fracture**. *Pathologic condition*. Break in an apophysis, usually from excessive pull by a ligament or muscle.

apophysis (uh-PAH-fuh-sus). *Anatomy*. Projection or outgrowth from a bone containing its own center of ossification; not adjacent to a joint. Example: iliac crest, greater trochanter of the femur. Plural: –es.

apophysitis (uh-pah-fuh-SI-tus). *Pathologic condition*. Inflammation of an apophysis
> **proximal humeral a., little league shoulder**. *Pathologic condition*. Stress fracture of the proximal humerus (upper growth plate of armbone) caused by repetitive throwing injury.

appendicular (ap-pen-DIK-yu-lur). *Anatomic description*. Refers to the extremities of the body (arms and legs). See also AXIAL.
> **a. skeleton**: the bones of the upper and lower extremities, including those of the pelvic and shoulder girdles; forms framework for the arms and legs. See also AXIAL SKELETON.

arachnodactyly (uh-rak-noh-DAK-tuh-lee). *Pathologic condition*. Elongated fingers that resemble spider legs; seen in Marfan's syndrome. Hereditary.

arcuate (AHR-kyu-it). *Anatomic description*. Shaped like an arc or bow.
> **a. line of Shenton, Shenton's line**: on a frontal x-ray view of the pelvis or hip, an imaginary arch formed by the underside of the femoral neck and lower edge of the pubic bone. May be disrupted in dislocation or subluxation of the hip. Used to identify subtle cases of developmental dysplasia of the hip.

arm. *Anatomy*. The upper extremity; generally refers to the area between the shoulder and the elbow. See also FOREARM.

Arnold Chiari syndrome /or/ **malformation**. *Congenital abnormality*. Bulging of the hindbrain into the hole at the base of the skull, resulting in hydrocephalus (water on the brain); may result in partial paralysis of the limbs.

arteriogram (ahr-TIR-ee-o-gram). *Radiologic test*. X-ray visualization of an artery after injection of a radiopaque dye. See also ANGIOGRAM.

arteriography (ahr-tir-ee-AHG-ruh-fee). *Radiologic test.* Radiographic study of arteries. See also ANGIOGRAM, ARTERIOGRAM.

arteriosclerosis (ahr-tir-ee-oh-skler-OH-sus). *Pathologic condition.* Chronic disease characterized by thickening and hardening of arterial walls resulting in loss of elasticity; may lead to decreased blood flow. See also ATHEROSCLEROSIS.

arteriovenous (AV) (ahr-tir-ee-oh-VEE-nus). *Anatomic description.* Relating to arteries and veins.

  fistula (FIS-tyu-luh). *Pathologic condition.* Abnormal connection of an artery to a vein; leads to rapid circulation of blood and greater demand on the heart.

  malformation (AVM). *Pathologic condition.* Configuration of twisted, curved blood vessels connecting arteries directly to veins; may lead to local dysfunction and malformation, increasing the demands on the heart.

artery. *Anatomy.* Blood vessel carrying blood away from the heart.

arthralgia (ahr-THRAL-jee-uh), **arthrodynia**. *Pathologic condition.* Pain in a joint.

arthrectomy (ahr-THREK-tuh-mee). *Surgical procedure.* Excision of a joint.

arthrempyesis (ahr-threm-pi-EE-sis). *Pathologic condition.* Pus in a joint.

arthritis (ahr-THRI-tus), **arthropathy**. *Pathologic condition.* Inflammation of a joint. Usually characterized by swelling, pain and restriction of motion.

  degenerative: loss of cartilage in the joints secondary to the physical wearing down or deterioration of a joint; also called OSTEOARTHRITIS.

  gonorrheal: due to gonorrheal infection.

  gouty: associated with hyperuricemia (elevated blood uric acid levels); inflammation is caused by crystals of uric acid in the joints.

  hemophiliac: results from repeated bleeding into a joint.

  hypertrophic: form of degenerative arthritis; large segments of exostoses (bony growths) around periphery of the joint.

  infectious: caused by infection.

  juvenile rheumatoid: occurs in childhood, with muscle and joint involvement. Elevated sedimentation rate; may be accompanied by a rash and fever.

    systemic onset (SOJRA), **Still's disease**: characterized by the onset of fever, chills, joint pain, and enlarged lymph nodes and spleen.

  osteo-: same as DEGENERATIVE (above).

  psoriatic: arthritis associated with psoriasis.

  purulent: full of pus; same as INFECTIOUS (above) or SUPPURATIVE (below).

  pyogenic: caused by a bacterial infection.

  rheumatoid (RU-muh-toyd): auto-immune disease that affects connective tissue, resulting in chronic inflammation, stiffness, swelling, and destruction of many joints, especially those of hands and feet; occurs more often in women.

  septic: same as INFECTIOUS (above).

  suppurative (SUP-ur-uh-tiv): full of pus; same as PURULENT (above).

arthrocentesis (ahr-thro-sen-TEE-sus). *Surgical procedure.* Surgical puncture of a joint, as to remove fluid.

arthrodesis (ahr-thro-DEE-sus), **artificial ankylosis**, **fusion**. *Surgical procedure.* Fusion of a joint by removing the cartilage and compressing the joint surfaces, allowing the bones on either side of the joint heal together; eliminates motion. See also ANKYLOSIS.

  Brittain: technique for fusing the femur (thighbone) and pelvis from outside the hip joint to eliminate hip motion, or the ulna (smaller forearm bone) to the humerus (upper armbone) to eliminate motion of the elbow.

compression: fusing a joint by holding the bone ends on either side in compression.

John C. Wilson: extra-articular fusion of the hip joint; a large segment of bone from the ilium is inserted into a segment of bone shaved off the greater trochanter.

Hibbs: hip fusion in which the femoral head is left undisturbed within the acetabulum (hip socket) and a strip of bone is slid down from the pelvis to the proximal aspect of the femur (thighbone).

Henderson: for hip fusion, a large bone segment is taken from the lateral wing of the ilium and placed between the trochanteric area and the ilium of the hip.

pantalar (pan-TAY-lur): fusion of the ankle (talonavicular) joint (between talus and naviculum) and subtalar joint (between talus and calcaneus) into a solid mass, usually for severe arthritis of the ankle and hindfoot.

sliding, **sliding inlay graft**: a segment of bone is removed from half the joint and replaced by a bone segment slid down from the adjacent bone.

thoracoscapular: for paralysis of scapular muscles; fusing the scapula (shoulderblade) to the thoracic wall to hold the scapula in correct position.

triple: fusion of the talus (top foot bone) to the calcaneus (heelbone), the navicular to the talus, and the cuboid to the calcaneus, eliminating three joints. Used to stabilize and/or correct deformity of the foot.

arthrodia, **gliding joint** (ahr-THRO-dee-uh). *Anatomy.* Type of joint that allows only for a slight sliding motion between two bones, as in the vertebrae. See also DIARTHROSIS.

arthrodynia (ahr-thro-DIN-ee-uh). *Pathologic condition.* Pain in a joint.

arthrography (ahr-THRAH-gruh-fee). *Radiologic test.* X-ray visualization of a joint after injection of a radiopaque dye.

arthrogryposis (ahr-thro-grih-POH-sus). *Congenital abnormality.* Group of congenital conditions characterized by limited joint movement at birth.

a. multiplex congenita (kun-JEN-ih-tuh), **amyoplasia congenita**: most recognized of the congenital contracture syndromes (arthropryposes); characterized by tubular joints with significant stiffness. Etiology unknown.

arthrokatadysis (ahr-throh-ka-tuh-DEE-sus), **Otto disease**, **Otto pelvis**, **protrusio acetabuli**. *Pathologic condition.* Protrusion of the acetabulum (hip socket) into the pelvis.

arthrolith (AHR-thro-lith). Obsolete term for joint mice (a loose body in a joint).

arthrolysis (ahr-THRAH-luh-sus). *Treatment.* Restoration of motion in a joint, as by manipulation.

arthroneus. See ARTHROPHYMA.

arthropathy (ahr-THRAH-puh-thee). *Pathologic condition.* Any disease or disorder involving a joint.

diabetic a.: destruction of a joint following loss of sensation in some diabetics; damage may go unnoticed until changes are severe.

arthrophyma (ahr-throh-FI-muh), **arthroneus**. *Pathologic condition.* Swelling or tumor of a joint.

arthroplasty (AHR-thro-plas-tee), **joint replacement**. *Surgical procedure.* Joint reconstruction by creation of an artificial joint or by the removal or reshaping of a joint.

ankle a., ankle replacement: resurfacing of the lower end of the tibia (shinbone) and the dome of the talus (upper foot bone) with metal and plastic so as to restore painless joint motion and function.

capsular a.: invaginating (folding within itself) of the capsule (joint lining) into the joint to cover areas of degenerated cartilage.

carpometacarpal joint a. /or/ **replacement** (kahr-poh-MET-uh-kahr-pul): reconstruction of a carpometacarpal joint, by joint replacement or by insertion of fibrous tissue between joints; for relief of arthritis symptoms.

ceramic a.: hip arthroplasty in which the femoral head component is made of ceramic; believed to last longer than metal in younger patients.

Charnley total hip a.: total hip joint replacement using components for cementing into the bone; designed by Sir John Charnley.

Colonna capsular a.: for congenital hip dislocations, the acetabulum (hip socket) is enlarged and deepened to cup shape; the capsule of the hip joint is then used to cover the femoral head, to act as a spacer between it and the acetabulum.

digital a.: same as FINGER A. (below).

elbow (total), elbow replacement: resurfacing the joint surfaces of the lower end of the humerus and upper end of the olecranon with plastic and metal, to restore painless joint motion.

femoral resurfacing a.: hemiarthroplasty technique in which only a small amount of the upper end of the femur is used to support the artifical surface. Designed to preserve bone for future arthroplasties in that patient.

finger a.: resurfacing adjoining surfaces of the finger bones with metal, plastic or silicone, to restore painless joint motion and function.

Goldthwaite: resection arthroplasty of the hip; the upper end of the femur is removed, leaving the patient without a hip joint.

hemiarthroplasty: replacement of only one of the two surfaces of a joint.

hip (total) (THA), total hip replacement: replacement of both the acetabular and femoral portions of the hip joint with other materials.

knee (total), total knee replacement: replacement of the joint surfaces of the lower end of the femur and upper end of the tibia, with or without resurfacing of the patella (kneecap).

metal on metal a.: hip arthroplasty in which articulating surfaces of the head of the femur and the acetabulum are made of metal; believed to last longer in the younger patient.

partial a.: same as HEMIARTHROPLASTY (above).

resection a.: excision of a joint. See also GIRDLESTONE PROCEDURE.

shoulder a. (total), shoulder replacement: resurfacing the upper end of the humerus and glenoid, to restore painless function and motion of the joint. If only humerus is resurfaced it is called a shoulder hemiarthroplasty.

silicone a.: joint reconstruction in which the material used is silicone.

unicompartmental knee a.: replacement of the inner or outer half of the lower end of the femur and the corresponding upper end of the tibia.

arthroscope (AHR-thruh-skope). *Instrument.* An endoscope (small camera for use in the body) for examining a joint space.

arthroscopy (ahr-THRAH-skuh-pee). *Surgical procedure.* Insertion of a small lighted camera (arthroscope) into a joint, for examination and evaluation.

arthrosis (ahr-THRO-sus). *Pathologic condition.* Any form of degenerative joint pathology; term sometimes used synonymously with osteoarthritis.

arthrotomy (ahr-THRAH-tuh-mee). *Surgical procedure.* Incising a joint for exploration or for removal of infected or loose material.

articular (ahr-TIK-yu-lur). *Anatomic description.* Refers to a joint.

cartilage. *Anatomy.* The smooth lining of a mobile joint.

facet (fuh-SET). *Anatomy.* Small joint surface, such as back part of a vertebra that connects with the vertebrae above and below, allowing motion in the spinal column. Each vertebra has two superior and two inferior facets.

fracture. *Pathologic condition.* Break involving the joint surface of a bone.

articulate (ahr-TIK-yu-layt). *Function.* To connect or join.

articulation. *Anatomic description.* Area where two bones are joined together. May be a movable joint, e.g., elbow or knee (diarthrosis), slightly moveable (amphiarthrosis), or nonmobile, e.g., between cranial bones (synarthrosis).

artifact (AHR-tuh-fakt). *Test finding.* Artificial abnormality caused by a technical problem or imperfection in a test (e.g., static electrical markings on an x-ray).

artificial ankylosis, **arthrodesis**, **fusion**. *Surgical procedure.* Fusion of a joint by removing the cartilage and compressing the joint surfaces, allowing the bones on either side of the joint to heal together into one bone; eliminates motion. See also ANKYLOSIS.

artificial limb, **prosthesis**. *Orthopedic appliance.* Artificial replacement for an amputated limb.

aseptic (ay-SEP-tik). *Description.* Without bacterial contamination. Sterile. See also ANTICEPTIC.

aseptic necrosis (ay-SEP-tik nek-ROH-sus), **avascular necrosis, osteonecrosis**. *Pathologic condition.* Bone death caused by loss of circulation to a bone, with no accompanying infection.

aspirate. 1. (ASS-pur-ayt). *Procedure.* Withdrawing material (e.g., fluid, air) by suction, usually with a needle, as from a joint or body cavity. 2. (ASS-pur-it). *Body fluid.* Material that has been removed from the body through the process of aspiration.

aspiration (ass-pur-AY-shun). *Procedure.* The removal, by suction, of a substance from a joint, bone, soft tissue or body cavity.

assistive equipment /or/ **device, adaptive equipment**. *Orthopedic appliance.* Any device used for aiding an individual in attaining highest functioning capability, e.g., a wheelchair.

asthenia (ass-THEE-nee-uh). *Pathologic condition.* Weakness, lack or loss of strength; debility.

astragalar. *Anatomic description.* Referring to the talus (astragalus).

astragalus (uh-STRAG-uh-lus), **talus**. *Anatomy.* The top foot bone. Bone in the ankle between the end of the tibia (shinbone) and the calcaneus (heelbone).

asymmetric (ay-sim-MET-rik). *Anatomic description.* In describing extremities, an inequality.

asymmetry (ay-SIM-uh-tree). *Description.* Unequal parts; lacking in symmetry.

asymptomatic (ay-simp-tuh-MAT-ik). *Clinical description.* Without symptoms or not producing symptoms.

asynergia, **asynergy** (ay-sin-UR-gee-uh, ay-SIN-ur-gee). *Pathologic condition.* Lack of coordination among muscle groups resulting in body parts not acting in unison, causing abnormality in motion. Frequently occurs in cerebral palsy.

Atasoy (AT-uh-soy), **advancement flap**. *Surgical technique.* Triangular flap of skin moved from an adjacent area to cover an amputated fingertip.

ataxia (ay-TAK-see-uh). *Pathologic condition.* Absence of muscular coordination.
   cerebellar: due to injury or disease of the cerebellum; causes gross gait abnormality with frequent loss of balance.
   spinal: due to injury or disease of the spinal cord; may be associated with syphilis or diabetes.

atelectasis (at-uh-LEK-tuh-sis). *Pathologic condition.* Collapse of parts of the lung; caused by mucus plugs in the smaller bronchi or by inadequate breathing.

atherosclerosis (ATH-ur-oh-skler-OH-sus). *Pathologic condition.* Chronic disease characterized by the deposition of fatty substances in the arteries, decreasing their diameter. May lead to obstruction and loss of circulation, as occurs in heart attack and stroke. See also ARTERIOSCLEROSIS.

atlantal (at-LAN-tul). *Anatomy*. Refers to the atlas, the 1st cervical (neck) vertebra.

    a. fracture. *Pathologic condition*. Break in the 1st cervical vertebra.

atlanto-axial (at-LAN-toh-AK-see-ul). *Anatomic description*. Refers to the area between the atlas (1st cervical vertebra) and axis (2nd cervical vertebra) or the area of the spine inhabited by the atlas and axis.

    fracture. *Pathologic condition*. A break that involves the 1st and 2nd cervical (neck) vertebrae (atlas and axis).

    joint. *Anatomy*. Joint between the 1st and 2nd cervical (neck) vertebrae (atlas and axis).

    rotary fixation (AARF) /or/ **displacement** /or/ **subluxation**. *Pathologic condition*. Condition characterized by partial (subluxation) to complete dislocation of the atlanto-axial joint. Usually occurs in children and is the most common cause of childhood torticollis. Of varying severity; usually self-resolving.

atlanto-occipital (at-LAN-toh-ahk-SIP-uh-tul). *Anatomic description*. Refers to the area between the atlas (1st cervical vertebra) and the base of the skull (the occiput) or to the area inhabited by these two structures.

    joint. *Anatomy*. Junction of the 1st cervical vertebrae (atlas) and the base of the skull; enables flexion/extension of the skull on the neck.

atlas. *Anatomy*. First cervical vertebra (C1); supports the skull. See also AXIS.

atonia (uh-TOH-nee-uh). See ATONY.

atonic (uh-TAH-nik). *Pathologic description*. Limp, flaccid (referring to atony).

    a. cerebral palsy: form of cerebral palsy characterized by flaccid and limp muscles and extremities.

atony (AT-uh-nee), **atonia**. *Pathologic condition*. Absence of muscle tone; state of complete muscle relaxation or flaccidity.

atrophy (AT-roh-fee). *Pathologic condition*. Wasting away of tissue, e.g., muscle; frequently from disuse or malnutrition.

attenuate (uh-TEN-yu-ayt). *Process*. To dilute, thin, reduce or weaken.

attenuation of tendons (uh-ten-yu-AY-shun). *Pathologic condition*. Stretching or thinning of connective tissue bands; may precede complete rupture.

attrition. *Pathologic condition*. Gradual wearing away, as of tendons. See also ABRASION, EROSION, PLANING.

atypical (ay-TIH-pih-kul). *Description*. Unusual, as in a finding or appearance.

Austin-Moore prosthesis. *Orthopedic appliance*. Replacement for the head of the femur (thighbone); used in hemiarthroplasty or in total hip replacement.

autogenous graft (ah-TAH-juh-nus), **autograft**. *Surgical implant*. A patient's own tissue implanted in another area of the body. See also ALLOGRAFT.

autograft. See AUTOGENOUS GRAFT.

autologous (ah-TAH-luh-gus). *Physiologic description*. Originating from the same person.

    a. blood. Blood taken from a patient prior to surgery, for the patient's own use during surgery.

    a. graft. *Surgical implant*. Tissue taken from one portion of a person's body to be implanted into another area of the body. See also AUTOGENOUS GRAFT.

autonomic nervous system (ANS), **visceral efferent nervous system**. *Anatomy*. Part of nervous system that maintains the resting function and state of readiness of the body and organ systems. Comprised of two generally antagonistic subsystems: the sympathetic and parasympathetic nervous systems.

avascular (uh-VAS-kyu-lur). *Description.* Refers to tissue that has no blood supply; may result from disease or may be normal as in certain forms of cartilage.

    a. necrosis (neh-KROH-sus), **aseptic necrosis, osteonecrosis**. *Pathologic condition.* Bone death caused by loss of circulation to a bone.

Avila approach. *Surgical technique.* Entry to the sacroiliac joint from the front of the pelvis.

avulsion (uh-VUL-shun). *Pathologic condition.* Pulling or tearing away of a bone, ligament or tendon from its attachment.

    a. fracture: break in a bone caused by a muscle or ligament pulling its point of attachment from the bone.

axial (AK-see-ul). *Anatomic description.* 1. Refers to or situated in the head and trunk. See also APPENDICULAR. 2. Refers to the 2nd cervical vertebra (axis).

    a. compression. *Force vector.* Pressure placed at the end of a bone in the direction of its length.

    a. fracture. *Pathologic condition.* Break of the axis (2nd cervical bone).

    a. line. *Anatomic description.* Refers to the central portion of the body in the vertical direction; the midline.

    a. plane, transverse plane. *Anatomic description.* Imaginary reference plane perpendicular to the length of the body or a body part (e.g., leg).

    a. skeleton. *Anatomy.* The bones of the vertebral column, thorax and skull; forms framework for the trunk and head. See also APPENDICULAR SKELETON.

axilla (aks-IH-luh). *Anatomy.* The armpit.

axillary (AKS-uh-lehr-ee). *Anatomic description.* Refers to the armpit (axilla) region.

    a. artery. *Anatomy.* Blood vessel that passes through the armpit.

    a. block. *Surgical procedure.* Injection of an anesthetic into the axilla (armpit) region to numb a part of the arm.

    a. incision. *Surgical procedure.* Surgical cut into the axilla (armpit), exposing the humerus (upper armbone) and front and center of shoulder joint.

    a. nerve. *Anatomy.* Nerve in the axilla (armpit) that circles the outside of the humerus (upper armbone) and supplies the deltoid (shoulder muscle).

    a. roll. *Surgical appliance.* Soft cylindrical roll, placed under the patient's axilla (armpit) during surgery as patient is lying on his/her side (lateral decubitus position). Serves to protect the brachial plexus.

    a. vein. *Anatomy.* Continuation of the brachial vein as it enters into the subclavian vein in the axilla (armpit).

axis. *Anatomy.* Second cervical vertebra (C2); supports the atlas (Cl).

axon, neuraxon. *Anatomy.* The long tail of a nerve cell; conducts nerve impulses away from the cell.

axonal response (aks-OH-nul). *Function.* Electrical response of a nerve cell to stimulation.

azotemia (az-oh-TEE-mee-uh), **uremia**. *Pathologic condition.* Higher-than-normal levels of urea or other nitrogenous compounds in the blood; may result in bone depletion among many other consequences.

azotemic osteodystrophy (az-oh-TEE-mik ahs-tee-oh-DIS-troh-fee). *Pathologic condition.* Bone depletion due to excessive calcium loss through the urine. Caused by kidney dysfunction.

B

Babinski reflex /or/ **response** /or/ **sign, extensor plantar response**.
   Clinical finding. Involuntary raising of the big toe when the bottom of the foot
   is firmly stroked from heel to toe. Sometimes called a positive Babinski. May
   indicate disease of the central nervous system (brain or spinal cord).
   Normal in an infant. See also PLANTAR REFLEX.

Bachelor technique. *Surgical procedure.* Method of fusing the talus (top foot
   bone) to the calcaneus (heelbone).

bacitracin (bas-ih-TRAY-sin). *Drug.* An antibiotic.

back-knee, genu recurvatum. *Pathologic condition.* Hyperextended (back-
   ward- bending) knee joint that occurs when standing or walking; caused
   by excessively flexible knee ligaments; gives the leg a backward curvature. See also EHLERS-DANLOS SYNDROME, MARFAN'S SYNDROME.

Badgley arthrodesis (ahr-thro-DEE-sus). *Surgical procedure.* Method for
   fusing the hip joint to stabilize it.

Badgley technique. *Surgical procedure.* Method of removing a portion of the
   iliac wing (one of the pelvic bones).

Bado classification (BAY-doh). *Fracture classification.* Identifies four groups
   of Monteggia fractures (broken ulna with dislocation of the proximal end
   of the radius).

Bailey and Dubow nail. *Surgical implant.* A telescoping intramedullary nail
   used in osteotomies; for osteogenesis imperfecta.

Bailey and Dubow procedure. *Surgical procedure.* Insertion of an elongating
   metal rod to realign bowed extremities while allowing lengthening of the
   affected bone.

Baker and Hill osteotomy (ahs-tee-AH-tuh-mee). *Surgical procedure.*
   Inserting a wedge of bone into the calcaneus (heelbone) to realign a foot
   that turns out (heel valgus).

Baker cyst, popliteal cyst. *Pathologic condition.* Sac located in the popliteal
   fossa (behind knee), filled with synovial fluid leaked from the knee joint.

balanced hemivertebrae. *Congenital abnormality.* Defective vertebral column with two half-vertebrae, mirror images of each other, that balance each
   other so that the overall alignment of the spine is preserved.

balanced suspension. *Treatment.* Type of traction in which the limb is held
   by pulleys and weights suspended above the bed.

Balkan frame, trapeze frame, trapeze bed. *Orthopedic appliance.* Metal struts
   attached to a bed frame to hold a splinted limb; provides handles the
   patient can grasp to move about the bed easier.

ball-and-socket joint. *Anatomic description.* Joint comprised of the large
   round end of a long bone fitting into the hollow part of another bone, to
   make swinging and rotating movements possible. Example: hips.

ballottable (buh-LAHT-uh-bul). *Description.* Refers to bouncy feeling of tissue
   as it responds to sudden pressure of a finger, indicating an abnormal collection of fluid, e.g., in the knee joint when the patella is pressed against
   the femoral condyles in the presence of a fluid collection (effusion) and
   springs back.

ballottment (buh-LAHT-munt). *Diagnostic test.* Bouncy feeling of tissue as it
   responds to sudden pressure of a finger, indicating an abnormal collection
   of fluid. Can occur in the knee joint when the patella is pressed against the
   femoral condyles (rounded ends of thighbone) and springs back.

bamboo spine. *Radiologic finding*. Spine having the appearance of bamboo on x-ray; occurs in advanced stage of ankylosing spondylitis.

bandage. *Orthopedic appliance*. Soft dressing applied to a part of the body in order to apply compression or to cover a wound.

bandylegs. See BOWLEGS.

Bankart lesion. *Abnormal condition*. Tear in the capsule at the front of the shoulder joint occurring after anterior dislocation of the humerus (upper armbone).

Bankart procedure. *Surgical procedure*. Reattachment of the shoulder joint capsule and glenoid labrum to the front rim of the glenoid (curved surface on edge of shoulderblade).

Bankart retractor. *Surgical instrument*. For moving the shoulder so the glenoid (curved surface on edge of shoulderblade) can be visualized during surgery.

Bardinet's ligament (bahr-din-AYZ). *Anatomy*. The posterior band of the ulnar collateral ligament; joins the humerus to the ulna on the inner side of the arm.

Barlow's disease. *Pathologic condition*. Childhood form of scurvy caused by lack of vitamin C. Characterized by the weakening of the soft tissues and bones along with weakness, bleeding gums, edema, and skin ulcerations.

Barlow test. *Clinical test*. For evaluating hip dislocation in a neonate (newborn). The hips are flexed and pressure is applied to the inner thigh in an attempt to force the femoral head out of the acetabulum (hip socket). See also DEVELOPMENTAL DYSPLASIA OF THE HIP.

Barton's fracture. *Pathologic condition*. Break at distal end of the radius (larger forearm bone), palmar side, with dislocation of the distal radioulnar joint (joint between the two forearm bones).

basal (BAY-sil). See BASILAR.

baseball elbow, **javelin thrower's elbow**, **little league elbow**. *Abnormal condition*. Repetitive stress injury of the medial condyle of the humerus (upper armbone) at the elbow joint.

baseball splint. *Orthopedic appliance*. Small metal moldable splint that protects and immobilizes the distal bone of a finger in extension.

baseline film *Radiologic procedure*. X-ray taken so that later changes can be compared on subsequent x-rays.

basilar (BAA-sih-lur, BAY-sih-lur), **basal**. *Anatomic description*. Relating to the base of a structure.

    b. impression /or/ **invagination**. *Pathologic condition*. Impression caused by the weight of the head pushing down on the cervical spine and resulting in the upper elements of the spine protruding into the foramen magnum (hole at base of skull).

    b. neck fracture. *Pathologic condition*. Break in the femur (thighbone) at the junction of the neck and the shaft.

basilic vein, **vena basilica** (buh-SIL-ik). *Anatomy*. Blood vessel that extends from the back of the hand to the armpit, where it joins the axillary vein.

Batchelor-Brown extra-articular arthrodesis. See BATCHELOR TECHNIQUE.

Batchelor technique, **Batchelor-Brown extra-articular arthodesis**. *Surgical procedure*. Method of fusing the talus (top foot bone) to the calcaneus (heelbone).

Bateman modification of Mayer trapezius transfer, **Bateman procedure**. *Surgical procedure*. Moving a segment of the trapezius muscle and a small portion of the scapula (wing bone) to the humerus (upper armbone). For treating paralysis of the deltoid (shoulder) muscle.

Bateman procedure. See BATEMAN MODIFICATION OF MAYER TRAPEZIUS TRANSFER.

Bateman prosthesis. *Orthopedic appliance*. Artificial replacement for the head of the femur (thighbone).

battered baby syndrome. *Pathologic condition*. Physical injuries (e.g., fractures, hematomas, contusions) resulting from gross abuse of a baby or young child.

Baumann's angle. *Radiologic measurement*. On an A.P. (anterior to posterior) x-ray projection, the angle formed between a line drawn along the physis (growth plate) of the capitellum (rounded joint surface of humerus that articulates with radius) and a line perpendicular to long axis of the shaft of the humerus (upper armbone).

bayonet apposition. *Anatomic description*. Appearance of a long bone when the broken ends have healed in a side-by-side position; compensates for overgrowth in a child. Gives appearance of a bayonet attached to a rifle.

beach chair position, Fowler's position. *Anatomic description*. Position of a patient reclining on his/her back against a backrest with knees slightly bent.

BE amputation (BEA). *Surgical procedure*. Removing the arm below the elbow joint.

bean bag. *Orthopedic appliance*. Deflatable, pellet-filled bag used in positioning a patient during surgery. When the air is sucked out of the bag, it becomes rigid, holding the patient in the desired position.

Bechterew's disease, ankylosing spondylitis, Marie-Strumpell disease, rheumatoid spondylitis. *Pathologic condition*. Autoimmune connective tissue disorder resulting in the gradual fusion of the joints between vertebrae; causes severe limitation of spinal motion, with back and hip pain.

Becker's muscular dystrophy. *Pathologic condition*. Milder form of muscular dystrophy similar to Duchenne's. Onset in latter half of first decade of life; patients can live into adulthood.

Beck's disease. Incorrect spelling of BOECK'S DISEASE.

Beck's syndrome, anterior spinal artery syndrome. *Pathologic condition*. Occlusion of the anterior spinal artery of the spinal cord, leading to motor abnormalities without sensory impairment.

bed sore, decubitus ulcer, pressure sore. *Pathologic condition*. Break in the skin caused by pressure and immobilization.

below knee amputation (BKA). *Surgical procedure*. Removing the leg below the knee joint.

bends, caisson disease, decompression sickness, diver's disease. *Pathologic condition*. Soft tissue and bone damage caused by nitrogen bubbles forming in the blood, associated with rapid decrease in pressure; may lead to avascular necrosis of bone. Symptoms include joint pain, skin lesions, respiratory and central nervous system dysfunction. Frequently occurs in divers who do not decompress on resurfacing from a dive.

benign (buh-NINE). *Description*. Does not threaten health or life, e.g., a lesion or tumor that is not malignant.

Bennett's fracture. *Pathologic condition*. A two-piece intra-articular (joint) break at the base of the metacarpal bone in the thumb.

Berndt and Hardy's classification. *Fracture classification*. Describes degree of displacement in osteochondral injuries about the talar dome (rounded part of talus that articulates with the tibia).

Bertin ligament, Bigelow's ligament, iliofemoral ligament, Y ligament. *Anatomy*. Connective tissue band at the front of the hip connecting the iliac spine to the femur between the neck and trochanters. Reinforces and stabilizes the hip joint. See also PUBOFEMORAL LIGAMENT.

Bextra. *Drug.* A trade name of valdecoxid, a COX-2 inhibitor.

biceps (BI-ceps). *Anatomy.* Large muscle with two heads (points of origin).

> **b. brachii** (BRAY-kee-eye): large muscle with two heads at the front of the upper arm; flexes and supinates the forearm (bends elbow and rotates forearm so that the palm points up).

> **b. femoris** (FEM-ur-us): large hamstring muscle on the back of the thigh; bends the knee.

> **b. groove, bicipital groove**: groove in the upper part of the humerus that holds the tendon of the long head of the biceps brachii muscle.

> **b. tuberosity, bicipital tuberosity** (tu-bur-AH-sit-ee): protrusion (bump) on the radius where the biceps brachii tendon attaches.

biceps reflex (BI-ceps). *Clinical test.* Sudden involuntary contraction of the biceps brachii muscle in response to a tap on the biceps tendon. See DEEP TENDON REFLEXES.

biceps tendinitis (BI-ceps ten-duh-NI-tus)**, bicipital tendinitis** /or/ **tenosynovitis**. *Pathologic condition.* Inflammation of the part of the biceps tendon that rests in the bicipital groove or attaches to the forearm.

bicipital (bi-SIP-ih-tul). *Anatomy.* 1. Having two heads (points of origin). 2. Of or relating to the biceps muscle.

> **b. groove**: see BICEPS GROOVE.

> **b. tendinitis**: see BICEPS TENDINITIS.

> **b. tenosynovitis**: see BICEPS TENDINITIS.

> **b. tuberosity**: see BICEPS TUBEROSITY.

Bïer block (beer)**, intravenous block**, **intravenous regional anesthesia**. *Treatment.* Type of regional anesthesia in which pain perception is blocked by injecting anesthetic into a vein whose circulation has been blocked through the application of a tourniquet.

bifid (BI-fid). *Anatomic description.* Divided into two parts by a median cleft. See also BIPARTITE.

> **thumb**. *Congenital abnormality.* Thumb with two segments side by side.

bifurcate (BI-fur-kayt). To divide into two branches or parts. Division may be anatomical, surgical, traumatic or pathological. Example: the trachea divides into right and left main bronchi.

> **b. ligament**. *Anatomy.* Strong, Y-shaped band of connective tissue attached to upper surface of the calcaneus (heelbone) and splitting to connect with the cuboid and navicular bones.

bifurcation. *Anatomic description.* The point of division of an artery or vein.

Bigelow's ligament, Bertin /or/ **iliofemoral** /or/ **Y ligament**. *Anatomy.* Connective tissue band at the front of the hip that connects the iliac spine to the femur between the neck and trochanters. Reinforces and stabilizes the hip joint. See also PUBOFEMORAL LIGAMENT.

bilateral. *Anatomic description.* Affecting or relating to two sides.

> **b. facet subluxation** (fuh-SET sub-lux-AY-shun). *Pathologic condition.* Malalignment in both of the posterior vertebral joints (between two vertebrae).

bimalleolar fracture (bi-mal-EE-oh-lur). *Pathologic condition.* Break in both the tibial (shinbone) and fibular (smaller lower leg bone) prominences of the ankle.

biocompatible. *Characteristic.* Refers to materials that are not toxic to the body or cause immune response or rejection.

biodegradable. *Material characteristic.* Capable of being broken down into simpler chemical compounds by biological means.

biomaterial. *Surgical implant*. Substance or compound intended for surgical implanation, e.g., artificial joint.

biopsy (BI-ahp-see). 1. *Surgical procedure*. Removal of tissue or fluid for laboratory examination. 2. *Test*. Laboratory examination of tissue or fluid to determine pathology.

>**bone marrow b**: removal of bone marrow through a large needle, usually from the pelvis.

>**closed b**: obtaining tissue without opening the tissue or skin; usually by needle aspiration.

>**needle b**: removal of tissue with a needle.

>**open b**: removing tissue after making an incision in skin and soft tissues.

bipartite. *Anatomic description*. Made up of two parts. Example: bipartite patella.

bipedicle flap (bi-PED-ih-kul). *Surgical technique*. Skin flap attached at two opposite poles, with blood supply provided by a pedicle or stem (attachment); often used to cover or fill a skin defect such as after removal of a tumor.

bipolar endoprosthesis. See BIPOLAR HEMIARTHROPLASTY, definition #2.

bipolar hemiarthroplasty (hem-ee-AHR-thro-plas-tee). 1. *Surgical procedure*. Type of femoral head replacement in which the artificial head has an extra, mobile extension allowing it to swivel on the stem. May have a lower dislocation rate and lower incidence of arthritis because of less friction between the artificial head and the patient's natural acetabulum (cup). See also UNIPOLAR HEMIARTHROPLASTY. 2. *Surgical implant*. Prosthesis with a mobile articulation between the head and neck of the implant, used to replace a femoral head and neck. Same as BIPOLAR ENDOPROSTHESIS.

Birbeck granules, Langerhans' granules. *Intracellular structure*. Racket-shaped structures found inside Langerhans' cells; function unknown.

bivalve cast (BI-valv). *Orthopedic appliance*. A cast that has been cut on two sides to allow it to spread, so as to allow for swelling.

blastoma (blas-TOH-muh). *Pathologic condition*. A tumor or growth made up of immature undifferentiated cells. Examples: neuroblastoma, from neural tissue; chondroblastoma, from cartilage tissue.

blastomycosis, **Gilchrist's disease** (blas-toh-mi-KOH-sus). *Pathologic condition*. Infectious fungal disease of the skin and mucus membranes; originates in the lungs, can spread to bone and soft tissues.

Bleck procedure. *Surgical procedure*. Method of elongating the iliopsoas tendon. Used in patients with cerebral palsy and gait abnormalities.

block. *Procedure*. Injection of an anesthetic drug to block the function of a nerve to an extremity or body part.

>**axillary b.**: injection of an anesthetic into the axilla (armpit) region to numb a part of the arm.

>**Bïer b.** (beer): type of regional anesthesia in which pain perception is blocked by injecting anesthetic into a vein whose circulation has been blocked through the application of a tourniquet.

>**intravenous b.**: same as BÏER BLOCK (above).

>**spinal b.**: injection of local anesthetic into the spine, to eliminate pain at a specific nerve area.

>**sympathetic b.**: injection of an anesthetic to the sympathetic nerve trunk to an extremity or body part. For treating pain conditions and autonomic disorders such as reflex sympathetic dystrophy.

blood urea nitrogen (BUN). *Blood test*. Indicates liver and kidney function by measuring waste products normally excreted by the kidneys; elevated BUN may indicate kidney failure.

Blount anvil retractor. *Surgical instrument*. One end (the anvil) is weighted to pull tissues to the side, providing exposure of a surgical wound.

Blount-Barber disease. See BLOUNT'S DISEASE.

Blount's disease, Blount-Barber disease, osteochondrosis deformans tibia. *Pathologic condition*. Stunting of growth at inner, upper portion of the tibial (shinbone) growth plate; produces bowlegs in children; progressively worsens.

Blount staple. *Surgical implant*. Heavy metal staple attached across the physeal plate (growth plate) of a growing long bone to prevent growth in that area; results in a change in alignment or length of the bone.

Blount's technique for epiphyseal stapling (ep-ih-FIZ-ee-ul). *Surgical procedure*. Placing Blount staples across the physeal (growth) plate to prevent further growth of a bone.

Blumensaat's line. *Anatomy*. A line visible along the posterior slope of the condylar notch of the femur, seen on a lateral view of the knee. With the knee bent to 30°, its shadow should touch the lower pole of the patella (kneecap). Determines relative position of the patella.

blunt dissection. *Surgical procedure*. Separating soft tissues with a blunt instrument or gloved finger. See also SHARP DISSECTION.

BMD. Abbreviation for BONE MINERAL DENSITY.

body cast. *Orthopedic appliance*. Cast applied to the trunk of the body, generally extending from above the nipple line down to the thigh or lower leg. For keeping the trunk and spine immobilized after surgery.

body jacket. *Orthopedic appliance*. Two-piece cast or brace, to maintain the trunk in a specific position.

Boeck's disease (beks), **Boeck's sarcoid** /or/ **sarcoidosis**. *Pathologic condition*. Chronic inflammatory disorder characterized by tiny soft nodules in the skin, lungs, liver, spleen and eyes. Affects most systems of the body. Unknown origin.

Boeck's sarcoid /or/ **sarcoidosis**. See BOECK'S DISEASE.

Böhler-Braun frame. See BRAUN FRAME.

bone. *Anatomy*. Hard connective tissue that comprises the skeleton and provides structural support to the body.

  cancellous b.: spongy, porous inner layer, with large latticework and a honeycomb appearance; filled with marrow.

  cortical b.: dense hard thick layer making up the outer surface of long bones; surrounds the spongy trabecular bone.

  flat b.: thin, flat shape. Example: scapula.

  irregular b.: lacks symmetry; has a peculiar or complex form. Example: calcaneus (heelbone).

  lamellar b.: layered.

  long b.: tubular bone with a growth plate at each end, from which normal growth occurs. Example: femur.

  short b.: cubical bone that grows on all sides rather than from a growth center. Example: cuboid.

  trabecular b.: same as CANCELLOUS BONE (above).

  Wormian b.: same as WOVEN BONE (below).

  woven b.: new or immature bone seen in the fetal skeleton and after a fracture in the area of healing; the collagen fibers of the matrix are arranged irregularly in the form of interlacing networks.

bone age. *Measurement*. Age assigned to a child's skeleton based on its degree of maturity as seen on x-ray. May not be the same as chronological age.

bone bank. *Medical facility.* Storage center of bones from live donors or cadavers.

bone block. *Surgical technique.* Bone graft that limits or stops joint motion.

bone cyst. *Pathologic condition.* Empty or fluid-filled cavity within a bone; benign process frequently accompanied by fractures of the thin bony wall.

    aneurysmal (ABC) (an-yur-IZ-mul): benign bone tumor containing abnormal anastamosing (communicating) hollow spaces filled with blood. The tumor has thin bony walls, resulting in a balloon-like appearance.

bone density, bone mineral density. *Measurement.* Amount of bone mineral (mainly calcium) in tested areas of the skeleton.

bone derivative. *Biologic implant.* A substance extracted from bone, such as bone morphogenic proteins (BMP).

bone dysostosis (dis-ahs-TOH-sus). *Abnormal condition.* Deformities caused by defective bone formation.

bone dysplasia (dis-PLAY-zjuh). *Abnormal condition.* Deformities caused by intrinsic metabolic disturbances; usually result in a decrease in stature.

bone dystrophy (DIS-truh-fee). *Abnormal condition.* Deformities caused by metabolic or nutritional deficiencies. Example: scurvy.

bone fixation. *Surgical procedure.* Attaching a metal device to bone, to bring two ends together.

bone graft. 1. *Biological material.* Bone taken from another area of patient (autograft), another individual (allograft), or a member of another species (xenograft), to supplement or speed healing. 2. *Surgical procedure.* Implanting bone material or segments into a diseased area to supplement or speed healing.

    free: segment of bone transferred from another area without vascular attachment, to act as a bridge.

    vascularized: segment of bone transferred with its feeding artery and vein so that it may remain alive during the incorporation and healing process. The artery and vein need to be attached to vessels in the recipient area so blood may flow to and from the graft.

bone infarction, avascular necrosis, osteonecrosis. *Pathologic condition.* Death of a small area of bone after its blood supply is lost.

bone inflammation, osteitis. *Pathologic condition.* Inflammatory process in bone, similar to that in soft tissue. May be secondary to infection or foreign material.

bone island. *Pathologic condition.* Localized area of dense bone visible on x-ray. Microscopically, there is an increase in calcium deposition.

bone lesion, bony lesion. *Pathologic condition.* General term for bone abnormality resulting from osteomyelitis, tumor, injury, or other cause. May appear on x-ray as a lucent (clear) or dense area.

bone marrow. *Anatomy.* Soft, spongy tissue filling the cavities in bones, which in youth are filled with blood-forming cells and in older adults with fat.

    biopsy (BI-ahp-see). *Surgical procedure.* Drilling a needle into a bone (usually the pelvis) to obtain bone marrow for microscopic examination.

    transplant. *Surgical procedure.* Implanting marrow from a donor in an attempt to induce formation of blood cells.

bone mass. *Measurement.* Total amount of bone in a skeleton or in a specific bone or region of a bone.

bone matrix. *Anatomy.* Framework of interlocking protein fibers made primarily of collagen; gives bone its capacity for relative flexibility.

bone mineral. *Biological material.* Primarily calcium and phosphorus. Provides rigidity and strength to the bone.

bone morphogenic protein. *Biologic material*. Protein found in demineralized bone that stimulates bone formation.

bone nippers, rongeur. *Surgical instrument*. Spring-loaded cutting tool for taking small bites from bone.

bone paste. *Orthopedic supply*. Cement-like material with a chemistry similar to bone that may be injected into a fracture; eventually replaced by natural bone.

bone remodeling. *Physiologic process*. Cyclic process of bone breakdown and formation that controls growth, maintenance, and repair of bone tissue.

bone scan. *Radiologic test*. Diagnostic nuclear imaging study of bone after injection of a radiopharmaceutical marker into the bloodstream that collects in the bones.

bone skid. *Surgical instrument*. Metallic device used to slide the end of a long bone into or out of its socket.

bone stimulation (electromagnetic). *Treatment*. Use of electrical and/or magnetic fields to stimulate fractured bones into healing. When applied externally, magnetic fields can stimulate growth. Direct stimulation can also be performed using electrodes placed directly within a fracture site to create a negative electrical charge across the fracture.

bone stimulator. *Treatment device*. For stimulating broken bones into healing via electrical fields (applied internally) or electromagnetic waves (worn externally).

bone tumor. *Pathologic condition*. A growth within or on bone; may be benign or malignant.

bone wax. *Orthopedic supply*. Mixture of wax, oil and antiseptic agents; stops flow of blood from bone by filling the open spaces.

bony ankylosis (an-kil-OH-sus). *Pathologic condition*. Abnormal bone growth that crosses a joint, preventing motion.

Borggreve operation. *Surgical procedure*. Outdated term for Van Nes procedure.

boss. *Pathologic condition*. A protuberance or rounded swelling.

bossing. *Pathologic condition*. Localized swelling or protuberance.

Boston brace. *Orthopedic appliance*. Molded chest brace used for controlling lower thoracic and lumbar scoliosis (curvature of the spine).

boutonnière deformity (bu-tun-YARE). *Pathologic condition*. Flexion deformity of the proximal interphalangeal joint and a hyperextension deformity of the distal interphalangeal joint of a finger. Caused by a tear in the extensor tendons of the finger.

boutonnière repair. *Surgical procedure*. Repair of a boutonnière deformity.

Bovie. *Surgical instrument*. Electrical device used to achieve electrocautery of bleeding vessels during surgery.

bowlegs, bandylegs, genu varum, genu varus, tibia vara. *Abnormal condition*. Legs whose knees point outward, remaining separated when standing with ankles together; results in a bowlike appearance.

bowler's thumb. *Pathologic condition*. Irritation of the ulnar digital nerve to the thumb, from repeated compression of the thumb while holding a bowling ball.

boxer's fracture. *Pathologic condition*. Break in the neck of the 5th metacarpus of the hand (knuckle), frequently after a punching blow.

Boyd amputation. *Surgical procedure*. Technique for removing the talus (top foot bone) and fusing the far end of the tibia (shinbone) to the top surface of the calcaneus (heelbone) through the ankle joint.

brace. *Orthopedic appliance*. Supporting device (orthosis) that maintains a correct position or immobilizes a part. May be made of plastic, leather, or metal.

Toronto b.: maintains legs in abduction, allowing movement of the hips. Used in the treatment of Perthes disease in the 1970s and early 1980s.

brachial (BRAY-kee-ul). *Anatomy.* Relating to the arm.

    b. artery: blood vessel that travels down the upper arm as a continuation of the axillary artery; divides at the elbow into ulnar and radial branches.

    b. plexus (BRAY-kee-ul): complex of nerves from the 5th, 6th, 7th and 8th cervical and the 1st and 2nd thoracic segments of the spinal cord, which interconnect in the region of the neck, shoulder and armpit; innervates part of the chest, shoulders and arms.

        injury. *Pathologic condition.* An injury to the area of the brachial plexus. Called an obstetrical palsy if it occurs during birth.

        neuropathy. *Pathologic condition.* Term used to describe injury to the nerves of the brachial plexus; may be birth injury.

    b. veins: two blood vessels that follow the brachial artery up the arm, eventually connecting with the axillary vein in the upper arm.

brachialgia (bray-kee-AL-jee-uh). *Pathologic condition.* Pain in the arm.

brachialis (bray-kee-AL-us). *Anatomy.* Muscle on front of arm, beneath the biceps, that connects the humerus and ulna; flexes the forearm (bends the elbow).

brachioradialis (BR) (bray-kee-oh-ray-dee-AL-us). *Anatomy.* Forearm muscle that connects the humerus and radius; pronates and supinates the forearm.

brachiotomy (bray-kee-AH-toh-mee). *Surgical procedure.* Outdated term: an incision into an arm; sometimes used to mean amputation of an arm.

brachydactylia. See BRACHYDACTYLY.

brachydactyly (bray-kee-DAK-til-ee-uh), **brachydactylia**. *Congenital abnormality.* Shortness of the fingers and toes.

Bradford frame. *Orthopedic appliance.* Rectangular metal frame with attached movable canvas strips onto which an extremity is laid.

Brailsford-Morquio disease (MOR-kee-oh), **Morquio's disease/syndrome**, **Morquio-Ullrich disease**. *Pathologic condition.* One of a series of hereditary chemical disorders called mucopolysaccharidoses. Results in normal appearing newborns who develop into short trunk dwarfs (final height 50 inches), with progressive hip disease, joint laxity, atlantoaxial instability and cloudy corneas, with normal faces and intellect.

Brand technique. *Surgical procedure.* Transfer of the extensor carpi radialis brevis tendon to the extensor tendons of the fingers, to restore extension to the fingers and wrist.

Braun frame, **Böhler-Braun frame**. *Orthopedic appliance.* Adjustable metal frame used for supporting the lower leg with the knee bent so that traction can be applied to the tibia (shinbone).

breastbone. *Anatomy.* Popular term for the sternum, large bone at the front of the chest where ribs attach.

breast stroker's knee. *Pathologic condition.* Strain on the medial collateral ligament of the knee frequently associated with a whipping type of kick used by competitive swimmers in the breaststroke.

bridging defects. *Surgical procedure.* Insertion of bone, a plate or fixation device between two ends of a bone in an attempt to create a functional extremity, after a severe fracture or other wound leaves a space between two ends of a bone.

brisement (BREEZ-munt, BREEZ-mawn). *Treatment.* Forcefully bending a joint held by adhesions. Closed manipulation of a stiff shoulder or knee.

Bristow technique, **Bristow-Helfet** /or/ **Bristow-Laterjet procedure**. *Surgical procedure.* Technique to stabilize recurrent anterior dislocation of the shoulder.

Brittain arthrodesis (ahr-thro-DEE-sus). *Surgical procedure.* Technique for fusing (1) the femur (thighbone) and pelvis from outside the hip joint to eliminate motion of the hip, or (2) the ulna (smaller forearm bone) to the humerus (upper armbone) to eliminate motion of the elbow.

brittle bones, fragilitas osseum congenita, osteitis fragilitans, osteogenesis imperfecta /or/ **imperfecta tarta**. *Pathologic condition.* Multiple system connective tissue disorder characterized by fragile bones that fracture easily. Involves the skeleton, eyes, ears, teeth, and vascular tissue. Hereditary.

Brodie's abscess. *Pathologic condition.* Localized infection in bone that has been walled off by the body's healing process.

Bröstrom procedure, anatomic ankle ligamentous construction. *Surgical procedure*. Technique for repair of ankle ligaments after sprain or injury. Involves supplementing the repair with a rotational graft from the extensor retinaculum.

Bröstrom technique for dye injection into the ankle, Gordon technique. *Injection technique.* Used for dye injection into the ankle, such as injecting radiographic contrast material into an ankle joint to evaluate an ankle sprain.

Brown-Séquard syndrome. *Pathologic condition.* Incomplete spinal cord injury involving motor loss on one side of the body, with pain and temperature loss on the opposite side.

brown tumor. *Pathologic condition.* Mass of fibrous tissue found in bones affected by severe hyperparathyroidism (hyperactive parathyroid glands). Brown color is imparted by blood breakdown product called hemosiderin.

Bruck's disease. *Pathologic condition.* Syndrome characterized by osteogenesis imperfecta, ankylosis of the joints, and muscular atrophy.

Brudzinski reflex /or/ **sign** (bru-JIN-skee). *Clinical sign.* Leg pain that occurs when the neck is passively flexed. Frequently associated with meningitis (inflammation of lining of brain or spinal cord).

bruise, contusion. *Pathologic condition.* Escape of blood into the tissues, with resultant discoloration. See also ECCHYMOSIS.

bruit (BRU-ee). *Clinical sign.* Abnormal blowing sound from a blood vessel or the heart. Caused by turbulent blood flow over the affected area. Associated with fistula, atherosclerotic vessel constriction, arteriovenous malformations. Sometimes heard in bones affected with Paget's disease.

Bryan and Morrey classification. *Fracture classification.* Defines fracture patterns of the capitellum (lower end of humerus that articulates with radius).

Bryant's sign. *Clinical sign.* Abnormal position of the axillary (armpit) folds; results from a dislocation of the shoulder.

Bryant traction. *Treatment.* Method of applying traction to lower limb without the use of pins or internal devices; patient lies with affected hip and knee bent. Used for infants and younger children with femur (thighbone) fractures.

bucket-handle fracture. *Pathologic condition.* Contiguous break in the periphery of the metaphyseal portion (flared end) of a long bone in a child. Thought to result from the violent shaking of a child during abuse-related violence. See also CORNER FRACTURE.

bucket handle tear. *Pathologic condition.* Tear or laceration in the central part of the meniscus (cartilage) of the knee, with both edges maintained in continuity; gives appearance of the handle falling against the edge of a bucket.

Buck's traction. *Treatment.* Longitudinal skin traction on the lower leg, applied through a soft boot.

Buerger's disease, thromboangitis obliterans. *Pathologic condition.* Inflammation of the inner wall of a blood vessel, leading to thrombosis (clot) in the vessel. Can result in gangrene.

bulbocavernosus reflex (bul-boh-kav-ur-NO-sus). *Clinical sign.* Spontaneous contraction of the rectal sphincter when the end of the penis is squeezed or tapped. Used in determining the end of spinal shock after spinal cord injury.

bulla. *Pathologic condition.* Fluid-filled blister. Plural: bullae.

BUN (blood urea nitrogen). *Blood test.* Indicator of kidney and liver function by measuring waste product normally excreted by the kidneys; elevated BUN may indicate kidney failure.

bunion, hallux valgus. *Pathologic condition.* Painful protrusion of the 1st metatarsophalangeal joint (main joint of big toe) at the inner side of the foot. Toe is deviated outward.

    tailor's b.: see BUNIONETTE.

bunionectomy (bun-yun-EK-toh-mee). *Surgical procedure.* Removal of a bunion.

bunionette, tailor's bunion. *Pathologic condition.* Inflammation and enlargement of the metatarsophalangeal joint of the little toe.

Bunnell crisscross stitch. *Surgical technique.* Suture devised to pull tendons together while maintaining a smooth exterior surface. The suture material is buried, so as to not interfere with gliding of the tendons.

Bunnell hand drill. *Surgical instrument.* Small drill used to insert Kirschner wires.

Bunnell suture. *Surgical technique.* Wire stitch inserted into a tendon with the end protruding from the wound; enables its withdrawal after the tendon has healed.

burner, stinger. *Pathologic condition.* Sudden jolt of pain across the arm after a blunt injury to the head and neck, most commonly in football players. Usually resolves spontaneously.

Burnett's syndrome, milk-alkali syndrome. *Pathologic condition.* Chronic disorder of the kidneys induced by long-term therapy of a peptic ulcer with alkalis and milk. Causes osteoporosis (porous bone).

burr. *Surgical instrument.* Designed to be used with a power drill, to shave or reshape bone.

bursa (BUR-suh). *Anatomy.* Sac or space in areas associated with friction, such as over bony prominences. Designed to diminish friction between closely apposed structures.

bursectomy (bur-SEK-tuh-mee). *Surgical procedure.* Removal of a bursa.

bursitis (bur-SI-tus). *Pathologic condition.* Inflammation of a bursa.

bursotomy (bur-SAH-tuh-mee). *Surgical procedure.* Incision into the wall of a bursa.

burst fracture. *Pathologic condition.* Break in a vertebra from excess pressure in a vertical direction. Usually results in an unstable fracture.

butterfly fracture. *Pathologic condition.* Fragmented break through a long bone; the pieces form a triangle that resembles a butterfly with outstretched wings.

buttocks. *Anatomy.* The fleshy back of the hip on which a person sits. The gluteal region.

buttonhole injury. *Pathologic condition.* Injury resulting in a piece of bone passing through a rent in the surrounding tissues, becoming entrapped. Resembles a button passed through its hole. Correction generally requires surgery.

buttress plate. *Surgical implant.* Metal device implanted in areas of fracture or osteotomy (cutting) to prevent one bone fragment sliding on another.

C

C. Abbreviation for CERVICAL VERTEBRA; used with specific number (C1– C7).

    C1. Abbreviation for the 1st cervical vertebra; the atlas.

    C2. Abbreviation for the 2nd cervical vertebra; the axis.

cable graft, **nerve graft**, **nerve cable graft**. *Surgical technique*. Transfer of a portion of a peripheral, expendable sensory nerve to repair a defect in an important nerve. A segment is removed from the nerve and sutured into the defect.

cable plate. *Orthopedic implant*. Plate designed to be attached to the bone with cables that wrap around the bone. Used in fixation of fractures where other implants such as artificial hip or shoulders lie within the bone impeding the passage of screws.

cable twister orthosis. *Orthopedic appliance*. Pelvic band attached to a plastic or steel cable fastened to a shoe or leg brace; rotating the cable changes position of the lower leg.

cadaver. A term generally applied to a dead human body or corpse.

café-au-lait spots (kuh-FAY-oh-LAY). *Pathologic condition*. Small patches of light brown discoloration of the skin. Occurs in various diseases, e.g., neurofibromatosis, fibrous dysplasia.

Caffey's disease /or/ **syndrome**, **Caffey-Silverman syndrome**, **infantile cortical hyperostosis**. *Pathologic condition*. Swelling of soft tissue around a bone (most commonly jaw and forearm), accompanied by fever, irritability, elevation in white count and sedimentation rate, and cortical bone thickening. Usually seen in children. Difficult to differentiate from a bone infection.

caisson's disease (KAY-sahnz), **bends**, **decompression sickness, diver's disease**. *Pathologic condition*. Soft tissue and bone damage caused by nitrogen bubbles forming in the blood, associated with rapid decrease in pressure; may lead to avascular necrosis of bone. Symptoms include joint pain, skin lesions, respiratory and central nervous system dysfunction. Frequently occurs in divers who do not decompress on resurfacing from a dive.

calcaneal (kal-KAY-nee-ul). *Anatomic description*. Relating to the calcaneus (heelbone).

    c. pad. *Orthopedic appliance*. Heel pad that relieves the pressure on a spur (bony outgrowth).

calcaneocavus deformity (kal-KAY-nee-oh-KAY-vus), **talipes calcaneocavus**. *Pathologic condition*. Foot with a dorsiflexed heel (pointed up) and plantarflexed forefoot and midfoot (pointed down). Arch of foot is abnormally high. Usually seen with certain forms of cerebral palsy.

calcaneocuboid (kal-KAY-nee-oh-KYU-boyd). *Anatomic description*. Relating to the calcaneus (heelbone) and cuboid bone (part of the ankle).

    c. bar. *Congenital abnormality*. Fusion of the calcaneus and cuboid.

    c. joint. *Anatomy*. Joint between the calcaneus and the cuboid.

    c. ligament. *Anatomy*. Connective tissue band that maintains stability between the calcaneus and the cuboid; part of the bifurcate ligament.

calcaneofibular ligament (kal-KAY-nee-oh-FIB-yu-lur). *Anatomy*. Connective tissue band that attaches the calcaneous (heelbone) to the lower tip of the fibula (smaller bone of lower leg). Adds to ankle joint stability.

calcaneovalgus deformity (kal-KAY-nee-oh-VAL-gus), **talipes calcaneovalgus**. *Pathologic condition*. High-arched foot that is deviated outward. Most commonly seen in an infant as a result of fetal malpositioning.

calcaneovarus deformity (kal-KAY-nee-oh-VEHR-us), **talipes calcaneovarus**. *Pathologic condition.* Combination of talipes calcaneus and talipes varus. Foot is flexed upward, inward and toward midline, turning in at both heel and toe, forming a C-shape; most weightbearing is on outer edge of foot.

calcaneus (kal-KAY-nee-us), **os calcis**. *Anatomy.* The heel or heelbone. Plural: calcanei.

calcar (KAL-cahr). *Anatomic description.* Dense area of bone. Also, a spur or osteophyte (bony outgrowth at the edge of a joint).

    c. femorale, medial c.: dense bone formation on the inner side of the neck of the femur (thighbone).

calcific tendinitis (kal-SIH-fik ten-dun-NI-tus). *Pathologic condition.* Calcification in tendons; most common in the rotator cuff, and Achilles, quadriceps and patellar tendons.

calcification (kal-suh-fih-KAY-shun). *Process.* Deposition of calcium salts, normal in bone and teeth, abnormal in soft tissue; visible on x-ray. See also OSSIFICATION.

calcinosis (kal-sin-OH-sus). *Pathologic condition.* Deposits of calcium salts in soft tissue. Often a sign of pseudogout. Plural: calcinoses.

    c. circumscripta (sur-kum-SKRIP-tuh): calcium salts deposits in soft tissues of skin and subcutaneous regions; frequently seen in dermatomyositis.

calcitonin (kal-sih-TOH-nun). *Hormone.* Regulates amount of calcium in the circulation and acts to slow the breakdown of bone. Released mainly by the thyroid gland.

calcium. *Mineral.* Metallic element found in nearly all living tissues; necessary for bone formation and muscle function, blood clotting and nerve impulse transmission.

    c. homeostatis. *Physiologic process.* Bodily function that maintains concentration of calcium disolved in body fluids within a tightly regulated range.

    c. pyrophosphate (pi-roh-FAHS-fayt). *Chemical.* Calcium-based crystal found in the body; excessive precipitation of this crystal is the underlying abnormality in calcium pyrophosphate deposition disease or pseudogout.

    c. pyrophosphate deposition disease, **pseudogout**. *Pathologic condition.* Abnormal precipitation of calcium pyrophosphate into crystals that deposit into the joints, most commonly the knee, resulting in pain and inflammation. Can be detected on x-ray. See also CHONDROCALCINOSIS.

calf. *Anatomy.* Portion of the back of the lower leg that includes the group of muscles at the back of the leg (gastrocnemius, solius, plantaris).

calipers (KAL-uh-purz). 1. *Instrument.* Measuring device with two adjustable arms; for determining thickness, diameter, or distance between two surfaces. 2. *Orthopedic appliance.* A brace.

callosity (kal-AH-suh-tee). See CALLUS.

callus (KAL-us), **callosity**. *Pathologic condition.* 1. A hard, thickened area on the skin, usually on the foot or hand, formed in response to pressure or friction. 2. Hard, calcified deposits of immature bone that form around the ends of fractured bones as part of the healing process.

Calvé-Kummel-Verneuil disease (kal-VAY), **vertebra plana**. *Pathologic condition.* Collapse and flattening of the vertebral body; most frequent in children 2–15 years of age. May be associated with eosinophilic granuloma (benign bone lesions).

Calvé-Perthes disease (kal-VAY PEHR-tayz), **Legg-Calvé-Perthes disease**, **osteochondritis deformans juvenilis** /or/ **juvenilis dorsi**, **Perthes disease**. *Pathologic condition.* Deterioration and flattening of the femoral head due to insufficient blood supply; may result in severe arthritic changes. No known cause; generally occurs between ages 4–8. See also <small>CATTERALL CLASSIFICATION</small>.

camptocormia (kamp-toh-KOHR-mee-uh), **camptospasm**. *Psychiatric condition*. An hysterical condition marked by forward bending of the trunk and sometimes accompanied by lumbar pain.

camptodactyly (kamp-loh-DAK-tuh-lee). *Congenital abnormality*. Permanent flexion of one or more finger joints.

camptospasm. See <small>CAMPTOCORMIA</small>.

Camurati-Engelmann, Engelmann's disease, diaphyseal /or/ **progressive diaphyseal dysplasia**. *Pathologic condition*. Type of dwarfism resulting from an abnormality in the growth of the long bones. Characteristics include abnormally short, wide long bones and early joint arthritis.

Canadian hip prosthesis. *Orthopedic appliance*. Artificial thigh and leg attached to a plastic cup and waistband; used after removal of a leg at the hip joint.

Canale modification of Hawkins classification. *Fracture classification*. Describes different severities of fracture involving the talus. Hawkins identifies three levels; Canale modification adds a fourth.

cancellous (KAN-sul-us, kan-SEL-us). *Anatomic description*. Refers to the inner layer of bone that has a porous, lattice-like, spongy structure.

    c. bone, trabecular bone. *Anatomy*. Type of porous bone with a spongy, honeycomb appearance; filled with marrow. See also <small>CORTICAL BONE</small>.

    c. screw. *Surgical implant*. Screw with large threads, better able to grip into the spongy latticework of cancellous bone.

cannula (KAN-yu-luh). *Surgical instrument*. Any tube-like device that can be inserted with a trocar (pointed pin) filling its lumen (central hollow part). The trocar can then be removed, leaving the cannula behind.

cannulated (KAN-yu-lay-ted). *Description*. Refers to any surgical device with a hollow center, such as a cannulated nail or cannulated screw, so that it may be inserted over a pin or trochar.

    nail. *Surgical implant*. Fixation device for holding bony fragments together; a hollow center allows placement over previously inserted guide pin.

capital epiphysis (uh-PIF-uh-sus). *Anatomy*. Growth area in upper femur (thighbone); begins to appear bony at about 6 months of age, fusing with the femur at the end of growth.

capital femoral epiphysiodesis /or/ **epiphyseodesis** (uh-pif-uh-see-oh-DEE-sus). *Surgical procedure*. Destruction of growth plate at the upper end of the femur (thighbone), or bridging with a bone or metal fixation device, to stop growth.

capitate (KAP-ih-tayt). *Anatomy*. Rounded bone in center of the wrist; part of the distal row of wrist bones and the largest of eight carpal (wrist) bones.

capitellum (kap-ih-TEL-um). *Anatomy*. A knob-like protuberance, especially at the end of a bone. Plural: capitella.

    c. humeri: knob-like protuberance at the end of the humerus (upper armbone); forms outer portion of elbow joint and articulates with the radius.

capitis femoris, fovea centralis. *Anatomy*. Notch in the femoral head where the ligamentum teres attaches to the femoral head and the acetabulum.

capsular (KAP-suh-lur). *Anatomic description*. Relating to the capsule, the fibrous sheath surrounding a joint.

    c. arthroplasty (AHR-throh-plas-tee). *Surgical procedure*. Invaginating (folding within itself) of the joint lining (capsule) into the joint to cover areas of degenerated cartilage.

    c. release. *Surgical procedure*. Cutting the joint lining (capsule) to allow increased motion.

capsule. *Anatomy*. Connective tissue sheath that surrounds and encloses the ends of bones that make up a joint.

capsulectomy (kap-suh-LEK-toh-mee). *Surgical procedure*. Removal of the joint lining (capsule), to increase motion of the joint.

capsulitis (kap-suh-LI-tus). *Pathologic condition*. Inflammation of the joint lining (capsule).

capsulodesis (kap-su-loh-DEE-sus). *Surgical procedure*. Tightening the capsule (joint lining) to prevent dislocation or to realign the articular surface.

capsuloplasty (KAP-su-loh-plas-tee). *Surgical procedure*. The reshaping of a capsule. See also CAPSULODESIS.

capsulorrhaphy (kap-suh-LOR-uh-fee). *Surgical procedure*. Suturing the joint lining (capsule).

capsulotomy (kap-suh-LAH-tuh-mee). *Surgical procedure*. Incision of a capsule (joint lining).

carpal bones (KAHR-pul). *Anatomy*. The eight bones forming the wrist; includes a proximal row containing the navicular, lunate and triquetrium, and a distal row containing the trapezium, trapezoid, capitate and hamate, and the pisiform. Correspond with the tarsal bones in the foot.

carpal ligaments (KAHR-pul). *Anatomy*. Connective tissue bands between the small bones of the wrist (carpal bones) that hold wrist bones in alignment.

carpalmetacarpal. Less preferred spelling for CARPOMETACARPAL.

carpal navicular, **scaphoid**. *Anatomy*. Boat-shaped bone in the wrist.

carpal tunnel (KAHR-pul). *Anatomy*. The canal running from the heel of the hand to the wrist, created by carpal bones at the back of the wrist and the transverse carpal ligament along the front, and through which pass the median nerve and nearly all the tendons from the forearm to the hand. Site of compression of the median nerve in cases of carpal tunnel syndrome.

　　release (CTR). *Surgical procedure*. Cutting the transverse carpal ligament (palmar surface of carpal tunnel), to release pressure on the median nerve in the canal.

　　syndrome (CTS). *Pathologic condition*. Pain, tingling, weakness, and wasting of the muscles in the thumb, and disturbance of sensation in the thumb, index and middle fingers; caused by pressure and/or compression of the median nerve in the carpal tunnel.

carpectomy (kahr-PEK-toh-mee). *Surgical procedure*. Removal of the carpal bones (wrist bones); for arthritis or deformity.

　　proximal row c: removal of the four wrist bones that directly articulate with the radius and ulna; for the treatment of arthritis or deformity.

carpometacarpal (kahr-poh-met-uh-KAHR-pul). *Anatomic description*. Refers to the joints between the distal row of the wrist bones (carpus) and the proximal ends of the hand bones (metacarpal bones).

　　c. joint arthroplasty (AHR-throh-plas-tee). *Surgical procedure*. Reconstruction of a carpometacarpal joint by joint replacement, removal, or by insertion of fibrous tissue between joints; for relief of arthritis symptoms.

carpus (KAHR-pus). *Anatomy*. Wrist. Plural: carpi.

carrying angle. *Anatomic description*. Angle formed at the elbow by the arm and forearm when the arm is extended in the anatomical position. The angle is generally greater in women and is often lost in supracondylar fractures. See also CUBITUS VARUS.

cartilage (KAHR-tuh-lidj). *Anatomy*. Fibrous connective tissue found throughout the body. Three types: elastic (ear, epiglottis, nose), fibrocartilage (intervertebral disc, pelvis), hyaline (wrist, fingers, elbows, ribs, fetus).

　　articular: the smooth lining of a mobile joint.

elastic: flexible connective tissue on the ends of long bones and ribs, also in the nose, trachea, external ear, skin and wrist.

fibro-: contains visible collagen fibers; frequently found in areas where hyaline cartilage has been damaged. Seen in menisci of the knee.

hyaline (HI-uh-leen): smooth, resilient, connective tissue on the ends of long bones that are part of the joint, such as at the shoulder, elbow or knee.

reticular: outdated term for fibrocartilage.

cartilage necrosis (KAHR-tuh-lidj nek-ROH-sus). *Pathologic condition.* Death of an area of connective tissue (cartilage), usually after trauma or infection.

cartilage space narrowing (KAHR-tuh-lidj). *Radiologic finding.* Decrease in joint space from wearing away of the cartilage (connective tissue) surface. On x-ray, joint space appears to be narrower, or lost, because the bones are either closer to each other or actually touching.

cartilaginous (kar-tuh-LAJ-uh-nus). *Anatomic description.* Composed of, relating to, or resembling cartilage (connective tissue).

c. joint. *Anatomy.* Type of articulation; ends of bones connected by a cartilage plate. Two types: synchondroses (in pelvis between ischium, pubis and ilium); symphyses (in center between the two pubic bones at front of pelvis).

c. hamartoma (hay-mahr-TOH-muh). *Pathologic condition.* Benign tumorlike lesion resulting from abnormal growth of cartilage. Usually seen in the chest wall.

cartwheel fracture, wagonwheel fracture. *Pathologic condition.* Break in the distal femur (thighbone) or proximal tibia (shinbone) in children. So named when children rode in carts and caught their leg in spoked wheels.

cast. *Orthopedic appliance.* Structure applied to a part of the body to prevent motion, or for immobilizing a diseased or broken part; usually formed from fiberglass, plastic, or linen impregnated with plaster of paris.

abduction boot: extends from upper thighs to feet, with a bar between the legs to keep hips and legs immobilized and hips in abduction.

arm cylinder: extends from the upper arm to the wrist, to keep the elbow immobilized while allowing for movement of the wrist and hand.

bivalve (BI-valv): cut on two sides to allow for swelling.

body: applied to the trunk, generally from above nipple line down to the thigh or lower leg; for keeping trunk and spine immobilized after surgery.

body jacket: two-piece cast or brace, to maintain the trunk in a specific position.

cylinder: spans the leg from upper thigh to the flare of the malleoli (tips of lower leg bones), not incorporating the foot, so as to allow for ankle movement. Usually applied with the knee in extension; commonly used in the nonoperative treatment of patella (kneecap) fractures.

extension body: applied to trunk to hold the back in an arched position.

flexion body: applied to trunk to hold the body in a flexed position.

gauntlet: forearm cast that incorporates part of the hand and fingers. Resembles a knight's glove.

gel: has gel incorporated in the gauze; used to prevent swelling and to treat skin ulcerations.

halo: consists of a vest with metal struts attached to a steel frame around the head, held in place with four pins strewed into the skull; for holding the head and neck in a rigid position.

hanging arm: extends from the upper arm to the hand, holding the elbow in a flexed position; used in the nonoperative treatment of humerus (upper armbone) fractures. The arm hangs freely within the cast so that its weight helps the humerus to realign itself.

hip spica: see SPICA (below).

leg cylinder: spans the leg from the upper thigh to the flare of the malleoli (tips of lower leg bones), not incorporating the foot, so as to allow for ankle movement. Usually applied with the knee in extension; commonly used in the nonoperative treatment of patella (kneecap) fractures.

long-arm (LAC): extends from the upper arm to the hand.

long-leg (LLC): extends from the upper thigh to the toes.

long-leg walking (LLWC): extends from the upper thigh to the toes and is reinforced at the bottom to allow for weightbearing.

Minerva jacket: body cast that includes the trunk and head, with ears and face left open; used for treating spine deformities.

Petrie: bilateral long leg casts held apart by two cross-beams so each hip is held in 45° of abduction and slight internal rotation; used in the nonoperative treatment of Legg-Calvé-Perthes disease.

plaster: made of plaster of paris.

Risser's: body cast used in scoliosis.

serial: regular (e.g., weekly) application of casts to stretch ligaments and joints; used in treatment of clubfoot and other deformities.

short-arm (SAC): extends from below the elbow to the hand, not including the fingers.

short-leg (SLC): extends from below the knee to the foot, not including the toes.

short-leg patella tendon bearing: spans from inner side of the lower leg to the foot. The front is molded so as to rest upon the lower tip of the patella (kneecap) so the patella and patellar tendon can absorb some of the load during weightbearing.

short-leg walking (SLWC): extends from the knee to the foot, with a reinforced plantar (bottom) surface to enable walking/weight bearing.

skelecast: consists of a series of thin, circumferential rings surrounding the affected areas of the body, connected by fortified struts. Allows for wide access to the immobilized segment.

slipper: small foot cast that encompasses the heel.

spica: applied to a section of the body and adjoining portion of a limb, or to the hand and an adjoining finger, in order to immobilize the encased appendage. Takes its name from its resemblance to an ear of wheat.

> **hip s.**: any body cast for immobilizing the hip joints and/or thighs.

>> **bilateral long-leg hip s.**: extends from nipple line, down both legs to and including the feet, with a bar between the legs to keep hips and legs immobilized.

>> **double hip s.**: extends from nipple line, down both legs, with a bar between the legs to keep hips and legs immobilizedt.

>> **one and one-half hip s.**: extends from the chest to the foot of one leg and to the knee of the other leg, with a bar between the legs to keep the hips and legs immobilized.

>> **short-leg hip s.**: extends from the chest to the thighs, not incorporating the knees.

> **shoulder s.**: encompasses arm and chest, immobilizing the shoulder.

> **thumb s.**: extends from the forearm to the hand and past the interphalangeal joint of the thumb.

turnbuckle: body cast with a turnbuckle that may be tightened to stretch or compress the body part under the cast.

univalve: cut on one side so it can spread to accommodate for swelling.

walking: see SHORT LEG WALKING CAST, LONG LEG WALKING CAST (above).

> **well-leg**: cast placed on a normal leg, either to exert traction on the opposite leg or to restrict patient movement.

> **windowed**: has a segment removed so the underlying skin or joint can be accessed.

cast boot. *Orthopedic appliance*. Rigid, boot-like device designed to immobilize the foot and ankle while allowing easy placement and removal.

cast brace. *Orthopedic appliance*. Cast with a hinged metal joint; allows joint motion while keeping the limb immobilized.

cast burn. *Pathologic condition*. Burn from heat generated as a plaster hardens.

cast shoe. *Orthopedic appliance*. Shoe fashioned to fit on the end of a cast, to allow walking without destroying the cast.

cast sock. *Orthopedic supply*. Stockinette material applied between skin and cast.

cast sore. *Pathologic condition*. A skin sore under the cast caused by abrasion or pressure.

Cataflam. *Drug*. A trade name of diclofenac, NSAID for treating pain and inflammation.

CAT scan. See CT SCAN.

Catterall classification. Describes extent and progression of Legg-Calvé-Perthes disease.

cauda (KAW-duh). *Anatomy*. Tail. Plural: caudae.

> **c. equina** (ee-KWI-nuh): cone-shaped structure making up the end of the spinal cord where the terminal nerves leave the cord at L1; resembles a horse's tail.

>> **syndrome**. *Pathologic condition*. Pattern of neurological defects resulting in loss of bladder and bowel control. Caused by abnormal compression or severing of nerves at the level of the cauda equina.

caudad (KAW-dad). *Location*. Toward the tail.

caudal (KAW-dul). *Anatomic description*. Pertaining to the tail or posterior end. See also CEPHALAD.

causalgia (kaw-SAL-jee-uh). *Pathologic condition*. Burning, pain, hypersensitivity and skin changes in an extremity resulting from injury to a peripheral nerve.

cauterization (kaw-tur-ih-ZAY-shun). *Treatment*. The use of electrical current, cold, hot iron, laser or caustic agent to destroy tissue and to control bleeding.

cauterize (KAW-tur-ize). *Process*. Using electrical current, cold, hot iron, laser or caustic agent to destroy tissue and to control bleeding.

cautery (KAW-tur-ee). *Instrument*. Device or agent (as a hot iron or caustic) used to burn, scar, or destroy tissue. See CAUTERIZATION.

cavernous hemangioma (hee-man-jee-OH-muh). *Pathologic condition*. Large vascular tumor composed of thin-walled vessels of large diameter.

cavovalgus deformity (kay-voh-VAL-gus), **talipes cavovalgus**. *Pathologic condition*. Abnormally high-arched foot that is flexed outward and away from the midline; weight is on the inside of the foot (false flatfoot). Associated with paralytic deformities.

cavus foot (KAY-vus), **claw foot**, **gampsodactyly**, **pes cavus**. *Pathologic condition*. Abnormally high-arched foot; usually with clawing of the toes. Associated with some forms of neurologic abnormality such as polio or Charcot-Marie-Tooth disease.

CBC (complete blood count). *Lab test*. A set of blood tests. Usually consists of white and red blood cell counts, differential count, hemoglobin, hematocrit, platelet count.

CE angle. See CENTER EDGE ANGLE OF WIBERG.

Celebrex. *Drug*. A trade name of celecaoxib, a COX-2 inhibitor.

cellulitis (sel-yu-LI-tus). *Pathologic condition*. Inflammation in the skin and subcutaneous tissue, associated with erythema (skin redness), edema (excessive water in the tissues), and heat.

cement. *Orthopedic substance*. Compound (e.g., polymethylmethacrylate) that binds two surfaces; used for attaching a prosthesis (artificial part) to the underlying bone.

    c. gun: device for mixing and directing cement into the central (medullary) cavity of a bone.

cemented hip replacement. *Surgical procedure*. Technique for replacing the hip using prostheses (artificial parts) designed to be cemented into position.

cementless /or/ **uncemented** /or/ **press-fit total hip replacement**. *Surgical procedure*. Technique for replacing the hip using prostheses (artificial parts) with porous rough surfaces that allow the bone to heal directly to them without cement.

center edge (angle of Wiberg), **CE angle, acetabular index** /or/ **angle**, **Wiberg angle**. *Radiologic measurement*. On a front view of the pelvis, the angle formed between a vertical line passing through the center of the femoral head and a second line from the center of the femoral head to the outer edge of the acetabulum. An angle greater than 25° is normal; less than 20° is suggestive of dysplasia.

centesis (sen-TEE-sus). 1. *Surgical procedure*. To pierce a cavity to remove fluid. 2. *Suffix*. Pierce or puncture (arthrocentesis: to pierce a joint to remove fluid).

central cord syndrome. *Pathologic condition*. Incomplete spinal cord injury that affects motor function of upper extremities more than ower extremities. Often seen in association with traumatic injury to the cord, ischemia (insufficient oxygen to the cord), or hemorrhage (bleeding into the cord).

central core disease. *Congenital abnormality*. Muscle disease characterized by muscular weakness or hypotonia in infancy due to impaired relase of calcium (needed for muscle contraction) by skeletal muscle. Hereditary.

central nervous system (CNS). *Anatomy*. Refers to the brain and spinal cord.

central slip of the extensor expansion. *Anatomy*. Tendon that extends from the extensor tendon of a finger to the large fibrous hood on the finger. Pulling on the tendon straightens the finger.

cephalad (SEF-uh-lad). *Location*. Toward the head. See also CAUDAD.

cephalic (suh-FAL-ik). *Anatomy*. Refers to the head.

    c. vein: blood vessel in front of the shoulder between the deltoid and pectoralis muscles; drains from the arm into the axillary vein (in armpit).

cerebellar ataxia (ay-TAKS-ee-uh). *Pathologic condition*. Loss of muscular coordination due to injury or disease of the cerebellum; causes gross gait abnormality with frequent loss of balance.

cerebral palsy (CP) (suh-REE-brul PAHL-zee). *Pathologic condition*. Group of non-progressive, chronic, central nervous system disorders that impair coordination, reflex and motor function. Associated with premature or difficult childbirth; may also be caused by congenital brain abnormalities.

    ataxic (ay-TAKS-ik): patient has problems with balance and coordination; may have hand tremors and speech irregularities.

    atonic (ay-TAH-nik): patient is flaccid, limp and listless.

    athetoid (ATH-uh-toyd): patient has slow, continuous, rhythmic, involuntary motion of the limbs, especially the arms.

    diplegic: partial paralysis of corresponding areas on both sides of the body, lower extremities more involved than upper extremities.

    dyskinetic: same as ATHETOID (above).

    flaccid: damage to nervous system results in limp muscles without tone.

    hypotonic: same as FLACCID (above).

spastic: hyperactive muscle activity leading to jerky, uncoordinated movements; most common form; four levels of involvement:

s. diplegia, **double hemiplegia**: involves principally two (usually lower) extremities.

s. hemiplegia: involves one side of the body.

s. monoplegia: involves one extremity.

cerebrospinal fluid (CSF) (sehr-EE-bro-SPI-nul). *Anatomy.* Clear, colorless liquid that bathes the spinal cord and brain, providing nutrients and acting as a shock absorber; produced in the ventricles of the brain. See also LUMBAR PUNCTURE.

cervical (SUR-vih-kul). *Anatomic description.* Refers to the neck.

c. disc. *Anatomy.* Fibro-cartilaginous (connective tissue) segment between cervical vertebrae that acts as a cushion and allows for motion.

c. dislocation. *Pathologic condition.* Displacement of a cervical vertebra relative to the vertebra above it, below it, or both.

c. dystonia, **spasmodic torticollis**. *Pathologic condition.* Disorder characterized by abnormal tension and activity across neck muscles, which can lead to abnormal posture and repetitive twisting movements. Can begin at any age but usually starts in 30s or 40s. No known cause or cure.

c. lordosis (lohr-DOH-sus). *Abnormal condition.* Characteristic posture of the cervical and lumbar spine (neck, lower back). Viewed from the side, the spine curves to the front, giving a hollow appearance to the back of the neck. If excessive or present in other areas of spine, can be pathologic.

c. myelogram (MI-loh-gram). *Radiologic test.* X-ray of the cervical spine (neck area) after injection of radiopaque dye.

c. nerves. *Anatomy.* Eight pairs of nerves that exit the spinal cord in the neck region.

c. neuritis (nu-RI-tus). *Pathologic condition.* Inflammation of nerves in the neck.

c. plexus. *Anatomy.* Network of nerves (plexus) exiting from the first four segments of the spinal cord in the neck.

c. ribs. *Anatomy.* Extra pair of ribs that articulate (loosely connect) with the 7th cervical vertebra; present in less than 1% of the population.

c. spine. *Anatomy.* The first seven spinal vertebrae.

c. spondylosis (spahn-duh-LOH-sus). *Pathologic condition.* Degenerative arthritic disorder of the spine affecting the vertebrae and intervetebral discs in the neck.

c. traction. *Treatment.* Traction or force applied to the head to pull the neck into a specific position. Used for relieving neck pain.

c. vertebrae. *Anatomy.* The seven bones that make up the neck region of the spine.

cervicothoracic area /or/ junction (sur-vih-koh-thor-ASS-ik). *Anatomy.* Junction between the 7th cervical (neck) and the 1st thoracic (chest) vertebrae.

Chaddock reflex/sign. *Clinical test.* Spontaneous raising or extending of the big toe as the skin over the outer side of the ankle is stroked. Indicates organic disease in the spinal cord.

chairback orthosis. *Orthopedic appliance.* Brace with rigid, vertical plastic or metal stays, for preventing motion in the lower thoracic and lumbar spine.

chalk bones, **Albers-Schönberg disease**, **ivory bones**, **marble bones**, **osteopetrosis**, **osteosclerosis fragilis**. *Pathologic condition.* Rare disorder characterized by extreme density and fragility of the bones and obliteration of marrow spaces. Symptoms include pathologic fractures, osteomyelitis of the mandible, cranial nerve palsy, enlargement of the spleen and liver, severe anemia, and possible deafness and blindness. Hereditary.

Chambers and Wilkins classification. *Fracture classification*. Identifies characteristic fracture patterns in the radial head.

chamfer. *Geometry*. A beveled edge; slanting or smoothing the edge of a cube, usually about 45°.

    c. reamer. *Surgical instrument*. A low-speed drill used for creating a chamfer cut in a bone.

Chandler arthrodesis. *Surgical procedure*. Technique for fusion of the hip joint, both from within and outside the joint.

Chance fracture. *Pathologic condition*. Break through a vertebra caused by combination of excessive flexion and distraction (pulling apart), as when a passenger in a car crash is wearing only the lap portion of a safety belt.

Charcot-Marie-Tooth disease (shar-KOH), **peroneal atrophy**. *Pathologic condition*. Progressive degeneration of the peripheral nerves, making ambulation difficult. Associated with certain foot deformities, weakness, muscle atrophy, reflex changes. Hereditary. See also HEREDITARY MOTOR SENSORY NEUROPATHY.

    type I, hypertrophic form, Roussy-Lévy syndrome: there is de-myelinization of peripheral nerves, with absence of deep tendon reflexes.

    type II, neuronal form: reflexes and conduction times for peripheral nerves remain normal. Generally slower in progression and milder than type I.

Charcot's disease (shar-KOHZ), **amyotrophic lateral sclerosis**, **Lou Gehrig disease**, **motor neuron disease**. *Pathologic condition*. Progressive degenerative disease of the spinal cord nerves that control motor function (the muscles); leads to gait and motor abnormalities and eventually death.

Charcot's joint (shar-KOHZ), **neurogenic fracture**. *Pathologic condition*. Joint that becomes injured and destroyed as a result of loss of sensation.

Charcot's syndrome (shar-KOHZ), **intermittent claudication**, **myasthenia angiosclerotica**, **vascular claudication**. *Pathologic condition*. Limping caused by insufficient blood supply to the leg muscles when blood vessels are constricted or obliterated, such as in diabetes or arteriosclerosis.

charley horse. *Pathologic condition*. Leg muscle pain generally associated with bruising or trauma.

Charnley screw. *Orthopedic implant*. Large screw used for the fixation of certain hip fractures. Has a compression screw that slides into a barrel and attaches to a side plate.

Charnley total hip arthroplasty. *Orthopedic implant*. Components for cementing into bone for total hip joint replacement; designed by Sir John Charnley.

cheilectomy (kee-LEK-toh-mee). *Surgical procedure*. Excision of an irregular piece of bone (osteophyte) at the edge of a joint, such as on top of the 1st metatarsophalangeal (big toe) joint. See also HALLUX RIGIDUS.

chemonucleolysis (kee-moh-nu-klee-oh-LI-sus). *Surgical procedure*. Injection of the chemical chymopapain into an intervetrebral disc to dissolve it (lysis), to treat lumbar disc herniation.

chemotherapy. *Treatment*. Use of chemicals to eliminate a tumor or decrease its size.

    adjuvant c.: use of chemicals to decrease the size of a tumor prior to surgical removal.

Chevron osteotomy. *Surgical procedure*. V-shaped cut made into the 1st metatarsal bone so it can be realigned. Used in treatment of bunions. See also HALLUX VALGUS.

Chiari procedure (kee-AHR-ee). *Surgical procedure*. Cutting through the innominate bone (hipbone) around the acetabulum (hip socket), to provide coverage for the femoral head.

chillblain, frostbite, pernio. *Pathologic condition*. Redness, itching, burning sensation of skin exposed to extreme cold; most frequently affects tops of fingers and toes. Tissue death can occur if circulation is not maintained.

Childress duck waddle test. *Clinical test*. Patient squats, first with legs rotated inward and then outward. The test is indicative of a meniscus tear if pain is elicited from the knees, if the patient is not able to fully squat secondary to knee pain, or if there is painful popping from the knee.

chip fracture. *Pathologic condition*. A break in which a small bone fragment is pulled away (or chipped off the edge) from the main body of a bone.

chiropodist (ki-RAH-poh-dist), **podiatrist**. *Health professional*. Doctor of podiatric medicine; trained and licensed to diagnose and treat foot problems.

choline magnesium trisalicylate. *Drug*. NSAID for treating pain and inflammation. Trade name: Trilisate.

chondr–, chondro–. *Prefix*. Cartilage (chondritis: inflammation of cartilage).

chondrectomy (kahn-DREK-tuh-mee). *Surgical procedure*. Removal of cartilage.

chondritis (kahn-DRI-tus). *Pathologic condition*. Inflammation of cartilage.

chondroblast (KAHN-droh-blast). *Anatomy*. Cartilage-forming cell.

chondroblastoma (kahn-droh-blas-TOH-muh), **Codman's tumor**. *Pathologic condition*. Benign cartilaginous tumor commonly seen in the epiphysis (growth area) of long bones, most frequently in the shoulder.

chondrocalcinosis (kahn-droh-kal-sin-OH-sus). *Pathologic condition*. Deposits of calcium in cartilage.

chondroclast (KAHN-droh-klast). *Anatomy*. Cartilage-absorbing cell.

chondrocyte (KAHN-droh-site). *Anatomy*. A cartilage cell.

chondrodysplasia (kahn-droh-dis-PLAY-zjuh), **chondystrophia calcificans congenita, chondrodysplasia punctata, congenita punctata, punctate epiphyseal dysplasia**. *Congenital abnormality*. Malformation of bones resulting in joint deformations and leading to a form of dwarfism. Characterized by limb deformities, spine abnormalities, varus deformation of the hips, difficulty walking, and x-ray appearance of stippled, calcified epiphyses. The stippling is present at birth, but usually disappears by one year of age. See also CONRADI-HUNERMANN DISEASE, RHIZOMELIC FORM.

chondrodysplasia punctata. See CHONDRODYSPLASIA.

chondystrophia calcificans congenita. See CHONDRODYSPLASIA.

chondrodystrophia fetalis (kahn-droh-dis-TROH-fee-uh fuh-TAL-us), **chondrodystrophy, achondroplasia, achondrodystrophy, osteosclerosis congenita, Parrot's disease**. *Congenital abnormality*. Abnormality of the growth cartilage of the extremities, resulting in a short-limbed dwarf, generally accompanied by an apparent enlargement of the front of the skull. Trunk length is normal. Hereditary.

chondrodystrophy. See CHONDRODYSTROPHIA.

chondroepiphysitis (kahn-droh-eh-pif-ih-SI-tus). *Pathologic condition*. Inflammation of the cartilage at the end of a long bone (the epiphysis).

chondrofibroma (kahn-droh-fi-BROH-muh), **chondromyxoid fibroma, chondromyxoma**. *Pathologic condition*. Benign bone tumor of cartilaginous origin.

chondroitin sulfate (kahn-DROY-tun). *Biologic chemical*. A mucopolysaccharide present in connective tissue. Excess amounts found in the urine in some pathological conditions. Also, used as a nutritional supplement for its analgesic and cartilage-protecting effects.

chondrolysis (kahn-droh-LI-sus). *Pathologic condition*. Loss or resorption of cartilage. Can be secondary to infection or autoimmune disease.

chondroma (kahn-DROH-muh). *Pathologic condition*. A benign cartilaginous tumor.
    juxta-cortical c.: beneath the periosteum against the bone's cortex.

chondromalacia (khan-droh-muh-LAY-shuh). *Pathologic condition.* Softening or degeneration of the articular cartilage.

    c. patella: softening of the articular (joint) surface of the patella (kneecap); an early stage in cartilage degeneration.

chondromatosis (synovial) (khan-droh-muh-TOH-sus), **osteochondromatosis, synovial osteochondromatosis.** *Pathologic condition.* Multiple small cartilaginous formations in the synovial membrane that may detach and fall into the joint as loose bodies (joint mice). Causes pain, swelling and stiffness.

chondromyxoid fibroma (khan-droh-MIKS-oyd). *See* CHONDROFIBROMA.

chondromyxoma (kahn-droh-miks-OH-muh). *See* CHONDROFIBROMA.

chondromyxosarcoma (kahn-droh-miks-oh-sahr-KOH-muh), **myxoid chondrosarcoma**. *Pathologic condition.* Malignant cartilaginous tumor containing mucus elements.

chondronecrosis (kahn-droh-nek-ROH-sus). *Pathologic condition.* Death of cartilage cells.

chondro-osteodystrophy deformans (kahn-droh-ahs-tee-oh-DIS-truh-fee). *Pathologic condition.* Refers to a number of bone and cartilage disorders that result in characteristic short stature and abnormal hips; most common is Morquio-Brailsford syndrome. See also MUCOPOLYSACCHARIDOSIS.

chondropathy (kahn-DRAH-puh-thee). *Pathologic condition.* Any disease of the cartilage.

chondrophyte (KAHN-droh-fite). *Pathologic condition.* Abnormal cartilage mass at the edge of a joint.

chondroplasty (KAHN-droh-plas-tee). *Surgical procedure.* Repair, realignment or trimming of cartilage.

chondrosarcoma (kahn-droh-sahr-KOH-muh). *Pathologic condition.* A malignant cartilaginous tumor.

    clear cell c.: rare type of malignant tumor of immature cartilage origin; tends to occur at upper ends of humerus (arm bone) and femur (thighbone).

chondrosarcomatosis (kahn-droh-sahr-koh-muh-TOH-sus). *Pathologic condition.* Multiple areas of sarcoma (malignant growth) of cartilaginous origin.

chondrotomy (kahn-DRAH-toh-mee). *Surgical procedure.* Division of cartilage.

Chopart amputation (sho-PAHR). *Surgical procedure.* Removal of the foot at the midtarsal joint.

chordoma (kor-DOH-muh). *Pathologic condition.* Malignant tumor of the spinal column, most frequently in the sacral or cervical spine.

chorea (koh-REE-uh). *Pathologic condition.* Involuntary, rhythmic movement of the extremities associated with diseases of the central nervous system.

    Huntington's c.: progressive deterioration of the central nervous system characterized by uncontrollable irregular movements of the limbs, trunk and face with attempts at voluntary movement. Accompanied by mental deterioration independent of the movement disorder. Most common form; begins between ages 35–40 (occasionally in childhood). Hereditary.

chronic (KRAHN-ik). *Description.* Of long duration, or frequent recurrence over a long time, often with a slow progressive course of indefinite duration. See also ACUTE.

cicatricial (sik-uh-TRISH-ul). *Description.* Scarlike.

cicatrix (SIK-uh-triks), **scar**. *Abnormal condition.* The fibrous tissue that forms over a wound during healing, replacing normal tissue.

cineplastic amputation (sin-uh-PLAS-tik). *Surgical procedure.* Amputation with preparation of the stump for suspending and activating a prosthesis with straps; most frequently in the arm.

cineplasty (SIN-uh-plas-tee). *Surgical procedure*. Forming a muscle into a loop covered with skin; for activating a prosthesis after amputation of an arm or leg.

circo-electric bed. *Appliance*. Motorized bed with a top and bottom frame that can be rotated to enable a patient to be turned from the back to the abdomen. See also FOSTER FRAME.

circumduction maneuver (sur-sum-DUK-shun). *Function*. Circular movement of an extremity or other part.

circumflex (SUR-kum-fleks). *Anatomic description*. Denoting an arc or circle. Often used in naming vessels or nerves that encircle a bone.

> **c. vessels**. *Anatomy*. Blood vessels that loosely wrap around a portion of bone. Usually named after the bones they surround, e.g., humeral circumflex artery and vein, iliac circumflex artery and vein.

Clarke procedure. *Surgical procedure*. For correction of congenital vertical talus.

claudication (klah-dih-KAY-shun). *Pathologic condition*. Limping.

> **intermittent**: occurs intermittently, usually in relation to effort or activity level. Most likely vascular in origin.

> **neurologic**: lower body pain and weakness related to position and relieved by change in posture; secondary to nerve root irritation.

> **vascular**: pain caused by cramping, from insufficient blood supply to the leg muscles as when blood vessels are constricted or obliterated, such as in diabetes or arteriosclerosis. Also called CHARCOT'S SYNDROME, MYESTHENIA ANGIOSCLEROTICA.

clavicle (KLAV-ih-kul), **collarbone**. *Anatomy*. Slender bone with a double curve. The round, inner end is attached to the sternum, and the flat, outer end is attached to the scapula.

claviculectomy (kluh-vik-yu-LEK-tuh-mee). *Surgical procedure*. Removal of the clavicle (collarbone).

> **distal c.**: removal of outer end of clavicle. See MUMFORD PROCEDURE.

claviculotomy. *Surgical procedure*. Division of the clavicle (collarbone).

clavus (KLAY-vus), **corn**. *Pathologic condition*. Callus (thickened, hardened area of skin with a hard core) induced by pressure over a bony area, frequently on the tops or sides of the toes.

> **c. durum**: occurs from pressure of a toe against the shoe.

> **c. mollum**: soft callus most frequently between the 4th and 5th toes.

claw foot, **cavus foot**, **gampsodactyly**, **pes cavus**. *Pathologic condition*. Abnormally high-arched foot; usually with clawing of toes. Associated with some forms of neurologic abnormality such as polio or Charcot-Marie-Tooth disease.

claw hand, **main en griffe**. *Pathologic condition*. Hyperextension of the metacarpophalangeal joints of the fingers and flexion of the middle and distal phalanges, giving a clawlike appearance. Frequently associated with neurological disorders and ulnar nerve lesions.

> **ulnar c. h.**: clawing of the 4th and 5th fingers, with decreased sensation, from injury or transection of the ulnar nerve.

claw toes. *Pathologic condition*. Hyperextension of the metatarsophalangeal joints of the toes and flexion of the proximal interphalangeal joints, giving a clawlike appearance. Frequently occurs in rheumatoid arthritis and Charcot- Marie-Tooth disease.

clay-shoveler's fracture. *Pathologic condition*. A break involving the spinous process of a lower cervical (neck) or upper thoracic (chest) vertebra; results from intense traction on the spinous process by the interspinous ligament.

clear cell chrondrosarcoma. See CHRONDROSARCOMA.

cleft foot, **lobster foot**. *Congenital anomaly*. Foot separated into two parts (like a lobster claw), possibly with missing parts such as metatarsal bones and toes.

cleft hand, lobster hand /or/ **claw, split-hand, main fourchee**. *Congenital anomaly.* Hand separated into two parts (like a lobster claw), associated with missing fingers and metacarpals.

cleidocranial dysostosis (kli-doh-KRAY-nee-ul dis-ahs-TOH-sus). *Congenital abnormality.* Absence of part of one or both clavicles (collarbones), resulting in extreme shoulder motion. May be associated with a bossing (prominence) at the front of the skull, scoliosis, and dental abnormalities. Hereditary.

clinodactyly (kli-noh-DAK-tuh-lee). *Abnormal condition.* Bending deformity of the small finger's distal phalanx. Rarely severe enough to treat. May be hereditary.

Clinoril. *Drug.* Trade name of sulindac, NSAID for treating pain and inflammation.

clonus (KLOH-nus). *Pathologic condition.* Rapid contraction and relaxation of a muscle, most frequently in the ankle; associated with central nervous system disease, e.g., cerebral palsy. Also normally seen at lighter depths of anesthesia.

closed amputation. *Surgical procedure.* Amputation in which the incision is covered by skin. See also OPEN AMPUTATION.

closed biopsy (BI-ahp-see). *Surgical procedure.* Obtaining tissue for exam, as by needle aspiration without cutting tissue or skin. See also OPEN BIOPSY.

closed dislocation. *Abnormal condition.* Joint displacement in which the affected bone does not communicate with the outside or surface area. See also OPEN DISLOCATION.

closed fracture, simple fracture. *Pathologic condition.* Break in which the bones do not exit the skin or damage the surrounding tissue.

closed hip reduction. *Treatment.* Manipulating the femoral head back into the hip socket (acetabulum) without opening the joint. See also OPEN HIP REDUCTION.

closed reduction. *Treatment.* Manipulating a dislocated or fractured bone back to its normal position without cutting the skin. See also OPEN REDUCTION.

closed suction irrigation. *Treatment.* With tubes placed in an infected wound and the tissues closed over them, antibiotic irrigation fluid is passed in one tube and pulled out the other by suction, continuously washing the wound. See also VACUUM ASSISTED CLOSURE (VAC) DRESSING.

closing wedge osteotomy (ahs-tee-AH-tuh-mee). *Surgical procedure.* Removing a wedge from one side of a long bone and straightening the bone, to realign a malunion or deformity. See also OPENING WEDGE OSTEOTOMY.

clothespin graft. *Surgical procedure.* Type of spinal graft: two wedges are cut from opposite ends of a graft so it can be held firmly between the spinous processes of adjacent vertebrae. Resembles a clothespin.

cloverleaf nail. *Surgical implant.* Intramedullary nail whose cross-section is in the shape of a cloverleaf. Designed to increase the nail's strength.

cloward spine fusion. *Surgical procedure.* Method of fusing the anterior cervical spine by removing the disc and/or vertebra and inserting a graft.

clubfoot, equinovarus, pes equinovarus, talipes equinovarus. *Congenital abnormality.* Rigid, inwardly rotated foot that bends down and in; if untreated, rests on outer edge and cannot be placed flat on the walking surface.

clubhand, radial clubhand, talipomanus. *Congenital abnormality.* Absence of the radius (larger forearm bone) and the thumb, with the wrist deviated toward the thumb side.

cluneal nerve (CLU-nee-ul). *Anatomy.* Small nerve that supplies the outer surface of the buttock and thigh; exits over the iliac crest.

CNS (central nervous system). Refers to the brain and spinal cord.

coalition. *Abnormal condition.* Abnormal union in the bones of the hand or foot.

coaptation splint (koh-ap-TAY-shun). *Orthopedic applicance.* Splint placed on both sides of a fracture, maintaining pressure against the fragments.

Cobb elevator. *Surgical instrument*. Long-handled tool used for stripping muscles and ligaments; has a flattened bulbous end with a narrow, curved sharp edge.

Cobb method. *Radiographic technique*. Used to measure size of a spinal curve.

cobra plate. *Surgical implant*. Used in hip fusion (arthrodesis); the upper part of the plate has a flared end that is bent, giving the appearance of a cobra.

coccidioidomycosis (cahk-sid-ee-oyd-oh-mi-KOH-sus). *Pathologic condition*. Fungal infection caused by the organism *Coccidioides immitis*, found in soil and inhaled in dust particles.

coccydynia (kahk-sih-DIN-ee-uh), **coccyalgia**. *Abnormal condition*. Pain in the coccyx (tailbone).

coccygectomy (kahk-sih-JEK-tuh-mee). *Surgical procedure*. Removal of the coccyx (tailbone).

coccyx (KAHK-siks), **tailbone**. *Anatomy*. The 3–5 fused rudimentary coccygeal vertebrae at the tip of the sacrum that represent the bony remnants of a tail.

cock-up splint. *Orthopedic appliance*. Plaster or metal splint that holds the wrist in a slightly dorsiflexed position; used for protecting the wrist.

Codman approach. *Surgical technique*. Approach to the shoulder; begins over the deltoid muscle at the front, crosses over the clavicle (collarbone), to the back of the shoulder.

Codman exercises. *Treatment*. Stretching exercises for improving the shoulder's range of motion.

Codman sign. *Clinical sign*. For rupture of the supraspinatus tendon; contraction of the deltoid muscle in the absence of a functional rotator cuff causes hunching of the shoulder.

Codman's triangle. *Radiologic finding*. X-ray finding of new bone deposited in a characteristic pattern when the periosteum is lifted by a tumor or infection; frequently seen in rapidly growing tumors such as osteogenic sarcoma and in osteomyelitis.

Codman's tumor, **chondroblastoma**. *Pathologic condition*. Benign cartilaginous tumor commonly seen in the epiphysis (growth area) of long bones, most frequently in the shoulder.

cogwheel sign, **cogwheel phenomenon**. *Clinical sign*. An irregular or jerky motion upon manipulation. Indicates central nervous system abnormality.

Coke and Jahss osteotomy. *Surgical technique*. Removing a wedge from the top of the foot at the level of the naviculocuneiform joint and bending the forefoot upward, to correct a cavus deformity.

Coleman block test. *Clinical test*. Test for rigidity of a cavus foot. Patient stands with a block placed under outer side of the foot. If the hindfoot varus corrects itself, the deformity is flexible; if it does not, then it is rigid.

Cole pull-out wire. *Surgical technique*. Wire passed through a tendon, to hold it temporarily while it heals.

collagen (KAHL-uh-jun). *Biologic material*. Protein that forms a major portion of the fibers of skin, tendons, cartilage, bone, and connective tissue.

> **c. vascular disease** (VAS-kyu-lur). *Pathologic condition*. Group of disorders with major involvement of connective tissues; caused by immune system malfunction. Example: rheumatoid arthritis.

collagenous (kuh-LAJ-un-us). *Description*. Made up of collagen.

collar and cuff sling. *Orthopedic device*. Strip of material used to immobilize an injured upper extremity. Runs around back of the neck and below the wrist.

collarbone. *Anatomy*. Popular term for the clavicle; slender bone with a double curve that attaches at one end to the sternum and the other to the scapula.

collar button abscess, **shirt-stud abscess**. *Pathologic conditon*. Collection of pus in the web space between the fingers. Begins on the palmar side and continues to the other, making two abscess cavities with a thin portion in between, giving the appearance of a collar button.

collateral ligaments. *Anatomy*. Connective tissue attachments on the sides of hinged joints (elbow, knee, wrist, fingers, toes); provide stability and support. See also CRUCIATE LIGAMENTS.

    medial (MEE-dee-ul): gives stability to the inner side of a joint.

    fibular: lateral collateral ligament of the knee. Runs along outer side of the knee; connects the femur (thighbone) to the tibia (shinbone). Acts as a stabilizer of the knee, keeping the tibia from rotating inward.

    lateral: gives stability to the outer side of a joint.

    radial: connective tissue band (1) along outer side of elbow, connecting humerus and ulna; acts as a restraining ligament of the elbow, keeping the ulna from rotating inward; (2) along the outer side of the interphalangeal and metacarpophalangeal joints of the fingers and thumb.

    tibial*: medial collateral ligament of the knee; connective tissue band along inner side of knee; connects the femur (thighbone) to the tibia (shinbone); acts as a stabilizer of the knee, keeping tibia from rotating outward.

Colles' fracture (KAHL-ees). *Pathologic condition*. Break in the distal end of the radius (larger forearm bone) in which the apex of the fracture points to the front, and the distal fragment is displaced to the back.

Colonna capsular arthroplasty (AHR-throh-plas-tee). *Surgical procedure*. Used in the treatment of congenital hip dislocations. The acetabulum (hip socket) is enlarged and deepened to a cup shape. The capsule of the hip joint is then used to cover the femoral head so that it may act as a spacer between it and the acetabulum.

Colton classification. *Fracture classification*. Identifies the four types of fractures of the olecranon (elbow).

comminuted fracture. *Pathologic condition*. Bone that is broken into more than two pieces.

common iliac arteries (IL-ee-ak). *Anatomy*. The two branches of the abdominal aorta (right and left); each then divides into internal (hypogastric) and external iliac arteries.

common iliac vein. *Anatomy*. Vein formed by the joining of the external and internal iliac veins of each upper leg; drains blood from the legs and pelvis into the heart.

common peroneal nerve (pehr-uh-NEE-ul). *Anatomy*. Branch of the sciatic nerve that wraps around the lateral fibula and splits into the deep and superficial peroneal nerves. These supply side and front of the lower leg.

compartment. *Anatomy*. A consistently identifiable segment of an extremity or body part containing multiple anatomic structures. With muscle compartments, the muscles are usually within sheaths of connective tissue. In addition to those listed below, there are muscle compartments in the foot and hand named after their respective muscles.

    adductor c. of the thigh: contains adductor muscles of the thigh; these include the adductor longus and gracilis muscles in a superficial layer, the adductor brevis in a middle layer and adductor magnus as a deep layer. All but the adductor magnus muscle are supplied by the obturator nerve.

    anterior antebrachial c.: compartment at the front or under surface of the antebrachium (forearm); contains flexor muscles of the wrist. Divided into a deep group (containing the flexor digitorum profundus, flexor pollicis longus and pronator quadratus muscles) and a superficial group (containing the pronator teres, flexor carpi radialis, palmaris longus, flexor carpi ulnaris and flexor digitorum superficialis muscles). Some texts add a "middle layer" that contains only the flexor digitorum superficialis.

anterior brachial c.: front compartment of upper arm; contains the biceps, brachialis and part of coracobrachialis muscles, the brachial vessels, the ulnar nerve and median nerve.

anterior c. of the thigh: contains quadriceps and sartorius muscles; innervated by the femoral nerve.

anterior crural c.: situated between tibia and anterior intermuscular septum; contains the tibialis anterior, extensor hallucis longus, extensor digitorum longus and peroneus tertius muscles. Innervated by the deep peroneal nerve and fed by the anterior tibial artery.

crural c.: see LATERAL CRURAL C., POSTERIOR CRURAL C. (below).

dorsal c. of the antebrachium: rear compartment of the forearm; contains the extensor muscles of the wrist. Innervated by the posterior interosseus nerve (branch of radial nerve). Divided into two groups: deep (containing the supinator, abductor pollicis longus, extensor pollicis brevis, extensor pollicis longus and extensor indicis muscles) and superficial (containing the brachioradialis, extensor carpi radialis longus, extensor carpi radialis brevis, extensor digitorum, extensor digiti minimi, extensor carpi ulnaris and anconeus muscles).

dorsal c. of the forearm: same as DORSAL C. OF THE ANTEBRACHIUM.

extensor c. of the brachium: rear compartment of the upper arm; contains the triceps muscle, the radial nerve and the deep brachial artery.

extensor c's of the wrist: six small tunnels made by the connective tissue septa connecting the extensor retinaculum of the wrist to the bones of the wrist. These tunnels maintain the extensor tendons of the wrist and hand in their respective positions as they make their way to their destination.

    1st: houses the abductor tendon of the pollicis longus and the extensor pollicis brevis tendon.

    2nd: houses tendons of extensor carpi radialis longus and brevis.

    3rd: houses the tendons of the extensor pollicis longus.

    4th: houses the tendons of the extensor digitorum.

    5th: houses the tendon of the extensor digiti minimi.

    6th: houses the tendon of the extensor carpi ulnaris.

flexor c. of the forearm: same as ANTERIOR ANTEBRACHIAL COMPARTMENT.

flexor c. of the brachium: same as ANTERIOR BRACHIAL COMPARTMENT.

lateral crural c.: situated at the outer aspect of the lower leg; contains the peroneus brevis and longus muscles. Innervated by the superficial peroneal nerve; does not have a dedicated artery.

lateral c. of the knee: articulation between the outer femoral condyle and outer tibial condyle; contains the lateral meniscus and popliteal tendon.

medial c. of the knee: articulation between the inner femoral condyle and inner tibial condyle; contains the medial meniscus.

medial c. of the thigh: same as ADDUCTOR COMPARTMENT OF THE THIGH.

patellofemoral c. of the knee: articulation between the front of the lower end of the femur (thighbone) and the patella (kneecap).

posterior antebrachial c.: same as DORSAL C. OF THE ANTEBRACHIUM.

posterior brachial c.: same as EXTENSOR COMPARTMENT OF BRACHIUM.

posterior c. of the thigh: houses the hamstring muscles. Supplied by the sciatic nerve.

posterior crural c.: situated at back of lower leg; houses muscles of the back of the lower leg. Divided into superficial (containing the gastrocnemius, soleus and plantaris muscles) and deep (containing the popliteus, flexor hallucis longus, flexor digitorum longus and tibialis posterior muscles) posterior crural compartments. Innervated by the tibial nerve and fed by the posterior tibial artery.

volar c. of the forearm: same as ANTERIOR ANTEBRACHIAL COMPARTMENT.

compartment syndrome. *Pathologic condition*. Increased pressure within the tight space of a fascial compartment of an arm or leg, impairing circulation to the muscles in the compartment; may cause pain, swelling, and death of the muscles.

compensatory curve. *Pathologic condition*. In scoliosis, the spinal curvature above and below the major curve, situated so that the head and neck remain centered over the pelvis.

Compere Vulpius gastrocnemius release (gas-trahk-NEE-mee-us). *Surgical procedure*. Lengthening the Achilles tendon by partially releasing it at the level where the gastrocnemius muscle converges onto the tendon (musculotendinous juncture).

complete blood count (CBC). *Lab test*. A set of blood tests. Usually consists of white and red blood cell counts, differential count, hemoglobin, hematocrit, platelet count.

complete fracture. *Pathologic condition*. A break in a bone that runs completely across the bone creating at least two separate fragments.

compound fracture, open fracture. *Pathologic condition*. Break in which the bone ends have protruded through the skin. Open fracture is the newer, preferred term.

compression arthrodesis (ahr-thro-DEE-sus). *Treatment*. Fusing a joint by holding the bone ends on either side in compression.

compression dressing. *Orthopedic device*. Type of dressing that acts as a circumferential pressure pad, giving equal pressure to all areas; useful in decreasing swelling or bleeding in an arm or leg.

compression fracture. *Pathologic condition*. A break resulting from the crushing of the bone (compressed toward the center of the bone); usually in a vertebra weakened from osteoporosis.

compression plate. *Orthopedic appliance*. Metallic internal fixation device for increasing pressure across a fracture or osteotomy site to promote stability, alignment and healing.

computed tomography, computerized tomography. See CT SCAN.

computerized axial tomography (CAT scan). See CT SCAN.

conduction time. *Test*. For nerve function; the time it takes for an impulse to travel from one spot along a nerve to another. Conduction time divided by the distance traveled results in the conduction velocity. See also NERVE CONDUCTION VELOCITY TEST.

conduction velocity. *Test*. A measure of nerve function; measures speed with which an impulse travels along a nerve (time divided by distance).

condylar fracture (KAHN-duh-lur). *Pathologic condition*. A break in the rounded flare at the end of a long bone.

condyle (KAHN-dile). *Anatomy*. Rounded end of a long bone.

congenital. *Description*. Present at birth.

c. anomaly. *Pathologic condition*. A physical abnormality present at birth. Generally refers to a specific deformity or malformation; may or may not be hereditary.

c. amniotic band, c. annular band /or/ **ring constriction**. *Congenital abnormality*. Constricting ring produced by a thin band of amniotic membrane that may encircle an arm, leg or digit in utero; may be deep so as to sever blood vessels and nerves. See also STREETER'S DYSPLASIA.

c. atonic pseudoparalysis. *Congenital disorder*. Neuromuscular disorder that in young children causes myotonia (muscle spasm) of the muscles innervated by the spinal nerves. See also AMYTONIA CONGENITA.

c. bars, tarsal coalition. *Congenital abnormality.* Fusion of two or more adjacent bones of the foot that are normally unconnected.

c. convex pes valgus. See CONGENITAL VERTICAL TALUS.

c. coxa vara (KAHKS-uh VEHR-uh). See COXA VARA.

c. disease. *Pathologic condition.* Any disease present at birth that began during fetal development; may or may not be hereditary.

c. dislocation of the hip (CDH), c. hip dysplasia. Obsolete terms; now called DEVELOPMENTAL DYSPLASIA OF THE HIP (DDH).

c. dysplasia of the hip (CDH) (dis-PLAY-zjuh), **acetabular dysplasia, developmental dysplasia of the hip**. *Pathologic condition.* Incomplete formation of the acetabulum (hip joint socket), leaving the head of the femur (thighbone) partially uncovered, with less-than-normal or no cartilage contact between the femoral head and the acetabulum. See also CRAIG ABDUCTION SPLINT, BARLOW TEST, ORTOLANI TEST.

c. elevation of the scapula, Sprengel's deformity. *Congenital abnormality.* Elevation and medial rotation of the scapula (shoulderblade). Motion is limited.

c. generalized fibromatosis (fi-broh-muh-TOH-sus), **infantile fibromatosis**. *Congenital abnormality.* Multiple benign fibromas (fibrous connective tissue) in soft tissues of many areas of the body. Usually presents in childhood; may result in progressive limb and spine abnormalities.

c. grooves. See CONGENITAL AMNIOTIC BANDS.

c. hypotonia (hi-poh-TOH-nee-uh). *Congenital abnormality.* Neuromuscular disorder that in young children causes lower than normal muscle tone. See also AMYTONIA CONGENITA.

c. indifference to pain. *Pathologic condition.* Varying degrees of insensitivity to normally painful stimuli, such as fractures, bruises. May be associated with congenital syphilis. See also FAMILIAL DYSAUTONOMA.

c. kyphosis (ki-FOH-sus). *Congenital abnormality.* An increase in the thoracic or lumbar arch of the spine secondary to partial absence or fusion of one or more vertebrae anteriorly; growth occurs only in posterior half of the vertebral column, causing the deformity to progress over time.

c. ring constriction. See CONGENITAL AMNIOTIC BAND.

c. rocker-bottom foot. See CONGENITAL VERTICAL TALUS.

c. sensory neuropathy. *Congenital abnormality.* Sensory nerve abnormality preventing the perception of pain. Usually first noted in late infancy with ulcerations and burn injuries. May be associated with anhydrosis and retinitis pigmentosa. Hereditary; recessive.

c. subluxation of the hip. Obsolete term; now called DEVELOPMENTAL DYSPLASIA OF THE HIP (DDH).

c. torticollis (tor-tuh-KAH-lus). *Congenital abnormality.* Head that is turned to one side and cocked to the other side, in response to contraction of neck muscles; may be secondary to contracture of the sternocleidomastoid during fetal development. May not be apparent until age 1 or 2.

c. vertical talus (TAY-lus), **c. convex pes valgus** /or/ **rocker-bottom foot**. *Congenital abnormality.* Foot deformity characterized by rigidity and rocker-bottom appearance: marked plantarflexion of the talus (foot bone connecting with ankle) and dorsiflexion of the forefoot.

congenita punctata, chrondrodysplasia, chondrodysplasia punctata, chondystrophia calcificans congenita, punctate epiphyseal dysplasia. *Congenital abnormality.* Malformation of bones resulting in joint deformations and leading to a form of dwarfism. Characterized by limb deformities, spine abnormalities, varus defomation of the hips, difficulty walking, and x-ray appearance of stippled, calcified epiphyses; stippling is present at birth, but usually disappears by age 1. See also CONRADI-HUNERMANN DISEASE, RHIZOMELIC FORM.

congruence angle. *Radiologic measurement.* On a tangential view of the knee (merchant's view), angle created by the intersection of a line connecting the apex of the sulcus angle and the lowest point of the patella (kneecap), and a second line bisecting the sulcus angle. If the line connecting the patella lies lateral to the bisector of the sulcus, the angle is considered positive; if medial, it is negative. The normal congruence angle is considered to be –6° with 95% of specimens having measurements within 11° of normal. An abnormal congruence angle (more than 4° positive) is considered a sign of patellar subluxation.

conjoined nerve root. *Congenital anomaly.* Two nerve roots that exit from the same canal within a single sheath; usually found in the lumbar region.

conjoined tendon. *Anatomy.* Tendon (e.g., iliopsoas) that divides into two or more parts, connecting two or more muscles to the same location on a bone.

conoid ligament (KOH-noyd). *Anatomy.* One of the connective tissue bands joining the clavicle (collarbone) to the scapula (shoulderblade).

Conradi-Hunermann disease. *Congenital abnormality.* Most common form of chondrodysplasia punctata. Autosomal dominant form with a high incidence of spontaneous mutation. Severity varies widely. Patients usually have a prominent forehead, wide-set eyes, flattened nose, thinning hair, heart abnormalities and, in severe cases, mental retardation.

constrained knee prosthesis (pros-THEE-sus) *Orthopedic appliance.* Artificial knee joint in which the femoral component is attached to the tibial component.

constricting annular groove (AN-yu-lur). See CONGENITAL AMNIOTIC BAND.

continuous passive motion machine (CPM). *Orthopedic appliance.* Used for applying continuous motion to a joint; used after surgery to restore motion.

contouring of bone. *Surgical procedure.* Shaving and patterning the ends of bones.

contraction. *Function.* Shortening of muscle fibers in normal movement.

contracture. *Pathologic condition.* Inability of a joint to complete its normal range of motion; secondary to tightness or thickening of the soft tissues.

> **extension c**: tightness prevents full flexion of the joint.
> **flexion c**: tightness prevents full extension of the joint.

contralateral. *Anatomy.* Refers to opposite side of the body. See also IPSILATERAL.

contralateral straight leg raising test, prostrate leg raising test, sciatic phenomenon, well leg raising test of Fajersztajn. *Clinical test.* With patient lying on his/her back, a leg is raised with the knee in extension. Pain in the opposite leg indicates irritation of the nerve as it exits the spine. Sign of herniated disc disease.

contrast bath. *Treatment.* Immersion of an extremity in ice water, then in warm water, then in ice water, etc. To stimulate blood circulation and reduce swelling when treating sprains and strains.

contrast medium. *Radiographic material.* Radiopaque dye injected into a vein or joint to outline the structure on x-ray.

control cable. *Orthopedic appliance.* Steel cable attached to a prosthesis that utilizes existing muscles to operate mechanical joints.

contusion, bruise. *Pathologic condition.* Escape of blood into the tissues, with resultant discoloration. See also ECCHYMOSIS.

conus medullaris (KOH-nus), **medullary cone**. *Anatomy*. The tapered lower end of the spinal cord as it separates into the cauda equina (nerve roots at tail end of spinal cord), between L1 and L2.

conventional NSAID (nonsteroidal anti-inflammatory drug). *Drug*. Any NSAID (pain-relieving drug that suppresses inflammation) that is not a COX-2 inhibitor.

Coopernail sign. *Clinical sign*. Bruising of the scrotum or labia; may indicate a fracture of the pelvis.

coracoid (KOR-uh-koyd), **coracoid process**. *Anatomy*. A beaklike projection on the front of the scapula (shoulderblade) to which is attached the short head of the biceps, pectoralis minor and coracobrachialis muscles, and the coracoacromial, coracohumeral, and coracoclavicular ligaments.

cord traction syndrome, filum terminale syndrome, tethered cord syndrome. *Congenital anomaly*. In patients with certain spinal defects (e.g., spina bifida), the conus medullaris (terminal end of spinal cord) becomes attached to the bone or scar tissue, preventing its upward migration with growth. Causes cord tension and can result in progressive paralysis of the bladder, bowel, and lower extremities.

corn, clavus. *Abnormal condition*. Thickened, hardened area of the skin with a hard core, induced by pressure over a bony area, frequently on the tops or sides of the toes.

    hard c., heloma durum: callus formed on or about a bony prominence or joint, caused by pressure.

    soft c., heloma molle: pressure area between the toes that results in the formation of a painful callosity. Usually macerated and softened from moistness between the toes.

coronoid process. *Anatomy*. Small triangular projection of bone at the proximal end of the ulna (smaller forearm bone); forms part of the elbow joint and provides attachment for the brachialis muscle.

cortex. *Anatomy*. Outer layer of an organ or structure. Plural: cortices.

cortical. *Anatomic description*. Refers to the cortex, the outer layer of an organ or structure.

    c. bone. *Anatomy*. Dense hard layer of bone making up outer surface of long bones; surrounds spongy trabecular bone. See also CANCELLOUS BONE.

    c. defect. *Pathologic condition*. Cavity in the cortex (hard outer surface of a bone) or missing piece of the cortex, such as in cases of trauma.

        fibrous, fibrocortical defect: benign asymptomatic fibrous bone lesion on the metaphysis of long bones; related to and smaller than nonossifying fibroma; usually seen in children.

    c. fracture. *Pathologic condition*. A break that involves the cortex (hard bone at the periphery of a bone).

    c. graft. *Biological implant*. Body tissue composed of the hard cortex (outer surface) of the donor bone.

    c. screw. *Surgical implant*. Screw with small threads that attaches a segment of cortical bone to a metal plate or another segment of bone.

corticosteroid, steroid. *Drug class*. Cortisone derivative; for treating inflammatory and allergic diseases.

cortisone. *1. Biologic substance*. Hormone produced by the adrenal gland. Serves as a metabolic enhancer and accelerator. *2. Drug*. Potent anti-inflammatory medication.

costal chondritis. *Incorrect spelling of COSTOCHONDRITIS*.

costochondritis (kahs-toh-kahn-DRI-tus), **costosternal syndrome**, **peristernal perichondritis**, **Tietze's syndrome**. *Pathologic condition*. Inflammation, pain and tenderness of the cartilage connecting the ribs to the sternum (breastbone). The pain is exacerbated with deep breathing.

costosternal syndrome (kahs-toh-STUR-nul). See COSTOCHONDRITIS.

costotransversectomy (kahs-toh-trans-vur-SEK-toh-mee). *Surgical procedure.* Incision through the back of the chest to gain side access to the vertebral column; part of the ribs and the transverse process (lateral projection) of the vertebra(e) are removed.

Cotrel cast technique. *Treatment.* Application of a cast using slings for traction on the head and pelvis; for correction of a spine deformity.

Cotrel derotation strap. *Orthopedic supply.* Strap used on a casting table to rotate the rib cage of a patient with scoliosis.

Cotrel-Dubousset (CD) (du-bu-SAY). *Surgical implant.* Series of hooks and cross-linked parallel rods surgically attached to the spine to correct fracture or a spinal deformity such as scoliosis.

cotton fracture. *Pathologic condition.* Trimalleolar break in the articular (joint) surface of the tibia (shinbone); involves the medial and lateral malleoli and the posterior distal tip of tibia.

counterextension. See COUNTERTRACTION.

countertraction, counterextension. *Treatment.* Traction pulling the weight of the body in the opposite direction from an extremity.

coxa (KAHKS-uh). *Anatomy.* Hip or hip joint. Plural: coxae.

    c. adducta. See COXA VARA.

    c. magna. *Pathologic condition.* Hip deformity: enlargement of the femoral head.

    c. plana (PLAN-uh). *Pathologic condition.* Hip deformity: flattening of the femoral head.

    c. valga (VAL-guh). *Pathologic condition.* Hip deformity: the neck angle of the proximal end of thighbone (femur) is increased (greater than 120°– 135°). May be congenital, acquired or developmental.

    c. vara (VEHR-uh), **coxa adducta.** *Abnormal condition.* Hip deformity: the neck shaft angle of the thighbone (femur) is decreased. May be congenital, acquired or developmental.

COX inhibitors. *Drug class.* Class of nonsteroidal anti-inflammatory drugs (NSAIDs) that works by inhibiting the cyclooxygenase (COX) enzyme.

    COX-1: NSAIDs that work primarily by inhibiting the action of the COX-1 enzyme. These are the conventional NSAIDs. Felt to have more side effects (e.g., gastrointestinal irritation) than the newer COX-2 inhibitors. See also CONVENTIONAL NSAID.

    COX 2: NSAIDs that work by inhibiting the COX-2 enzyme. Felt to have more specialized effects at controlling inflammation than COX-1 inhibitors, but have potential heart side effects. Trade names: Bextra, Celebrex, Vioxx.

coxodynia (kahks-uh-DIN-ee-uh). *Pathologic condition.* Pain in the hip joint.

Craig abduction splint. *Orthopedic appliance.* Splint that maintains reduction of a congenitally dislocated hip by abducting the legs.

cranial halo. *Orthopedic appliance.* Ring placed around the skull for maintaining alignment or stability of the neck; held in place with four pins screwed into the skull.

Crawford-Adams cup. *Surgical implant.* Type of metal cup used in total hip replacement, to replace the hip's natural cup (acetabulum).

creatinine phosphokinase (CPK) (kree-AT-in-in fas-foh-KI-nays). *Biologic substance.* An enzyme present in cardiac and skeletal muscles and in the brain. After an injury or in some pathological conditions, a higher level of CPK is released into the bloodstream indicating the severity of injury or disease.

crepitus (KREP-uh-tus). *Clinical finding.* Grating, cracking sensation of a joint when flexed and extended or when bone ends rub against each other at a fracture site.

crescentic osteotomy. *Surgical procedure.* Cutting either end of a long bone into a semi-circle so that alignment can be correct in all three dimensions.

crescent sign. *Radiologic sign.* On x-ray, a clear (lucent) line (crack) underneath the articular joint surface at the edge of a bone. Seen in avascular necrosis of the femoral head.

cretinism (KREE-tin-iz-um). *Congenital abnormality.* Hypothyroidism in an infant. Causes delay in physical and mental development.

cross-finger flap. *Surgical procedure.* Technique for grafting skin from one finger to an adjacent finger.

cruciate ligaments (KRU-shee-ut). *Anatomy.* Bands of connective tissue in the knee connecting the thighbone (femur) to the shinbone (tibia) and giving stability to the knee joint. See also COLLATERAL LIGAMENTS.

    anterior: connects the distal lateral femoral condyle (thighbone) to the front part of the tibia (shinbone) across the knee joint; prevents the tibia from slipping forward on the femur.

    posterior: joins the femur (thighbone) to the tibia (shinbone) within the knee joint; prevents the tibia from slipping backward on the femur.

cruciform ligament of the atlas. *Anatomy.* Cross-shaped connective tissue connecting the axis (2nd neck vertebra) to the atlas (1st neck vertebra).

crura (KRU-ruh). *Anatomy.* Plural of CRUS.

crural. *Anatomic description.* Pertaining to the crus, portion of leg between the knee and the ankle.

    c. compartment. See COMPARTMENT.

crus. *Anatomy.* Portion of the leg between the knee and the ankle. Pl: crura.

crush fracture. *Pathologic condition.* 1. Fracture resulting from a crushing force; usually causes the bone to collapse into itself. 2. A collapsed vertebra.

crust, scab. *Pathologic lesion.* Hardened dried secretions (e.g., blood, plasma, pus) that form over a wound.

crutches. *Orthopedic appliance.* Supports (used singly or in pairs; can be made from wood or metal) extending from the armpits to the floor; used to assist in walking and balance.

Crutchfield tongs. *Surgical implant.* Tongs that are imbedded in the skull for applying traction to the neck.

CT scan (computed tomography), CAT scan. *Radiologic test.* Low dosage x-rays coupled with computers to generate film showing tissue detail in three dimensions.

cubital, triquetral bone, triquetrum. *Anatomy.* Wrist bone in the 2nd row of carpal bones, on the outer side of the wrist between the pisiform and lunate.

cubital tunnel. *Anatomy.* Fibro-osseous (made of ligament and bone) tunnel in the inner side of the elbow through which runs the ulnar nerve, which can be the location of irritation and compression (cubital tunnel syndrome). Since the ulnar nerve lies so close to the skin here, direct impact or trauma to the cubital tunnel area can irritate the ulnar nerve, sending unpleasant electrical sensations to the hand. See also FUNNY BONE.

    syndrome. *Pathologic condition.* Pain, numbness and weakness to the ulnar side of the hand (about the pinky and ring finger) resulting from excessive compression of the ulnar nerve at the cubital tunnel in the elbow.

    release. *Surgical procedure.* Opening the cubital tunnel to alleviate the constriction of the ulnar nerve within the tunnel. Usually performed along with an ulnar nerve transposition. Used in treatment of cubital tunnel syndrome. Also called ULNAR NERVE RELEASE.

cubital vein (KYU-bit-ul). *Anatomy.* The large vein in the front of the elbow.

cubitus (KYU-bit-us), **elbow**. *Anatomy.* Hinged joint comprised of the distal end of the humerus (upper armbone) and the proximal end of the radius and ulna (two forearm bones).

    c. valgus: larger-than-normal angle formed by the upper armbone (humerus) and the forearm; elbow joint deviates away from the midline.

    c. varus, gun stock deformity: smaller-than-normal angle formed by the upper armbone (humerus) and the forearm; the elbow joint deviates toward the midline.

cuboid (KYU-boyd). *Anatomy.* Tarsal bone on outer side of foot that connects with the calcaneus, lateral cuneiform, and 4th and 5th metatarsal bones.

cuneiforms (kyu-NEE-uh-formz). *Anatomy.* Three small wedge-shaped bones (medial, middle, lateral, also referred to as 1st, 2nd and 3rd, respectively) in the midfoot that articulate with the 1st, 2nd and 3rd metatarsal bones (small bones of the midfoot) and with the navicular bone.

curettage (kyur-uh-TAHJ). *Treatment.* The scraping and removal of bone and tissue from an area of infection, fracture or tumor.

cutaneous (kyu-TAY-nee-us). *Anatomic description.* Pertaining to the skin.

    c. nerve. *Anatomy.* Any of the nerves supplying sensation to the skin.

cuticle. *Anatomy.* 1. Epidermis, skin. 2. Popular term for the skin that partly covers the base of a fingernail or toenail. Also called EPONYCHIUM, PERIONYCHIUM.

cyanosis (si-an-OH-sis). *Pathologic condition.* Dark blue or purplish skin color resulting from lack of oxygen in the blood.

cylinder cast. *Orthopedic appliance.* Cast that spans the leg from upper thigh to the flare of the malleoli (tips of lower leg bones), not incorporating the foot, so as to allow for ankle movement. Usually applied with the knee in extension; commonly used in the nonoperative treatment of patella (kneecap) fractures.

cylindrical reamer gauge. *Instrument.* Device used during surgery to determine depth of hip socket (acetabulum) in preparation for total hip replacement.

cyst (sist). *Pathologic condition.* Closed sac that contains fluid. Usually abnormal.

    aneurysmal c. (an-yur-IZ-mul): benign bone tumor containing abnormal anastamosing (communicating) hollow spaces filled with blood. Thin bony walls result in a balloon-like appearance.

    Baker's c.: cyst in the back of the knee; represents a protrusion of synovial (joint) fluid through the back of the knee joint; sometimes enlarges to the point where it is palpable (perceptible through touch).

    bible c.: cyst found in the back of the wrist; named for antiquated treatment of striking it with a large book, or bible, to rupture it.

    bone c.: cyst (empty or fluid-filled) within a bone; benign process may be accompanied by fractures of the thin bony wall.

    ganglion c. (GANG-lee-un): fluid-filled sac protruding from the synovial sheath (lining) of a tendon or the capsule of a joint.

    inclusion c.: abnormal formation of material under skin or within tissue.

    synovial c.: cyst found about a joint and filled with synovial (joint) fluid.

    unicameral c. (yu-nih-CAM-ur-ul): benign single-cavity cyst most commonly found in the humerus (upper armbone).

cystic (SIS-tik). *Pathologic description.* Containing or composed of one or more fluid filled or fibrous sacs (cysts) in a cavity or structure of the body.

    c. angiomatosis of bone (an-jee-oh-muh-TOH-sus). *Pathologic condition.* Bone having, and eventually weakened by, multiple cysts (sacs) composed of blood vessels or lymphatic vessels. Rare.

    c. lesion. *Clinical/radiologic finding.* A fluid-filled lesion.

D

Dacron tape. *Surgical implant*. Tape made of Dacron; used for holding two parts of a ligament together or to hold metal to bone.

Dameron and Rockwood classification. *Fracture classification*. Identifies fractures to the distal end of the clavicle in children.

Darrach-Hughston-Milch fracture (DEHR-uh), **Piedmont fracture**, **Galeazzi's fracture**. *Pathologic condition*. Break in the distal third of the radius (larger forearm bone); associated with dislocation of the distal radioulnar joint (between the two forearm bones).

Darrach procedure (DEHR-uh). *Surgical procedure*. Removal of the distal end of the ulna when there is destruction of the joint between the radius and ulna (two forearm bones) at the wrist.

Das Gupta technique. *Surgical procedure*. Removal of part of the scapula (shoulder blade), leaving the glenohumeral joint intact.

Dawbarn sign. *Clinical sign*. Dissipation of pain in the subacromial bursa (outer edge of shoulder) when the arm is passively abducted (elevated to the side by the examiner); indicates that pressure has been taken off the bursa. Sign of subacromial bursitis.

Daypro. *Drug*. Trade name of oxaprozin, NSAID for treating pain and inflammation.

debride (duh-BREED). *Surgical procedure*. To remove dead tissue and/or foreign matter from a wound.

debridement (duh-BREED-munt). *Surgical procedure*. Removal of dead tissue and/or foreign matter from a wound.

debridement and irrigation (D & I). *Surgical treatment*. Cleansing of a wound with saline or antibiotic solution followed by the removal of dead or infected tissue and foreign material.

decalcification (dee-kal-sih-fih-KAY-shun). *Pathologic process*. Removal of calcium from bone, leaving the basic cellular structure intact. May be a disease process, or a laboratory process performed on surgical specimens.

decalcify (dee-KAL-sih-fi). *Process*. To remove calcium from a bone.

decompression (dee-kum-PRESH-un). *Surgical procedure*. Elimination of pressure on an area, e.g., by removing bone that is pressing on a nerve.

  d. laminectomy (lam-in-EK-tuh-mee). *Surgical procedure*. Removing the lamina (posterior elements of spinal cord) to alleviate pressure on the spinal cord or nerve root.

  d. sickness, **bends**, **caisson's disease**, **diver's disease**. *Pathologic condition*. Soft tissue and bone damage caused by nitrogen bubbles forming in the blood, associated with rapid decreases in pressure; may lead to avascular necrosis of bone. Symptoms include joint pain, skin lesions, respiratory and central nervous system dysfunction. Frequently occurs in divers who do not decompress on resurfacing from a dive.

decortication (dee-kor-tih-KAY-shun). *Surgical procedure*. Removal of the cortex (outermost layer of bone). Most often used during spinal fusion or in treatment of nonunions.

decubitus (de-KYU-bit-us). *Anatomic description*. Lying down.

  dorsal d.: patient lying on his/her back. See also SUPINE.

  lateral d.: patient lying on his/her side (may be left or right).

  ventral d.: patient lying on his/her stomach. See also PRONE.

decubitus ulcer (duh-KYU-bih-tus), **bed sore**, **pressure sore**. *Pathologic condition*. Skin lesion caused by pressure and immobilization.

deep femoral artery (FEM-ur-ul), **profunda femoris**. *Anatomy*. Branch of the femoral artery, which supplies upper and inner thigh regions.

deep peroneal nerve (pehr-uh-NEE-ul), **anterior tibial nerve**. *Anatomy*. Branch of the common peroneal nerve that travels around the back of the fibula (smaller lower leg bone) and innervates muscles at the front of the leg and the area between the first and second toes and the skin at the dorsum of the foot.

deep tendon reflex (DTR). *Physiologic function*. Reflex (involuntary contraction of a muscle) elicited by tapping or sudden pulling of a muscle or its tendon. Most commonly used during physical examination of the biceps (front of elbow), patella (knee), Achilles (back of ankle), triceps (back of elbow) or brachioradialis (wrist) tendons.

deep vein thrombosis (DVT) (thrawm-BOH-sus). *Pathologic condition*. Blood clot formation in a vein deep within the leg or abdomen; common source of pulmonary embolism. See also SUPERFICIAL VEIN THROMBOSIS.

defervescence (def-ur-VES-ents). *Physiologic function*. Reduction of an elevated temperature to normal.

deformans tibia, **Blount-Barber disease**, **Blount's disease**, **osteochondrosis tibia**. *Pathologic condition*. Depressed or stunted growth at the inner, upper portion of the tibial (shinbone) growth plate inhibiting growth in the inner half of the knee, while the lateral growth plate of the tibia continues to grow; produces bowlegs in children; progressively worsens.

degenerative arthritis, **arthrosis**, **degenerative joint disease**, **osteoarthritis**. *Pathologic condition*. Loss of cartilage in a joint secondary to age, obesity, or their abnormal use or function. Inflammation of a joint. Usually characterized by swelling, pain and restriction of motion.

degenerative disc disease. *Pathologic condition*. Destruction of the intervertebral discs (between the vertebrae), causing pain, potential pressure on the spinal cord, and loss of normal spine resiliency. Caused by aging or trauma.

degenerative joint disease. *See* DEGENERATIVE ARTHRITIS.

dehiscence (dee-HISS-ents). *Pathologic condition*. Opening of a wound along a suture line.

Déjérine's disease (day-zhur-EENZ). See DEJERINE-SOTTA DISEASE.

Déjérine's sign (day-zhur-EENZ). *Clinical sign*. Increase in pain in the lower leg caused by coughing, sneezing or straining at stool. Indicative of spinal nerve root irritation (radiculitis).

Déjérine-Sotta disease /or/ **syndrome** (day-zhur-EEN so-TAH), **familial interstitial hypertrophic neuritis**, **hypertrophic interstitial neuritis**. *Pathologic condition*. Type III hereditary motor sensory neuropathy, a syndrome characterized by progressive degeneration of the peripheral nerves. Weakness in the hands and feet are associated with localized swelling of the peripheral nerves and sensory changes in the extremities; results in hand and foot deformities. Hereditary; detected in late infancy. See also CHARCOT-MARIE-TOOTH disease.

delayed flap. *Surgical technique*. Skin graft done in successive stages over several weeks, to maintain blood supply.

delayed primary closure. *Surgical technique*. Repairing a wound after it has been left open. Used in treatment of some infections or in closing some large open wounds.

delayed union. *Pathologic condition*. Refers to a fracture that has not healed in the normal time period. See also NONUNION.

Delbet classification (del-BAY). *Fracture classification.* Identifies four types of femoral hip fractures in children.

DeLee classification. *Fracture classification.* Identifies different age-related break patterns of transphyseal fractures of the distal humeral physis (growth plate).

deltoid (DEL-toyd). *Description.* Triangular in shape; resembling the Greek letter delta.

    d. ligament. *Anatomy.* Triangular band running from the medial malleolus (prominence on inside of ankle), to the talus (top foot bone) and the navicular bone.

    d. muscle. *Anatomy.* Triangular shoulder muscle that raises, rotates and abducts the arm. Attaches in front to the clavicle (collarbone), behind to the acromion (lateral portion of shoulder blade), and to the deltoid tuberosity (middle lateral side of humerus).

    d. splitting approach. *Surgical technique.* Cutting the upper part of the deltoid muscle along the length of its fibers to expose the shoulder joint.

    d. sprain. *Pathologic condition.* Partial tear of the deltoid ligament in the ankle.

demineralization. *Pathologic condition.* Loss of mineral salts in bone, decreasing the strength of the bone and giving a washed out appearance on x-ray.

dendritic cells. *Anatomy.* Part of the immune system; cells that scour the tissues exposed to the outside of the body (e.g., skin), looking for foreign material (e.g., bacteria). Named for their long projections called dendrites.

denervation fibrillation potentials. *Lab finding.* Spikes of electrical activity seen on electromyography (electrical testing) after a nerve has been cut. Indicates laceration of the nerve.

Denis Browne bar /or/ **brace** /or/ **splint, abduction bar** /or/ **bar splint, Fillauer bar, Tarso abduction bar.** *Orthopedic appliance.* Metal bar that holds a pair of shoes together, positioning the feet. Used to control leg rotation in infants.

Denis classification of sacral fractures. *Fracture classification.* Identifies three types of fractures of the sacrum.

Denis classification of vertebral fractures. *Fracture classification.* Describes three types of vertebral fractures based on whether the fracture involves the front, back and/or middle portion of a vertebra. See also BURST FRACTURE.

Denis-Weber classification, Weber classification. *Fracture classification.* Defines three types of ankle fractures based on their level on the distal fibula.

dens fracture. *Pathologic condition.* A break involving the toothlike projection (dens process) of the 2nd cervical vertebra.

densitometry (den-suh-TOHM-uh-tree). *Radiologic test.* Used to measure the density (amount of bone mineral, mainly calcium) in a bone segment. Considered an indirect indicator of bone mineral density (BMD).

dens process, odontoid process. *Anatomy.* Projection of the 2nd cervical vertebra toward the skull; fits within the ring of the 1st cervical vertebra, in front of the spinal cord.

dentinogenesis imperfecta (den-tin-oh-JEN-uh-sis im-pur-FEK-tuh). *Pathologic condition.* Defective formation and calcification of the teeth, causing irregular and blue or brown appearance. Characteristic of osteogenesis imperfecta.

dependent. *Location.* Refers to areas of the body that are generally closer to the ground (or downhill).

    d. drainage. *Pathologic condition.* Fluid that has accumulated and drained out through the lower parts of the body (downhill). Term can be used to describe how an infection spreads or to explain swelling.

    d. edema. *Pathologic condition.* Swelling in the lower parts of the body under the influence of gravity (e.g., the feet, at the end of the day).

depressed fracture. *Pathologic condition*. 1. Break in which part of the bone is driven into surrounding bone or soft tissue. 2. Refers to the sunken position of a fragment in an articular (joint) fracture.

de Quervain's disease (day-kur-VAYNZ), **de Quervain's tenosynovitis**. *Pathologic condition*. Inflammation of abductor pollicis longus and extensor pollicis brevis tendons of the thumb due to chronic overuse. See also FINKELSTEIN TEST.

de Quervain's release (day-kur-VAYNZ). *Surgical procedure*. Opening the sheath holding the abductor pollicis longus and extensor pollicis brevis tendons of the thumb, to relieve pain.

derangement (dee-RAYNJ-munt). *Pathologic condition*. Abnormality in the regular alignment or arrangement of a structure, e.g., a joint.

dermatan sulfate. *Biologic substance*. A mucopolysaccharide found in the urine of patients with various diseases, e.g., Maroteaux Lamy syndrome, Scheie's syndrome. See also MUCOPOLYSACCHARIDOSIS.

dermatofibroma (dur-MAH-toh-fi-BROH-muh), **fibroxanthoma**, **sclerosing hemangioma**. *Pathologic condition*. Type of slow-growing, benign, fibrous skin nodule; usually affects lower extremities.

dermatomal patterns (dur-muh-TOH-mul). *Anatomic description*. Reproducible patterns of nerve innervation to different parts of the skin.

dermatome (DUR-muh-tohm). 1. *Anatomy*. Area of skin supplied by a single nerve or nerve root. 2. *Surgical instrument*. Cutting device for shaving off skin in various thicknesses for making skin grafts.

    d. distribution: see DERMATOME (above), definition no. 1.

dermatomyositis (dur-muh-toh-mi-oh-SI-tus). *Pathologic condition*. Progressive autoimmune disease of connective tissue; characterized by muscle weakness, a typical (purplish) skin rash, edema (fluid in the tissues), and calcification of the tissues.

dermis. *Anatomy*. The skin. See also EPIDERMIS.

derotation osteotomy (dee-roh-TAY-shun ahs-tee-AH-tuh-mee). *Surgical procedure*. Cutting a long bone into two segments, then rotating one into alignment. Both segments held in the new position with a plate or fixation device.

derotation strap (Cotrel). *Orthopedic supply*. Strap used on a casting table to rotate the rib cage of a patient with scoliosis.

-desis. *Suffix*. Binding or fusing (epiphysiodesis: surgical closure or fusion of the epiphysis).

desmo-. *Prefix*. Connecting band or ligament between two structures (desmoplastic: characterized by the growth of fibrous tissue).

desmoid (DEZ-moyd). *Pathologic condition*. Firm, agressive tumor comprised of fibroblasts (fibrous cells). Most common in abdominal muscles of women who have had children.

developmental dysplasia of the hip (DDH) (dis-PLAY-zjuh), **acetabular dysplasia, congenital dysplasia of the hip**. *Pathologic condition*. Incomplete formation of the acetabulum (hip joint socket), leaving the head of the femur (thighbone) partially uncovered, with less-than-normal or no cartilage contact between the femoral head and the acetabulum.

dexter. *Location*. Right; to the right; on the right side.

dextrorotary scoliosis, **dextrorotoscoliosis**, **dextroscoliosis**. *Pathologic condition*. Curvature of the spine with direction of the curve to the right.

diabetic arthropathy. *Pathologic condition*. Destruction of a joint following loss of sensation; may go unnoticed until changes are severe. Seen in some diabetics.

dial lock. *Orthopedic appliance*. Locking hinge attached to a brace to stabilize a joint at a particular angle; can be changed to allow for increasing or limiting range of motion.

dial osteotomy (ahs-tee-AH-tuh-mee). *Surgical procedure.* Method of cutting the acetabulum (hip socket) from the pelvis, to allow its redirection.

diaphyseal (di-uh-FIZ-ee-ul). *Anatomic description.* Refers to the diaphysis (shaft of a long bone).

    d. dysplasia (di-uh-FIZ-ee-ul dis-PLAY-zjuh), **Camurati-Engelmann**, **Engelmann disease**, **progressive diaphyseal dysplasia**. *Pathologic condition.* Type of dwarfism resulting from an abnormality in the growth of the long bones. Characteristics include abnormally short, wide long bones and early joint arthritis.

    d. fracture. *Pathologic condition.* Break through the shaft of a long bone.

    d. lengthening. *Surgical procedure.* Cutting a long bone at the diaphysis (shaft) and adding a distraction device to increase its length. Most commonly performed at the femur (thighbone).

    d. shortening. *Surgical procedure.* Removal of a segment from the diaphysis (shaft) of a long bone and joining the two remaining ends, usually with a metal device added for stability; shortens length of the bone.

diaphysectomy (di-uh-fiz-EK-toh-mee). *Surgical procedure.* Removing a portion of the diaphysis (shaft) of a long bone.

diaphysial (di-uh-FIZ-ee-ul). Incorrect spelling of DIAPHYSEAL.

diaphysis (di-AF-uh-sis). *Anatomy.* Shaft (area between ends) of a long bone.

diarthrosis (di-ahr-THROH-sus), **synovial joint**. *Anatomy.* Freely movable joint with a synovial lining (fluid secreting membrane), e.g., knee, wrist.

Dias and Tachdjian classification (tah-KID-ee-an). *Fracture classification.* Describes different ankle fracture patterns in children.

diastasis (di-ASS-tuh-sis). *Pathologic condition.* Separation of two normally joined bones, e.g., between the tibia and fibula in the ankle joint.

diastematomyelia (di-as-stem-at-oh-mi-EE-lee-uh). *Congenital abnormality.* Spinal cord split longitudinally by a band of cartilage. Often associated with spina bifida. See also DIPLOMYELIA.

diastrophic dwarf (di-us-TROH-fik). *Congenital abnormality.* Individual suffering from diastrophic dysplasia.

diastrophic dysplasia (di-us-TROH-fik). *Congenital abnormality.* Severe form of dwarfism characterized by short arms and legs, frequently with clubfeet, abnormal ears and cleft palate.

diathermy (DI-uh-thur-mee). *Treatment.* High frequency electricity, ultrasonic waves, or microwaves used to raise temperature of skin and tissues; used for treating muscle aches and sprains.

    microwave d.: elevating temperature within tissues with microwaves.

    short wave d.: ultrasonic wave used in physical therapy to elevate temperatures in a small area of tissue.

Dickson-Diveley procedure. *Surgical procedure.* Removal of a portion of the proximal phalanx of a lesser toe with tendon transfer; to correct clawing.

diclofenac (di-KLO-fen-ak). *Drug.* NSAID for treating pain and inflammation. Trade names: Voltaren, Cataflam.

didactylism (di-DAK-til-iz-um). *Congenital abnormality.* Having only two fingers on a hand and/or two toes on a foot.

die-punch fracture. *Pathologic condition.* An intra-articular (joint) fracture in which a central part of the joint surface has been propelled into the bone. Most commonly applied to certain distal radius (forearm bone) and proximal tibia (shinbone) fractures.

diffuse infantile familial sclerosis, **globoid cell leukodystrophy**, **Krabbe's disease**. *Pathologic condition.* Infantile condition characterized by rapid deterioration of the central nervous system (leukodystrophy). Death usually occurs by age 2. Hereditary; most likely autosomal recessive.

diflunisal (di-FLU-nih-sal).*Drug.* NSAID for treating pain and inflammation. Trade name: Dolobid.

digit (DIH-jit). *Anatomy.* A finger or toe.

digital prosthesis (DIH-jit-ul prahs-THEE-sus). *Orthopedic implant.* Material used (plastic or metallic) in the replacement of the finger joints, that allow motion. Used in the treatment of arthritis.

diplegia (di-PLEE-jee-uh). *Pathologic condition.* Paralysis of corresponding parts on both sides of the body.

> **spastic:** jerky, uncoordinated movements involving both sides of the body.

diplomyelia (dip-loh-mi-EE-lee-uh). *Congenital abnormality.* Duplication of the spinal cord, its dural sacs and nerve roots, usually with loss of function below the separation. Often associated with spina bifida. See also DIASTEMATOMYELIA.

Disalcid. *Drug.* Trade name of salsalate, NSAID for treating pain and inflammation.

disarticulation (dis-ahr-tik-yu-LAY-shun), **exarticulation**. *Surgical procedure.* Amputation through a joint.

disc, **intervertebral disc**, **vertebral disc**. *Anatomy.* A disk of cartilage between adjacent vertebrae; absorbs shocks and permits movement of the spine. Named after the vertebrae they reside between (e.g., C4, C5 refers to the disc between the 4th and 5th cervical vertebrae).

> **d. degeneration**. *Pathologic process.* The loss of the structural and functional integrity of a disc.

> **herniated d.**, **herniated nucleus pulposus**, **slipped disc**. *Pathologic condition.* Extrusion of the cartilaginous tissue in the nucleus pulposus (center of disc), which can place pressure on a nerve and result in leg or arm pain, numbness, tingling or weakness (neuropraxia).

> > **slipped d.**: See HERNIATED DISC (above).

> **d. space infection**. See DISCITIS.

> **d. space narrowing**. *Radiographic finding.* Decrease in space between two vertebrae due to wearing away of the intervertebral disc. On x-ray, this space appears to be narrower, or lost.

discectomy (dis-KEK-toh-mee). *Surgical procedure.* Removal of an intervertebral disc or disc fragment.

discitis (dis-KI-tus), **disc space infection**. *Pathologic condition.* Inflammation or infection of an intervertebral disc.

discogenic pain (dis-koh-JEN-ik). *Pathologic condition.* Pain originating from a disc.

discogram (DIS-koh-gram). *Radiologic test.* X-ray of a disc taken after it has been injected with a radiopaque dye.

discography (dis-KAH-gruh-fee). *Radiologic test.* Injection of a radiopaque dye into an intervertebral disc to make it visible on x-ray.

discoid lateral meniscus (DIS-koyd, muh-NIS-kus). *Pathologic condition.* Abnormally shaped lateral meniscus (cartilage between tibia and femur) that covers the whole outer joint surface of the tibia rather than only its periphery; gives the meniscus a round shape (as opposed to its usual half-moon shape).

disect. Incorrect spelling of DISSECT.

disk. Alternate spelling of DISC.

dislocation, **luxation**. *Pathologic condition.* 1. Movement of a part from its normal position. 2. Loss of the normal relationship of one bone to the other at a joint.

acute d.: of recent occurrence.

central d.: in the hip joint, protrusion of the femoral head into the pelvis.

closed d.: joint displacement in which the affected bones do not communicate with the outside or surface area.

congenital d.: occurs in utero; present at birth.

habitual d.: occurs recurrently; most frequently encountered in the kneecap or shoulder. Has a volitional component.

open d.: joint dislocation that has ruptured the skin, exposing bone and tissues to the air.

recurrent d.: continues to occur at the same joint; most frequently the shoulder or patella (kneecap).

dismemberment. *Abnormal condition.* Amputation of a limb.

displaced fracture. *Pathologic condition.* Break in which a bony fragment shifts from its natural position.

displasia. Incorrect spelling of DYSPLASIA.

dissect. *Surgical procedure.* To separate soft tissues of the body.

dissection. *Surgical procedure.* Process of separating soft tissues.

blunt d.: using a blunt instrument or a gloved finger.

sharp d.: using a knife.

scissors d.: using scissors.

distal (DIS-tul). *Anatomy.* Away from the center of the body or proximal part of an area; a distal fracture of the tibia is closer to the ankle than the knee.

d. clavicular resection, Mumford procedure. *Surgical procedure.* Removal of the outer end of the clavicle (collarbone); to treat pain from acromioclavicular arthritis.

d. interphalangeal (DIP) fusion (in-tur-fal-an-JEE-ul). *Surgical procedure.* Fusion of the joint between the proximal and distal phalanges (bones) of the finger.

d. interphalangeal (DIP) joint (in-tur-fal-an-JEE-ul). *Anatomy.* Articulation between the last two phalanges (finger or toe bones). Does not exist in the thumb or the great toe because they have only two phalanges.

d. palmar crease. *Anatomy.* The crease across the palm of the hand at the level of the metacarpal heads (opposite the knuckles).

d. phalanx (FAL-unks). *Anatomy.* The farthest bone of a finger or toe.

distend (diss-TEND). *Pathologic finding.* To expand or fill with fluid or gas. After injury, a joint (e.g., knee) may be distended with blood. See also EFFUSION.

distonia. Incorrect spelling of DYSTONIA.

distraction. *Treatment.* Pulling bones or parts of a joint apart so they no longer touch.

d. osteotomy. *Surgical procedure.* Cutting a bone so it may be pulled apart, to heal in a lengthened position.

diverticulum (di-vur-TIK-yu-lum). *Abnormal condition.* Outpouch from the lining of a joint.

dog-ears. *Description.* Triangular ends formed in the uneven closure of a wound or in the closure of a round wound.

Dolobid. *Drug.* Trade name of diflunisal, NSAID for treating pain and inflammation.

dome fracture, talar dome fracture. *Pathologic condition.* Break in the rounded surface (top) of the talus (top foot bone).

donor site. *Location.* Area from which a graft is removed.

donor tissue, graft. *Biological implant.* Body tissue (e.g., bone, skin) removed from an individual to be transferred from one area or one person to another.

Doppler ultrasound. *Test.* Noninvasive sound technique that uses the sound of blood as it passes through an artery or vein to measure blood flow.

dorsal (DOHR-sul), **posterior**. *Anatomy*. Back of the body or body part in the anatomic position; the dorsal surface of the hand is opposite the palm. Opposite: VENTRAL.

    d. hood, extensor aponeurosis, extensor hood. *Anatomy*. Band of connective tissue at the back of a finger or toe that gives attachment to extensor muscles and provides stability to the straightened fingers/toes.

    d. interossei muscles (in-tur-AH-see-i). *Anatomy*. Four small muscles on the back of the hand or top of the foot that flex (bend) and abduct (spread) the fingers/toes.

    d. scapular nerve (SKAP-yu-lur). *Anatomy*. Nerve arising from the 5th cervical (neck) nerve roots; innervates the rhomboid major and minor muscles (pulls up on the scapula) and sends a branch to provide part of the innervation to the levator scapula muscle (pulls up on the scapula).

    d. wedge osteotomy (ahs-tee-AH-tuh-mee). *Surgical procedure*. Cutting a bone, with a wedge taken from the back so the base is directed to the back.

dorsalis pedis artery (dor-SAL-us PEE-dus). *Anatomy*. Continuation of the tibialis anterior artery on the front of the leg as it courses over the ankle and top of the foot.

dorsalis pedis pulse (dor-SAL-us PEE-dus). *Function*. Pulsations of the dorsalis pedis artery; felt when palpating the top of the foot.

dorsiflexion (DOR-suh-flek-shun). *Function*. Bending wrist backward (opposite: palmar flexion, volar flexion) or the foot upward (opposite: plantar flexion).

    d. osteotomy of the first ray. *Surgical procedure*. Cutting a wedge of bone from the 1st ray of the foot (metatarsal and toe) inclusive of the 1st tarsometatarsal joint and fusing the joint in an upwardly bent position (dorsiflexion). For treating forefoot pain from excessive weight across the 1st ray.

dorsum. *Location*. Posterior side of a structure or body.

double I-beam nail. *Surgical implant*. Intramedullary nail (driven down the center of a long bone) shaped like two steel girders, perpendicular to each other, as used in construction. Used to stabilize a fracture or osteotomy.

double innominate osteotomy (in-AH-mun-ut ahs-tee-AH-tuh-mee). *Surgical procedure*. Cutting through the pelvic bones in the area of the ilium and ischium or between the ilium and pubis, to direct the acetabulum (hip joint cup) in a more favorable direction. Used in treatment of hip dysplasia.

dowager's hump, humpback. *Abnormal condition*. A protuberance of the upper back (kyphosis) like that caused by collapsing of the vertebrae in osteoporosis. See also KYPHOSIS.

dowel graft. *Surgical technique*. Use of a bone segment for a graft; resembles a dowel.

Down syndrome, mongolism, trisomy 21. *Congenital abnormality*. Presence of three #21 chromosomes; associated with mental retardation, hyperelasticity, heart disease, oblique eyelids, flat skull and flattened facial features.

drain. *Surgical implant*. Rubber, plastic, or cotton material that allows blood or infected material to flow from a wound or cavity.

drainage. 1. *Process*. Drawing off fluids from a wound or body cavity by means of gravity or suction. 2. *Biologic material*. The fluid that is drained from a wound or surgical site.

    dependent d. *Biologic material*. Fluid that has accumulated and drained out through the lower parts of the body (downhill). Term can be used to describe how an infection spreads or to explain swelling.

drawer sign. *Clinical sign*. With the knee flexed at 90°, excessive motion elicited by pulling the tibia (shinbone) forward or backward on the femur (thighbone) at the knee; indicates instability or tear of the cruciate ligaments of the knee.

> **anterior**: forward tibial slide; indicates anterior ligament rupture.

> **posterior**: backward tibial slide; indicates posterior ligament rupture.

drill guide. *Surgical tool.* Hollow device that directs a drill into a specific region, for drilling a hole in a precise direction.

driver/extractor. *Surgical tool.* Used to insert or remove a plate, screw or rod from a bone or sleeve.

drop foot, foot drop. *Pathologic condition.* Inability to raise the foot at the ankle. The foot falls downward, causing the toes to strike the ground during ambulation; occurs in paralysis or absence of the muscles on the front of the leg.

drop-lock ring. *Orthopedic appliance.* Part of a brace; used for preventing motion across a joint.

dual onlay graft. *Surgical procedure.* Laying strips of bone on the outside of a fracture or osteotomy. Used to provide stability and to stimulate healing. See also INLAY GRAFT.

dual x-ray absorptiometry (DEXA) (ab-sorb-she-AHM-uh-tree). *Radiologic test.* Measurement of the amount of x-ray absorption by a bone, to gain an idea of its density. Used in the diagnosis and evaluation of osteoporosis.

Duchenne-Erb paralysis (du-SHEN), **Erb's palsy** /or/ **paralysis**. *Congenital abnormality.* Paralysis of shoulder muscles and those that flex the elbow; occurs during birth when the shoulder is unable to progress through the pelvic canal and there is stretch on the upper part of the brachial plexus (nerves to the arm).

Duchenne's muscular dystrophy (DMD) (du-SHENZ), **Duchenne's paralysis**, **muscular dystrophy**, **pseudohypertrophic dystrophy**. *Pathologic condition.* Progressive weakness of the voluntary muscles. Onset generally before age 3, with frequent falls, difficulty getting up, and enlargement of the calf muscles. Hereditary, sex-linked (males); females are carriers. Death before age 25. See also BECKER'S MUSCULAR DYSTROPHY.

Duchenne's paralysis (du-SHENZ). See DUCHENNE'S MUSCULAR DYSTROPHY.

duck waddle test, **Childress duck waddle test**. *Clinical test.* Patient is asked to squat, first with the legs rotated internally and then externally. If pain is elicited from the knees, if the patient is not able to fully squat secondary to knee pain, or if there is painful popping from the knee, the test is considered positive and indicative of a meniscus tear.

Dunlop traction. *Treatment.* Skeletal traction technique used in the treatment of supracondylar fractures (just above the elbow).

Duplay disease, **subacromial bursitis**. *Pathologic condition.* Inflammation of the bursa of the shoulder causing pain with arm elevation.

Dupuytren's contracture (du-pwe-TRAHNZ), **palmar fibromatosis**. *Pathologic condition.* Loss of motion due to contracture of the connective tissues underneath the skin of the palm, caused by a proliferation of fibroblasts (necessary in production of scar tissue). Nodules and cords form, causing loss of motion in the finger joints.

Dupuytren's fracture (du-pwe-TRAHNZ). *Pathologic condition.* Break in the iliac (wing bone) of the pelvis.

Dupuytren's signs (du-pwe-TRAHNZ). *Clinical signs.* 1. Crepitus (grating, cracking joint sensation) on palpation of a bone; seen in certain kinds of sarcoma. 2. In congenital dislocation, excessive movement of the hip when pushed or pulled; indicates instability of the femoral head in the hip socket.

dura, **dura mater** (DUR-uh MAH-tur). *Anatomy.* Outermost covering of the spinal cord and brain; comprised of connective tissue.

DuVries technique. *Surgical procedure*. 1. Removing a spur (extra bone) from the inner side of the 1st metatarsal bone. Used in surgical treatment of hallux valgus (bunion). 2. Sliding a piece of the back of the fibula (outer bone of ankle), to keep the peroneal tendons (outer ankle tendons) from displacing from behind the fibula. See also PERONEAL SNAPPING SYNDROME.

dwarf. *Congenital anomaly*. Person with abnormally short stature and related abnormalities. See also CONRADI'S SYNDROME, DYSPLASIA.

    achondroplastic d.: normal trunk, large skull, short extremities.

    diastrophic d.: individual suffering from diastrophic dysplasia, who has short arms and legs (trunk approximates normal), frequently with clubfeet, abnormal ears, cleft palate.

    idiopathic d.: has no apparent cause or pathology.

    metatropic d. (met-uh-TROH-pik): characterized by changing body proportions with growth.

    micromelic d. (mi-kroh-MEE-lik): associated with short arms.

Dwyer calcaneal osteotomy. *Surgical procedure*. Cutting the heelbone to realign the back portion of the foot (hindfoot).

Dwyer instrumentation. *Surgical implant*. Staples designed to be implanted in the front of the spine, along the vertebral bodies. Used to correct certain spinal deformities.

dynamic compression plate (DCP). *Surgical implant*. Metallic plate with offset screw holes. When the screws are tightened, the fractured ends of the bone are compressed together, aiding in union.

    low-contact (LCDCP): same as DCP except that the plate's surface is indented between holes so there is little contact between plate and bone. Minimizes bone tissue damage from the plate resting against the bone.

dynamic orthosis. *Orthopedic appliance*. A brace that allows motion, to aid in walking.

dynamic splint. *Orthopedic appliance*. Splint that allows function by motion of joints or accessory tendons. Example: wrist-driven hand splint allows quadriplegics to have motion in the paralyzed hand.

dynamic tendon transfer. *Surgical procedure*. Moving a tendon from one place to another, to give function in a new position.

dynamometer (di-nuh-MAH-muh-tur). *Test instrument*. Measures the extent of muscular power.

-dynia. *Suffix*. Pain (coccydynia: pain in the coccyx).

dys- *Prefix*. Difficult or bad (dysplasia: an abnormal joint, not completely formed).

dysautonomia (dis-ah-toh-NOH-mee-uh), **familial dysautonomia**, **Riley Day syndrome**. *Pathologic condition*. Abnormality of the autonomic nervous system, causing numerous difficulties including difficulty controlling body temperature, insensitivity to pain, motor uncoordination, lack of tearing, intolerance to anesthetics. Hereditary.

dysbaric osteonecrosis (dis-BAHR-ik ahs-tee-oh-neh-KRO-sis). *Pathologic condition*. Form of avascular necrosis (bone death) caused by the choking off of the microscopic blood vessels to the bone by nitrogen bubbles that form after prolonged exposure to compressed air. See also BENDS.

dyschondroplasia (dis-kahn-droh-PLAY-zjuh), **enchondromatosis**, **Ollier's disease**. *Pathologic condition*. Multiple benign cartilage tumors, usually within the metaphyses of long bones. Called Maffucci's syndrome when associated with multiple hamartomas (benign blood vessel tumors).

dyskinesia (dis-kin-EE-zjuh). *Abnormal function*. Uncoordinated voluntary movement. Frequently occurs in neurologic diseases such as Parkinson's and cerebral palsy.

dysmetria (dis-MET-ree-uh). *Abnormal function.* Inability to stop muscle movement at a chosen point.

dysmorphia (dis-MOHR-fee-uh). *Pathologic condition.* Abnormal shape.

dysmyotonia (dis-mi-oh-TOH-nee-uh). *Pathologic condition.* Abnormality in muscle tone; may be greater (hypertonic) or less (hypotonic).

dysostosis (dis-ahs-TOH-sis). *Pathologic condition.* Malformation of bones, as seen in mucopolysaccharidosis.

　　d. multiplex, Hurler's syndrome: syndrome characterized by scoliosis, contractures of the joints, progressive coarsening of facial features, corneal clouding, and enlargement of spleen and liver. Usually diagnosed by age 2, with death before age 10 from heart and lung deterioration. Hereditary. See also GARGOYLISM.

dysplasia (dis-PLAY-zjuh). *Congenital abnormality.* Abnormality in growth and development of bones resulting in a short stature and characteristic deformities. Most forms of dwarfism can also be referred to as dysplasias (e.g., diastrophic dysplasia, achondroplastic dysplasia). See also DWARF.

　　achondroplastic d.: abnormality of growth cartilage of the extremities, resulting in a short-limbed dwarf, generally accompanied by an apparent enlargement of the front of the skull. Trunk length is normal. Hereditary.

　　diastrophic d.: severe form of dwarfism characterized by short arms and legs, frequently with clubfeet, abnormal ears and cleft palate.

　　epiphyseal d. (ep-ih-FIZ-ee-ul): group of hereditary abnormalities involving the development of long bones, usually resulting in joint deformities, difficulty in walking, development of early degenerative arthritis and short limb dwarfism. See also CONRADI'S SYNDROME, EPIPHYSEAL MULTIPLEX.

　　d. epiphysealis, epiphyseal osteochondroma, hemimelica, tarso-epiphyseal aclasia, Trevor disease: abnormal development of osteochondromas, usually involving multiple bones in one limb. Three variations: localized (involves one epiphysis); classic (involves more than one bone in a single limb); and generalized (involves multiple bones in more than one limb).

　　d. epiphysealis multiplex (eh-pih-fiz-ee-AL-iss), **multiple epiphseal d.**: abnormality at ends of long bones, causing difficulty in walking, joint deformities and pain, short stubby fingers, short limb dwarfism. The condition tends to spare the spine. Two types: I. Fairbank; 2. Ribbing, less severe. Hereditary.

　　d. epiphysealis punctata (eh-pih-fiz-ee-AL-iss), **Conradi's disease** /or/ **syndrome, chondrodysplasia congenita punctata, stippled epiphysis**: abnormality of ends of the long bones, causing difficulty in walking, joint deformities and short limb dwarfism. On x-ray, the epiphyses (growth areas) are stippled with small centers of calcification. Hereditary. See also CONRADI-HUNEMANN DISEASE.

　　fibrous d.: lesion in bone made up of disorganized connective tissue; can lead to significant deformities or fracture. See also MCCUNE-ALBRIGHT SYNDROME.

　　idiopathic d.: has no apparent cause or pathology.

　　metatropic d. (met-uh-TROH-pik): characterized by changing body proportions with growth.

　　micromelic d. (mi-kroh-MEE-lik): associated with short arms.

　　monostotic d.: form of fibrous dysplasia: only a single bone is affected.

　　multiple epiphyseal d. (eh-pih-FIZ-ee-al): same as DYSPLASIA EPIPHYSEALIS MULTIPLEX (above).

　　spondyloepiphyseal d. (spahn-dul-oh-uh-pif-uh-SEE-ul): syndrome characterized by short trunk dwarfism, delayed deposition of bone in the vertebrae and proximal femur, and coxa vara. Hereditary.

Streeter's d.: syndrome of numerous constricting rings produced by thin bands of amniotic membrane that may encircle an arm, leg or digit in utero; may be deep so as to touch the bone and sever blood vessels and nerves. See also AMNIOTIC BAND.

dysplastic hip. *Pathologic condition*. Abnormally shaped hip. May be congenital or acquired.

dysraphism (dis-RAY-fiz-um). *Anatomic defect*. A failure of tissue fusion in an embryo, e.g., cleft palate. See also MYELODYSPLASIA, MYELOMENINGOCOELE.

dystonia. *Pathologic condition*. State of abnormal tension across soft tissues or muscles.

cervical d. (SUR-vih-kul), **spasmodic torticollis**: disorder characterized by abnormal tension and activity of the neck muscles, which can lead to abnormal posture and repetitive twisting movements. Can begin at any age but usually starts in the 30s or 40s. No known cause or cure.

dystrophia adiposogenitalis, Frölich's adiposogenital dystrophy /or/ **appearance** /or/ **syndrome, Launois-Cleret syndrome.** *Pathologic condition*. Obesity and delayed secondary sexual characteristics, sometimes seen with a pituitary tumor; occasionally associated with slipped capital femoral epiphysis.

dystrophic myotonia (dys-TROH-fik mi-uh-TOH-nee-uh), **myotonic dystrophy, Steinert's disease**. *Pathologic condition*. Hereditary weakness of the muscles of the face, neck and distal extremities. Patients usually present with a weakness of the hands and difficulty walking or tendency to fall. Many individuals die young from pulmonary-cardiac failure; they are especially at risk during anesthesia.

dystrophy (DIS-truh-fee). *Pathologic condition*. Refers to a series of disorders in metabolism leading to abnormal function. When muscles are affected, the condition is referred to as muscular dystrophy.

Becker's muscular d.: milder form of muscular dystrophy similar to Duchenne's. Onset in latter half of first decade of life; patients can live into adulthood.

Duchenne's muscular d. (DMD) (du-SHENZ): progressive weakness of the voluntary muscles. Onset generally before age 3, with frequent falls, difficulty getting up, and enlargement of the calf muscles. Hereditary, sex-linked (males); females are carriers. Death before age 25. .

fascioscapulohumeral d. (fash-ee-oh-skap-yu-loh-HYU-mur-ul), **Landouzy-Dejerine disease**: mild, common form of muscular dystrophy; results in loss of arm strength, especially around the shoulder, with wasting of the shoulder girdle muscles; also affects muscles of the face, which may lead to inability to generate facial expressions such as smiling.

muscular d.: progressive weakness of the voluntary muscles. Onset generally before age 3, with frequent falls, difficulty getting up, and enlargement of the calf muscles. Hereditary, sex-linked (males); females are carriers. Death before age 25.

oculocerebrorenal d. (OCRL), Lowe syndrome: autosomal recessive abnormality resulting in kidney dysfunction and failure, congenital eye disorders such as cataracts and glaucoma, and severe mental retardation. Death often occurs in childhood.

eburnation (eh-bur-NAY-shun). *Pathologic condition.* Extreme denseness and smoothness of subchondral (under cartilage) bone that occurs when it is subjected to abnormal pressures, as in degenerative joint disease (osteoarthritis).

ecchondroma (ek-ahn-DRO-muh), **ecchondrosis**. *Pathologic condition.* An overgrowth of cartilage that protrudes into the joint. See also ENCHONDROMA.

ecchymosis (ek-ee-MO-sus). *Clinical finding.* Purple discoloration of the skin resulting from injury to or bleeding within underlying tissues. See also BRUISE.

ecchymotic (ek-ee-MAH-tik). *Description.* Having a bruised appearance.

ecto- *Prefix.* On the outside (ectoblast: an external membrane or cell wall).

edema (eh-DEE-muh). *Pathologic condition.* Excessive accumulation of fluid in cells, tissues or spaces; swelling.

> **dependent e.**: development of swelling in the lower parts of the body under the influence of gravity (e.g., feet toward the end of the day).

effusion (eh-FYU-zjun). *Pathologic condition.* A collection of fluid within a joint; the fluid may be bloody, inflammatory or infectious.

Egawa sign. *Clinical sign.* With the back of the hand placed flat on the table, patient attempts to bend the long (middle) finger and then move it from side to side; inability to do this indicates dysfunction of the ulnar nerve to the hand.

Eggers' plate. *Surgical appliance.* Metal plate with screw-holes; used for holding bony fragments in place.

Ehlers-Danlos syndrome. *Pathologic condition.* Connective tissue disorder characterized by marked hyperelasticity of joints, skin and ligaments. Hereditary.

elastic cartilage (KAHR-tuh-lidj). *Anatomy.* Flexible connective tissue on ends of long bones and ribs, also in nose, trachea, external ear, skin and wrist. Has more elastic fibers than hyaline or fibrocartilage.

elastic tourniquet. *Orthopedic appliance.* Tight elastic band placed around an extremity to cut its circulation. Easier to apply than inflatable tourniquet; also has absence of expensive instrumentation. See also INFLATABLE TOURNIQUET.

elastofibroma (ee-las-toh-fi-BROH-muh). *Pathologic condition.* Benign tumor, usually of lower part of the scapula (shoulderblade); usually in the elderly.

elbow, cubitus. *Anatomy.* Hinged joint comprised of distal end of the humerus (upper armbone) and proximal ends of the radius and ulna (forearm bones).

> **e. disarticulation** (dis-ahr-tik-yu-LAY-shun). *Surgical procedure.* Amputation of the arm through the elbow joint.

electrical potentials. *Test.* Visualized component of an electromyogram (EMG). Represents the voltage of electrical currents across nerve or muscle cells.

electric stimulation. *Treatment.* Generally refers to mild electrical shock to the muscles of an extremity or the back, causing them to contract. Used for preventing atrophy or weakening of a muscle after injury to the nerve.

electrocautery (eh-lek-troh-KAH-tur-ee). 1. *Surgical device.* Electrical device used to cauterize (burn) small blood vessels, to stop bleeding during surgery. 2. *Surgical procedure.* Control of bleeding during surgery using an electrical current.

electromagnetic field. *Treatment.* Used for inducing bone healing in fractures or osteotomies.

electromagnetism. *Treatment.* Use of electromagnetic waves to stimulate fractured bones into healing. Applied through an externally worn device called a bone stimulator.

electromyogram (EMG) (eh-lek-troh-MI-oh-gram). *Diagnostic test*. Recording of the general health of muscle with respect to its electrical activity. With electrodes placed in the muscles, electrical potentials are visualized on a screen (oscilloscope) and recorded. See also NERVE CONDUCTION TEST.

electromyography (eh-lek-troh-mi-AH-gruh-fee). *Test*. Method of measuring and recording the electrical activity of muscles. See also ELECTROMYOGRAM.

Ellis and Edwards classification, modified by Leach. *Fracture classification*. For tibial shaft fractures, combines different degrees of displacement, comminution (fragmentation), wound size and energy (degree of violence) associated with the injury.

embolism (EM-boh-liz-um). *Pathologic condition*. Sudden obstruction of a blood vessel by an embolus, an abnormal floating particle (such as an air bubble, blood clot, cholesterol plaque, clump of tumor cells, marrow of broken bones). If large and affecting a crucial organ (e.g., lung or brain), may result in death.

embolus (EM-boh-lus). *Pathologic structure*. Fragment of matter (blood clot, tumor cells, debris, fat, etc.) free-floating within the bloodstream; depending on its size, can obstruct a blood vessel and prevent normal blood flow and cause death of (infarct) a tissue or organ. Plural: emboli. See also THROMBUS.

eminence. *Anatomy*. Bony prominence.

  e. fracture: abridged term for TIBIAL EMINENCE FRACTURE.

enchondroma (en-kahn-DROH-muh), **enchondrosis**. *Pathologic condition*. Benign cartilaginous growth arising from the metaphysis and/or diaphysis of a long bone. See also ECCHONDROMA.

enchondromatosis (en-kahn-droh-muh-TOH-sus), **dyschondroplasia**, **Ollier's disease**. *Pathologic condition*. Multiple benign cartilage tumors, usually within the metaphyses of long bones. Called Maffucci's syndrome when associated with multiple hamartomas (benign blood vessel tumors).

enchondrosis. See ECCHONDROMA.

Ender's nail. *Surgical implant*. Solid, flexible metal rod passed into the central (medullary) canal of a broken long bone to fasten it together.

endogenous (en-DAH-jen-us) *Description*. Arising within or derived from the body.

endoprosthesis (en-doh-prahs-THEE-sus) 1. *Orthotic device*. Artificial extremity having an internal supporting portion and an outside covered with soft foam. 2. *Surgical implant*. Any prosthetic device that replaces a joint or part of a bone.

  bipolar e.: for replacing a femoral head and neck; contains a mobile articulation between the head and neck portions of the prosthesis.

  unipolar e.: for replacing a femoral head and neck that does not have a mobile articulation between the head and neck of the implant

endoscope (EN-doh-skope). *Instrument*. Device used for looking inside the body.

endosteum (en-DAHS-tee-um). *Anatomy*. Thin layer of connective tissue lining the medullary canal (marrow cavity) of a bone.

endothelial myeloma (en-do-THEE-lee-ul mi-uh-LOH-muh), **Ewing's sarcoma**, **Ewing's tumor**. *Pathologic condition*. Malignant bone tumor; usually occurs between ages 10–20. X-ray shows irregular bone destruction and periosteal new bone formation.

Engelmann disease, Camurati-Engelmann, diaphyseal dysplasia, progressive diaphyseal dysplasia. *Pathologic condition*. Type of dwarfism resulting from an abnormality in the growth of the long bones. Characteristics include abnormally short, wide long bones and early joint arthritis.

enolic acids. *Drug*. Class of NSAIDs (nonsteroidal anti-inflammatory drugs).

enthesis (en-THEE-sis). *Anatomy*. Place of attachment of a tendon onto a bone.

enthesitis (en-thee-SI-tis). *Pathologic condition*. Inflammation of point of attachment of a tendon onto a bone. Frequently found in ankylosing spondylitis.

enthesopathy (en-thee-AHP-uh-thee). *Pathologic condition.* Disease, inflammation or wearing down of the attachment of a tendon onto a bone.

entrapment syndrome. *Pathologic condition.* Loss of normal function of a nerve, vessel or tendon that is trapped in scar tissue or under a tight fibrous or bony structure.

enucleate (ee-NU-klee-ayt). *Surgical procedure.* To remove in one piece.

eosinophilic granuloma (ee-oh-sin-oh-FIL-ik). *Pathologic condition.* Most common, benign form of Langerhans' cell histiocytosis; characterized by a solitary lytic (hole-like) bone lesion in the skull or spine. Onset between ages 5–10. Hereditary. See also HAND-SCHULLER-CHRISTIAN DISEASE, LETTERER SIWE DISEASE.

epiarticular (ep-ee-ahr-TIK-yu-lur). *Anatomic description.* Refers to the edge of a joint.

epibasal fracture. *Pathologic condition.* Break at the base of the thumb or 5th (little finger) metacarpal bone, just above the joint surface.

epicondylar (eh-pih-KAHN-dih-lur). *Anatomic description.* Refers to small prominences on the medial (inner) and lateral (outer) sides of some long bones, e.g., the distal humerus (armbone) at the elbow joint or the femur (thighbone) at the knee joint.

    e. fracture. *Pathologic condition.* Break at edge of the flare of the femur (thighbone) or humerus (armbone).

epicondyles (eh-pih-KAHN-diles). *Anatomy.* Small prominences at the ends of some long bones to which muscles or ligaments attach; most prominently noted on the distal humerus (armbone) and distal femur (thighbone).

    lateral e.: small prominence on the outer side of some long bones.

    medial e.: prominence on the inner side of some long bones.

epicondylitis (eh-pih-kahn-duh-LI-tus). *Pathologic condition.* Inflammation of one of the small prominences and the adjoining tissues at the elbow joint.

    lateral e., tennis elbow: inflammation of the extensor tendons where they attach to the capitellum and lateral condyle of the humerus (upper armbone), from repetitive motion in dorsiflexion of the wrist.

    medial e., golfer's elbow: inflammation of the small bony protuberance at the elbow joint, where flexor muscles of the forearm are attached. Caused by overuse or trauma; pain may occur with muscle contraction.

epidermis. *Anatomy.* The outer layer of skin. See also DERMIS.

epiphyseal (eh-pih-FIZ-ee-ul). *Anatomic description.* Refers to the epiphysis (growth center of a long bone).

    e. cartilage (KAHR-tuh-lidj). *Anatomy.* See EPIPHYSEAL PLATE.

    e. dysplasia. *Pathologic condition.* Group of hereditary abnormalities involving the development of long bones, usually resulting in joint deformities, difficulty in walking, development of early degenerative arthritis and short limb dwarfism. See also CONRADI'S SYNDROME, EPIPHYSEAL MULTIPLEX.

    e. exostosis (ex-ahs-TOH-sus). *Pathologic condition.* Bony cartilaginous growth from the region of the epiphysis.

    e. fracture. See FRACTURE.

    e. hyperplasia (hi-pur-PLAY-zjuh). *Pathologic condition.* Overgrowth of the cartilage of the epiphysis (growth center of a long bone), leading to irregularity of the growth plate.

    e. line. *Anatomy.* Marks site of EPIPHYSEAL PLATE (below) of a long bone.

    e. osteochondroma, dysplasia epiphysealis, hemimelica, tarso-epiphyseal aclasia, Trevor disease. *Congenital abnormality.* Abnormal development of osteochondromas, usually involving multiple bones in one limb. Three variations: localized (involves one epiphysis); classic (involves more than one bone in a single limb); and generalized (involves multiple bones in more than one limb).

e. plate, **epiphyseal cartilage**, **growth plate**, **physis**. *Anatomy.* In a long bone, the layer of cartilage between the epiphysis (growth center) and the metaphysis, where growth in length occurs.

epiphysiodesis (eh-pif-iz-ee-AH-dis-is). *Surgical procedure.* Destruction of a bone's growth plate (physis or epiphyseal plate), to prevent further growth that might result in a limb length abnormality or angular deformity.

epiphysiolysis (eh-pif-uh-see-oh-LI-sus). *Pathologic condition.* Loosening or separation of the epiphysis (growth area) from the diaphysis (shaft) of a bone.

epiphysis (eh-PIF-uh-sis). *Anatomy.* Segment at the end of a long bone that contains the growth center.

epiphysitis (eh-pif-uh-SI-tus). *Pathologic condition.* Inflammation of the epiphysis (growth area of a long bone).

epitrochlea (ep-uh-TROH-klee-uh). *Anatomy.* Medial (inner) epicondyle (prominence) at the distal end of the humerus (upper armbone) by the elbow.

eponychium (ep-uh-NIK-ee-um), **cuticle**, **perionychium**. *Anatomy.* The skin that partly covers the base of a fingernail or toenail. Plural: eponychia.

Epstein classification. *Fracture classification.* Describes different types of anterior dislocations of the hip.

equinovalgus, talipes equinovalgus. *Congenital abnormality.* Plantarflexed (bends downward) foot that turns outward.

equinovarus (ee-kwi-noh-VEHR-us), **clubfoot, pes equinovarus**, **talipes equinovarus**. *Congenital abnormality.* Rigid, inwardly rotated foot that bends down and in; if untreated, rests on outer edge and cannot be placed flat on the walking surface.

equinus deformity (ee-KWI-nus), **talipes equinus**. *Congenital abnormality.* Plantarflexed foot (hindfoot points downward as if on tiptoes); can lead to a toe walking deformity or can be part of a rocker-bottom foot.

Erb's palsy /or/ **paralysis**, **Duchenne-Erb paralysis**. *Congenital abnormality.* Paralysis of shoulder muscles and those that flex the elbow; occurs during birth when the shoulder is unable to progress through the pelvic canal and there is stretch on the upper part of the brachial plexus (nerves to the arm).

Erichsen sign. *Clinical finding.* Pain in the sacroiliac joint when the iliac crests are compressed toward each other; indicates sacroiliac joint disease.

erosion. *Pathologic condition.* Wearing away of an area of tissue by inflammation, ulceration or trauma. See also ABRASION, ATTRITION, PLANING.

erythema (ehr-ih-THEE-muh). *Pathologic condition.* Redness; associated with injury, inflammation, infection or trauma.

erythrocyte sedimentation rate (ESR) (uh-RITH-roh-site), **sed rate**, **sedimentation rate**. *Lab test.* Rate (in mm per hour) at which red blood cells settle to the bottom of a tube of unclotted blood. Nonspecific test used for measuring presence or progress of various systemic inflammatory diseases.

eschar (ES-kahr). *Pathologic lesion.* A scab, especially after a burn; the covering of dead tissue that forms over skin that has been burned or corroded.

Esmarch bandage (ESH-mark), **Martin bandage**. *Orthopedic supply.* Elastic band used to squeeze the blood out of an extremity.

Essex-Lopresti classification. *Fracture classification.* Identifies heel fractures according to the pattern of the fracture fragments.

Essex-Lopresti fracture. *Pathologic condition.* Break in the calcaneus (heelbone) that involves the subtalar joint (between the calcaneus and the talus).

etiology (ee-tee-AHL-uh-jee). Cause(s) of a disease or abnormal condition.

etodolac (ee-TOH-doh-lak). *Drug.* NSAID for treating pain and inflammation. Trade name: Lodine.

Evans and Jensen classification. *Fracture classification.* Classifies intertro-chanteric femur (thighbone) fractures.

eversion. *Function.* Turning inside out, as turning eyelid over to allow examination of the undersurface; the turning or rotating outward of a foot.

e. stress test. *Clinical test.* The inner side of the foot is pushed to force it to the outside; instability reveals a tear in the deltoid ligament of the ankle. See also TALAR TILT TEST.

Ewing's sarcoma /or/ **tumor, endothelial myeloma**. *Pathologic condition.* Malignant bone tumor that usually occurs between ages 10–20; x-ray shows irregular bone destruction and periosteal new bone formation. Often fatal.

exacerbation (eks-ass-ur-BAY-shun). *Pathologic process.* Flare-up or worsening of a previously existing disease or condition. See also REMISSION.

exarticulation (eks-ahr-tik-yu-LAY-shun), **disarticulation.** *Surgical procedure.* Amputation through a joint.

excise (eks-SIZE), **resect.** *Surgical procedure.* To remove or cut out. See also INCISE.

excision (eks-SIH-zjun), **extirpation, resection.** *Surgical procedure.* Cutting out; removing. Partial or complete removal or surgical destruction of bone, muscle, tumor, or other organ. See also INCISION.

excoriation (eks-kor-ee-AY-shun). *Pathologic condition.* Abrasion or wearing off of skin, as from severe scratching.

exogenous (ex-AH-jen-us). *Description.* Arising outside of the body.

exostectomy (eks-ahs-TEK-tuh-mee). *Surgical procedure.* Removal of an exostosis (protrusion of bone).

exostosis (eks-ahs-TOH-sus). *Pathologic condition.* Benign tumor covered with cartilage at ends of long bones, always pointing away from the nearest joint. See also OSTEOCHONDROMA.

multiple e.: large bony protuberances occuring around joints; slight chance of becoming malignant. Hereditary.

extension body cast. *Orthopedic appliance.* Cast applied from chest to groin, to hold the back in an arched position. See also FLEXION BODY CAST.

extensor (eks-TEN-sur). *Anatomy.* Muscle that causes a joint to straighten. See also FLEXOR.

e. carpi radialis brevis (ECRB) (KAHR-pee ray-dee-AL-us): short wrist and forearm muscle that raises the wrist and dorsiflexes (extends) the hand.

e. carpi radialis longus (ECRL): long muscle on back of the forearm that extends and abducts the hand, raising it toward the thumb.

e. carpi ulnaris (ECU) (ul-NEHR-us): wrist and forearm muscle that extends and adducts the hand, raising the wrist toward the little finger.

e. digiti minimi (EDM), e. digiti quinti: slender muscle that extends the little finger.

e. digitorum brevis (EDB) (dij-uh-TOR-um): small muscle on top of foot that extends the toes.

e. digitorum communis (EDC) (kum-MYU-nus): large muscle on the back of the forearm that extends the fingers and wrist.

e. digitorum longus (EDL): ankle muscle that raises the four small toes and dorsally flexes and pronates the foot.

e. hallucis brevis (EHB) (HAL-uh-sus): small muscle on top of foot that raises the big toe.

e. hallucis longus (EHL): long thin muscle on the shin that extends the big toe and dorsiflexes and supinates the foot.

e. indicis (EI), e. indicis propius: muscle in back of forearm; arises from the ulna in the more distal part of forearm and extends index finger.

e. pollicis brevis (EPB) (PAHL-uh-sus): muscle on back of forearm that raises and straightens the thumb and adducts the hand.

e. pollicis longus (EPL): long muscle on top of forearm that raises the thumb and abducts the hand.

extensor aponeurosis. See EXTENSOR HOOD.

extensor compartments of the wrist, extensor tunnels of the wrist. *Anatomy.* A series of compartments at the back of the wrist separating the different extensor tendons that cross the wrist into six distinctly separate groups; numbered from radial (thumb side) to ulnar (pinky side).

> 1st: houses the e. pollicis brevis and abductor pollicis longus.
>
> 2nd: houses the e. carpi radialis longus and e. carpi radialis brevis.
>
> 3rd: houses the extensor pollicis longus.
>
> 4th: houses extensor indicis propius and extensor digitorum communis.
>
> 5th: houses the extensor digitorum minimi.
>
> 6th: houses the extensor carpi ulnaris.

extensor hood, extensor aponeurosis, dorsal hood. *Anatomy.* Band of connective tissue at the back of a finger or toe that gives attachment to extensor muscles and provides stability to the straightened fingers/toes.

extensor plantar response, Babinski reflex /or/ **response** /or/ **sign.** *Clinical finding.* Involuntary raising of the big toe when the bottom of the foot is firmly stroked from heel to toe. Sometimes called a positive Babinski. May indicate disease of the central nervous system (brain or spinal cord). Normal in an infant. See also PLANTAR REFLEX.

extensor tendon. *Anatomy.* Cconnective tissue band of an extensor muscle.

external fixation. *Surgical procedure.* Use of pins fixed in a rigid frame that enter from outside the skin and hold a fragment or fracture in alignment.

external oblique muscle. *Anatomy.* One of the superficial muscles of the abdominal wall; running in an oblique direction, from lateral to medial.

extirpation (eks-tur-PAY-shun). See EXCISION.

extra-articular arthrodesis (ahr-throh-DEE-sus). *Surgical procedure.* Fusion of a joint outside the capsule (fibrous lining of a joint) by means of a bone graft or cartilage removal.

extra-articular fracture. *Pathologic condition.* A break in a bone that does not involve the joint surface.

extracapsular ankylosis (an-kil-OH-sus). *Pathologic condition.* Fusion of a joint caused by rigidity of structures outside the capsule (fibrous lining of a joint).

extracapsular fracture. *Pathologic condition.* A break in a bone outside the capsule (fibrous lining of a joint).

extremity, limb. *Anatomy.* An arm or leg.

> **lower e.**: refers to the area between the knee and ankle.
>
> **upper e.**: refers to an arm.

extrusion (eks-TRU-zjun). *Pathologic condition.* Projection of muscle, bone, or other tissue out of its confined space.

exudate (EKS-yu-dayt). *Pathologic condition.* Fluid that forms in response to irritation, inflammation or infection; composed of serum, fibrin, and white blood cells. See also TRANSUDATE.

FAbER sign, Patrick's test, figure-4 test. *Clinical sign/test*. Acronym for Fusion, Abduction, External Rotation. With patient lying on his/her back, the thigh and knee are bent, and the foot is placed above the patella (kneecap) of the opposite leg. The knee on the affected side is then depressed. Pain indicates an abnormality of the hip joint or sacroiliac joint.

facet (fuh-SET). *Anatomy*. Smooth area at the end of a bone.

    articular f.: small joint surface, such as the back part of a vertebra that connects with the vertebrae above and below, allowing motion in the spinal column. Each vertebra has two superior and two inferior facets.

facetectomy (fas-uh-TEK-toh-mee). *Surgical procedure.* Removal of the joint (articular) surfaces at the back of the spine.

facilitation (fuh-sil-uh-TAY-shun) *Function.* Reinforcement of an activity, such as a reflex, by repeated stimulation.

Fajersztajn test (FAH-zjur-stine), **contralateral straight leg raising test, prostrate leg raising test, sciatic phenomenon, well-leg raising test of Fajersztajn**. *Clinical test*. With patient lying on his/her back, a leg is raised with the knee in extension. Pain in the opposite leg indicates irritation of the nerve as it exits the spine. Sign of herniated disc disease.

fallen arch, flatfoot, pes planus, splayfoot, talipes planus. *Abnormal condition*. A foot whose metatarsal arch, which runs from the heel to the ball of the foot, is flattened or collapsed. May be congenital or developed over time.

familial dysautonomia (dis-ah-toh-NOH-mee-uh), **dysautonomia, Riley Day syndrome**. *Pathologic condition*. Abnormality of the autonomic nervous system, causing numerous difficulties including difficulty controlling body temperature, insensitivity to pain, motor uncoordination, lack of tearing, intolerance to anesthetics. Hereditary.

familial interstitial hypertrophic neuritis, Déjérine-Sotta disease /or/ **syndrome, hypertrophic interstitial neuritis**. *Pathologic condition.* Type III hereditary motor sensory neuropathy, a syndrome characterized by progressive degeneration of the peripheral nerves. Weakness in the hands and feet are associated with localized swelling of the peripheral nerves and sensory changes in the extremities; results in hand and foot deformities. Hereditary; detected in late infancy. See also CHARCOT-MARIE-TOOTH disease.

familial lymphedema (lim-fuh-DEE-muh). *Pathologic condition*. A permanent edema (swelling from fluid in tissues); causes pitting in the legs. Two types: Milroy's disease, which is congenital, and Meige's, which is acquired.

fan sign. *Clinical sign*. Stroking the outer portion of the foot causes the toes to spread apart; sign of neurological deficit.

fascia (FASH-uh). *Anatomy*. A sheath (band of connective tissue) that encloses and connects organs, structures and muscles and helps keep them in place.

    f. lata (LAH-tuh): sheet of fibrous tissue that extends from the iliac crest of the pelvis, down the outer side of the thigh, to the knee joint.

        tensor fascia lata (TFL): muscle that flexes and abducts the thigh; originates from the lateral aspect on the ilium (pelvis) and attaches to the proximal anterolateral tibia (shinbone) via the iliotibial band.

palmar f.: connective tissue underneath the skin of the palm. Gives rigidity to the skin, to avoid slipping or bunching.

plantar f., aponeurosis: tight connective tissue band on sole of foot that forms part of the arch.

fascicle (FAS-ih-kul). *Anatomy*. Bundle of fibers (nerve or muscle) surrounded by a thin connective tissue sleeve.

fasciculation. 1. *Pathologic condition*. Fine, involuntary, ripple-like muscular contractions. 2. *Anatomy*. Tissue that has been organized into fascicles.

fasciectomy (fash-ee-EK-toh-mee). *Surgical procedure*. Removal of a fascia.

fasciitis (fash-ee-I-tus). *Pathologic condtion*. Inflammation of the fascia.

fascioscapulohumeral dystrophy (fash-ee-oh-skap-yu-loh-HYU-mur-ul DIS-truh-ee), **Landouzy-Déjérine disease**. *Pathologic condition*. Mild, common form of muscular dystrophy; results in loss of arm strength, especially around the shoulder, with wasting of the shoulder girdle muscles; also affects the muscles of the face, which may lead to inability to generate facial expressions such as smiling.

fasciotome (FASH-ee-oh-tohm). *Surgical instrument*. Knife-like instrument for cutting fascia to be transplanted.

fasciotomy (fash-ee-AH-toh-mee). *Surgical procedure*. Incision of a fascia to relieve pressure in a compartment; used in some cases of violent trauma. See also COMPARTMENT SYNDROME.

fat embolism (EM-boh-liz-um). *Pathologic condition*. Blockage of small blood vessels from release of fat droplets into the bloodstream. Disorientation and pulmonary difficulties result, and sometimes death. Associated with multiple fractures.

fatigue fracture, **stress fracture**. *Pathologic condition*. Break in a bone caused by prolonged repetitive activity, such as running or marching.

fat pad. *Anatomy*. Accumulation of fat in certain areas of the body.

retropatellar (ret-tro-puh-TEL-ur): fat segment behind and below the patella, external to the knee joint capsule.

fat pad sign. *Radiologic sign*. Layer of fat that becomes detectable on x-ray following injury secondary to swelling. May indicate a fracture.

Feiss line. *Clinical finding*. A line drawn from the medial malleolus to the base of the bottom of the 1st metatarsophalangeal joint. With the patient seated, the naviculum should fall within the line; falling below the line is indicative of pes planus. Then with patient standing, if the naviculum falls below the line but was inside the line with patient sitting, it is indicative of flexible pes planus.

Feldene. *Drug*. Trade name of piroxicam, NSAID for treating pain and inflammation.

felon (FEL-un), **whitlow**. *Pathologic condition*. Purulent soft tissue infection at the end of a finger.

Femister. Incorrect spelling of PHEMISTER.

femoral (FEM-ur-ul). *Anatomic description*. Refers to the femur (thighbone).

f. anteversion (an-tee-VUR-zjun). *Function*. Rotation of the neck of the femur (thighbone) to the front, about its long axis. If excessive could be considered abnormal. See also FEMORAL RETROVERSION (below).

f. artery. *Anatomy*. Major artery supplying legs; branch of the external iliac artery.

deep: branch that supplies upper and inner thighs.

f. circumflex artery. *Anatomy*. Supplies the area around the neck and outer side of the femur (thighbone). Two branches: lateral and medial.

lateral: exits laterally off the deep femoral artery; supplies part of the femoral head and neck. It and its branches connect with the branches of the medial femoral circumflex artery to completely encircle the upper part of the femur.

medial: exits medially off the deep femoral artery; supplies part of the femoral head and neck. It and its branches connect with the branches of the lateral femoral circumflex artery to completely encircle the upper part of the femur.

f. collateral ligaments. *Anatomy.* Connective tissue attachments that give stability to the knee joint in medial and lateral motion.

f. condyle (KAHN-dile). *Anatomy.* Rounded ends of the femur that articulate with the tibia (shinbone). Part of the knee.

f. epiphysiodesis (eh-pif-iz-ee-oh-DEE-sus). *Surgical procedure.* Destruction of the growth plate of the distal femur to prevent growth or to control the length and angular alignment of the leg.

f. epiphysis (uh-PIF-uh-sus). *Anatomy.* One of two growth plates of the femur: capital (below the femoral head) and distal (at lower end of femur).

capital f. epiphysis: growth area in the upper femur; begins to appear bony at about 6 months of age, fusing with the femur at the end of growth.

f. head. *Anatomy.* Ball-shaped area at the top of the femur.

f. jig. *Surgical tool.* Used to cut the proximal or distal femur (thighbone) for insertion of a prosthesis or artificial joint.

f. neck. *Anatomy.* Short curved area between the head of the femur (top of thighbone) and its shaft.

f. nerve. *Anatomy.* Large nerve that enters the leg at the front of the thigh.

f. retroversion. *Abnormal function.* Posterior rotation of the neck of the thighbone (femur) about the long axis of its shaft, causing the feet and legs to turn out. See also FEMORAL ANTEVERSION.

f. vein. *Anatomy.* Major blood vessel in the leg that drains the lower leg; accompanies the femoral artery.

femur (FEE-mur). *Anatomy.* The thighbone. Largest bone in the body; joins the hip to the knee.

fenamic acids. *Drug.* Class of NSAIDs (nonsteroidal anti-inflammatory drugs).

fenestra (fuh-NES-truh). *Anatomy.* 1. Opening in bone or fascia. 2. An opening or window in a cast. Plural: fenestrae.

fenoprofen (fen-oh-PRO-fen). *Drug.* NSAID for treating pain and inflammation. Trade name: Nalfon.

Fexicam. *Drug.* A trade name of piroxicam, NSAID for treating pain and inflammation.

fiberglass (FG). *Chemical substance.* Material used in casting and splinting. Preferred for its light weight, ease of application and resistance to water.

fibril (FI-bril). *Anatomy.* Small nerve or muscle fiber. See also MYOFIBRIL, NEUROFIBRIL.

fibroblast (FI-broh-blast). *Anatomy.* Type of cell in connective tissue that forms collagen (a protein).

fibrocartilage (fi-broh-KAHR-tuh-lij). *Anatomy.* Type of connective tissue that contains visible collagen fibers and is frequently found in areas where hyaline cartilage has been damaged. Also seen normally in the menisci of the knee. See also ELASTIC CARTILAGE, HYALINE CARTILAGE.

fibrocortical defect, fibrous cortical defect. *Pathologic condition.* Benign asymptomatic fibrous bone lesion, usually in children in the metaphysis of long bones.

fibrocyte (FI-broh-site). *Anatomy.* Collagen-forming cell (fibroblast) when it is not actively producing collagen.

fibroma (fi-BROH-muh). *Pathologic condition.* Benign tumor comprised of fibrous connective tissue.

aponeurotic (ay-pahn-yu-RAH-tik): occurs within an aponeurosis (fibrous tissue); most frequently seen in the hands and feet as a slow-growing and painless nodule.

juvenile: occurs in children, within certain fibrous tissues (aponeuroses); most frequently in the hands or feet as a slow-growing and painless nodule.

fibromatosis (fi-broh-muh-TOH-suhs). *Pathologic condition.* Multiple fibromas (benign tumors), most frequently in the hands or bottom of feet. Can cause pain and contracture (inability of a joint to complete normal range of motion).

congenital generalized f.: multiple fibromas occur in the soft tissues in many areas of the body; usually presents in childhood and may result in progressive limb and spine abnormalities.

infantile f.: same as CONGENITAL GENERALIZED FIBROMATOSIS.

palmar f., Dupuytren's contracture: loss of motion in the connective tissues underneath the skin of the palm, caused by a proliferation of fibroblasts (necessary in production of scar tissue). Nodules and cords form, causing loss of motion in the finger joints.

plantar f, Ledderhose's disease: scarring of the plantar fascia resulting in painful nodules along the bottom of the foot.

fibromyalgia (fi-broh-mi-AL-gee-uh). *Pathologic condition.* Disease characterized by pain in the fibrous or connective tissue in muscle.

fibrosarcoma (fi-broh-sahr-KOH-muh). *Pathologic oondition.* Malignant tumor composed primarily of connective tissue with many reproducing fibroblasts (oollagen forming cells).

fibrosis (fi-BROH-sus). *Pathologic process.* Formation of fibrous tissue as a reaction to injury or disease.

fibrositis (fi-bro-SI-tus). *Pathologic condition.* Inflammation of fibrous tissue.

fibrous (FI-brus). *Anatomic description.* Refers to tissue composed of connective tissue fibers and fibroblasts (collagen forming cells).

f. ankylosis (an-kuh-LOH-sus). *Pathologic condition.* Immobilizaton of two bones from extensive fibrous tissue. See also BONY ANKYLOSIS.

f. cortical defect. See FIBROCORTICAL DEFECT.

f. dysplasia (dis-PLAY-zjuh). *Pathologic condition.* Lesion in bone made up of disorganized connective tissue. Can lead to significant deformities or fracture. See also MCCUNE-ALBRIGHT SYNDROME.

monostatic: only a single bone is affected.

f. hamartoma (hay-mahr-TOH-muh). *Pathologic condition.* Fibrous malformation, generally found in upper arm or shoulder of children under age 2.

f. histiocytoma (his-tee-oh-si-TOH-muh). *Pathologic condition.* Tumor made of histiocytes in a fibrous tissue background.

malignant f. histiocytosis (MFH): tumor derived from primitive and fast-growing fibrous cells; most frequently found in the femur (thighbone) and tibia (shinbone). Often fatal.

f. nonunion. *Pathologic condition.* Fracture whose fragments are held together by fibrous tissue instead of bone.

fibroxanthoma (fi-broh-zan-THOH-muh), **dermatofibroma**, **sclerosing hemangioma**. *Pathologic condition.* Type of slow-growing, benign, fibrous skin nodule; usually affects lower extremities.

fibroxanthosarcoma (fi-broh-zan-thoh-sahr-KOH-muh). *Pathologic condition.* A fibroma (benign tumor) that has become malignant as evidenced by rapid duplication of abnormal cells.

fibula (FIB-yu-luh), **peroneal bone**, **peroneus** *Anatomy.* The smaller of the two bones of the lower leg; articulates with the talus (top foot bone) below, and the tibia (shinbone) above.

fibular (FIB-yu-lur). *Anatomic description*. Refers to the fibula.

    f. collateral ligament *Anatomy*. Connective tissue band (1) running along outer side of the knee and connecting the femur to the tibia; acts as a stabilizer of the knee, keeping the tibia from rotating inward; (2) running along outer side of interphalangeal and metatarsophalangeal joints of the toes.

    f. hemimelia (hem-ee-MEE-lee-uh). *Congenital abnormality*. Absence of part or all of the fibula; associated with short femur (thighbone) and absence of the lateral two or three metatarsals (bones in foot).

    f. neck. *Anatomy*. Narrow part of the fibula near its attachment to the tibia at the knee.

    f. strut graft. *Biologic implant*. Segment of fibula transferred to another area, generally to the femoral neck for avascular necrosis of the femur. May be transferred alive (vascular) or nonliving (avascular).

Fielding's classification. *Fracture classification*. Identifies types of subtrochanteric fractures (area just below the hip).

figure 8 harness. *Orthopedic appliance*. Harness that pulls the shoulders into extension, to treat a fracture of the clavicle (collarbone); looks like a figure 8.

figure-4 test, Patrick's test, FAbER sign. *Clinical sign/test*. With patient lying on his/her back, the thigh and knee are bent, and the foot is placed above the patella (kneecap) of the opposite leg. The knee on the affected side is then depressed. Pain indicates an abnormality of the hip or sacroiliac joint.

Fillauer bar, **Fillauer abduction bar**, **abduction bar** /or/ **bar splint, Denis Browne bar** /or/ **brace** /or/ **splint, Tarso abduction bar**. *Orthopedic appliance*. Metal bar that holds a pair of shoes together, positioning the feet. Used for controlling leg rotation in infants.

filum terminale syndrome (FI-lum tur-min-AL-ee), **cord traction** /or/ **tethered cord syndrome**. *Pathologic condition*. In patients with certain spinal defects (e.g., spina bifida), the conus medullaris (terminal end of spinal cord) becomes attached to the bone or scar tissue, preventing its upward migration with growth. Causes cord tension and can result in progressive paralysis of the bladder, bowel, and lower extremities.

finger. *Anatomy*. One of the five appendages of the hand. Anatomically, the thumb is not considered a finger.

    f. trap, Chinese f. trap. *Orthopedic appliance*. Cylindrical mesh used to secere the fingers while they are being pulled by a weight. Used in the acute treatment of certain displaced fractures.

fingertip flaps. *Surgical technique*. The flaps that close the end of a finger after its amputation; made from the skin along the side of the finger.

fingertip pinch test, Jeanne's sign. *Clinical test*. Strength tested by pressing fingertip to thumb. Loss of strength or inability to perform a pinch is indicative of ulnar nerve dysfunction.

Finkelstein sign/test. *Clinical test*. Pain felt on the radial side (thumb side) of the wrist when it is bent toward the small finger by the examiner while the patient clasps his/her thumb in his palm; indicative of tendonitis of the abductor of the thumb. See also DE QUERVAIN DISEASE.

fishmouth amputation. *Surgical procedure*. Technique of fashioning soft tissues at the tip of an amputated part in the shape of a fish's mouth so the wound may be closed.

fisial. Incorrect spelling of PHYSEAL.

fisis. Incorrect spelling of PHYSIS.

fissure (FISH-ur). *Pathologic condition*. A deep slit, crack, or cleft.

fissure fracture, linear fracture. *Pathologic conditon.* A break that extends along the length of a bone rather than across it.

fistula (FIS-tyu-luh). *Pathologic conditon.* Abnormal passage from an abscess or hollow organ to the body surface or from one hollow organ to another.

   arteriovenous f.: joining of an artery and a vein; may be congenital or acquired; blood flows from the artery into the vein. Can result in heart failure.

fixation (bone). *Surgical procedure.* Attaching a plate or other device to bone, so as to immobilize a fracture or osteotomy site. See also FIXATOR.

   external: metal pins inserted through slits in the skin and into a fractured bone; attached to a frame outside the body. Designed to be temporary, generally removed after about 5 to 6 weeks.

   internal: screws and/or plates surgically placed inside or along a fractured bone and contained completely within the body; designed to remain in the body indefinitely. Refers also to the materials used.

fixator. *Orthopedic appliance.* Support device, generally made of metal, used to help immobilize a fracture.

   external: pins fixed in a rigid frame that enter from outside the skin and hold a fragment or fracture in alignment.

fixed curve. *Anatomic deformity.* Rigid spinal curve that cannot be straightened through normal means; usually refers to scoliosis, lordosis or kyphosis.

fixed flexion contracture, flexion contracture. *Pathologic condition.* Inability of a joint to achieve full extension because of dense scar tissue or shortening of the soft tissues about the bone making up the joint; cannot be corrected by gentle stretch.

flaccid (FLASS-id). *Anatomic description.* Limp; without tone.

   f. cerebral palsy, hypotonic cerebral palsy. *Pathologic condition.* Form of cerebral palsy: damage to the nervous system results in a very loose muscle group with little or no tone.

flail. *Clinical finding.* Floppy; without rigidity or tone. Refers to a limb without muscular control; a badly fractured segment where the bone is unable to maintain the limb's structural integrity; or in reference to a segment of a fractured rib cage that moves independently of the bones surrounding it, keeping the rib cage from properly expanding the lungs.

flap. *Anatomy.* A projection or tongue of tissue and/or bone.

   advancement f., Atasoy. *Surgical technique.* Triangular flap of skin moved from an adjacent area to cover an amputated fingertip.

   bipedicle f. (bi-PED-ih-kul). *Surgical technique.* Skin flap attached at two opposite poles, with blood supply provided by a pedicle or stem (attachment); often used to cover or fill a skin defect such as after removal of a tumor.

   cross-finger f. *Surgical procedure.* Technique for grafting skin from one finger to an adjacent finger.

   delayed f. *Surgical technique.* Skin graft done in successive stages over several weeks, to maintain blood supply.

   groin f. *Surgical technique.* Large flap of skin and subcutaneous tissue removed from the groin and reattached with its veins and arteries to another site, to cover a large wound.

   iliofemoral f. Same as GROIN FLAP (above).

   pedicle f. *Surgical technique.* Flap of transplanted tissue that maintains its circulation with a long pedicle; may include muscle, fascia and even bone that share the same vascular stalk.

   rotational f. *Surgical procedure.* Section of skin cut with its blood supply intact, rotated to cover or fill a skin defect as after removal of a tumor or scar.

skin f. Tongue-shaped segment of skin that has been cut (surgically or traumatically) so its blood supply remains intact; often used in surgery to cover or fill a skin defect, such as after removal of a tumor or scar.

flat bones. *Anatomy.* Subclassification of bones that are thin (e.g., scapula). See also IRREGULAR BONES, LONG BONES, SHORT BONES.

flatfoot, fallen arch, pes planus, splayfoot, talipes planus. *Abnormal condition.* Foot whose metatarsal arch, which runs from the heel to the ball of the foot, is flattened or collapsed. May be congenital or developed over time.

> **flexible**: a foot whose metatarsal arch collapses when weight is applied and resumes its arched position when the weight is removed.

> **rigid**: a foot whose metatarsal arch is constantly flat.

flebo-. Incorrect spelling of many words beginning with PHLEBO.

flex. *Function.* To bend at a joint.

flexion. *Function.* Bending at a joint

flexion contracture. See FIXED FLEXION CONTRACTURE.

flexor. *Anatomy.* Muscle that causes attached part to bend. See also EXTENSOR.

> **f. carpi radialis (FCR)** (KAHR-pee ray-dee-AL-us): in the forearm; bends the wrist toward the thumb side.

> **f. carpi ulnaris (FCU)** (KAHR-pee ul-NEHR-us): in the forearm; attaches to the wrist; bends the wrist down and toward the little finger.

> **f. digiti minimi** (DIJ-it-ee MIN-ah-mee): in the sole of the foot; bends the little toe.

> **f. digiti quinti** (DIJ-it-ee KWIN-tee): in the palm of the hand; bends the little finger.

> **f. digitorum brevis** (dij-uh-TOH-rum BREV-us): on the sole of the foot; bends the toes; also in the hand.

> **f. digitorum longus (FDL)** (dij-uh-TOH-rum): in the back of the leg below the knee; bends the toes; also in the hand.

> **f. digitorum profundus (FDP)** (dij-uh-TOH-rum pro-FUN-dus): in the forearm, on the side of the palm; bends all fingers but the thumb.

> **f. digitorum sublimus (FDS)** (dij-uh-TOH-rum sub-LI-mus): in the forearm, on the side of the palm; bends the fingers at the first joint.

> **f. hallucis brevis** (HAL-uh-sus BREV-us): on the bottom of the foot; bends the big toe.

> **f. hallucis longus** (HAL-uh-sus): muscle and corresponding tendon in back of leg, between knee and ankle; bends the big toe at its distal joint.

> **f. pollicis brevis** (PAHL-uh-sus BREV-us): in the palm near the thumb; bends the thumb at the base.

> **f. pollicis longus (FPL)** (PAHL-uh-sus): in the forearm; bends the thumb.

flexor retinaculum (ret-in-AK-yu-lum). *Anatomy.* Sheath of fascia (connective tissue) across the wrist that acts as a pulley, giving better strength to the flexor muscles.

flexor sheath. *Anatomy.* Narrow channel of connective tissue that holds a tendon.

flexor tendon. *Anatomy.* Connective tissue band that attaches a flexor muscle to bone.

floating ribs. *Anatomy.* Lowest two ribs (11th, 12th), so named because they do not attach at the front to the sternum (breastbone).

floating traction. *Treatment.* Traction incorporating a pulley system, to allow limited movement in bed without displacing the fracture.

floppy baby syndrome. *Abnormal condition.* Poor muscle tone and decreased movement in a newborn. Several possible causes. See also AMYOTONIA CONGENITA.

flurbiprofen (flur-BI-proh-fen). *Drug.* NSAID for treating pain and inflammation. Trade name: Ansaid.

fluoroscopy (flohr-AHS-kuh-pee). *Radiologic technique.* Method of viewing x-ray images as they are taken, in single frame or motion. Used during surgery.

focomelia. Incorrect spelling of PHOCOMELIA.

foot drop, drop foot. *Pathologic condition.* Inability to raise the foot at the ankle. The foot falls downward, causing the toes to strike the ground during ambulation; occurs in paralysis or absence of the muscles on the front of the leg.

foramen (for-AM-un). *Anatomy.* Hole; a natural opening or passage in bone. Plural: foramina.

foraminal stenosis (stuh-NOH-sus) *Pathologic condition.* Narrowing of the neural foramen (bony opening in spine through which nerve roots exit to the body) causing compression and irritation of the affected nerve root(s).

foraminotomy (for-am-in-AHT-uh-mee). *Surgical procedure.* Opening a foramen by cutting a membrane or scar tissue.

forearm, antebrachium. *Anatomy.* The part of the arm between the elbow and the wrist; comprised of two bones, radius and ulna.

forefoot. *Anatomy.* That portion of the foot distal to the cuneiform bones (midfoot).

    f. abductus. *Pathologic condition.* Same as FOREFOOT VALGUS (below).

    f. adductus. *Pathologic condition.* Same as FOREFOOT VARUS (below).

    f. equinus (ee-KWINE-us). *Pathologic condition.* Foot that points downward at the tarsal and metatarsal joints.

    f. valgus (VAL-gus). *Pathologic condition.* Foot with toes and metatarsals that point outward.

    f. varus (VEHR-us). *Pathologic condition.* Foot with toes and metatarsals that point inward.

foreign body (FB). *Pathologic condition.* Any object (e.g., needle, bullet, prosthesis) within the tissues that is not produced by the body.

forequarter amputation, interscapulothoracic amputation. *Surgical procedure.* Removal of the arm through the shoulder.

fosfolipid. Incorrect spelling of PHOSPHOLIPID.

fossa (FAH-suh). *Anatomy.* Depression or cavity in a bone (e.g., acetabular fossa: the hip socket).

Foster frame. *Orthopedic appliance.* Type of bed frame that allows patient to be turned (side to side) without lifting. See also CIRCOELECTRIC BED.

four-point gait. *Description.* Method of walking with crutches so that one leg and one crutch is always in contact with the floor.

four-poster orthosis. *Orthopedic appliance.* Brace with four posts, two in front and two in back, to immobilize the neck.

Fowler's position, beach chair position. *Anatomic description.* Position of patient reclining on his/her back against a backrest, with knees slightly bent.

fovea centralis (FOH-vee-uh sen-TRA-lus), **capitis femoris.** *Anatomy.* Notch in the femoral head where the ligamentum teres attaches to the femoral head and the acetabulum.

fracture. *Pathologic condition.* Break in a bone.

    angulated: the bone is bent at the point of fracture.

    apophyseal (uh-pah-fuh-SEE-ul): break in a traction growth plate (where muscles or ligaments attach), usually from excessive pull by a ligament or muscle.

    articular: involves the articular (joint) surface.

    atlantal: a break in the 1st cervical (neck) vertebra.

    atlantoaxial: involves the 1st and 2nd cervical (neck) vertebrae.

    avulsion: caused by the effect of a muscle or ligament that pulls its point of attachment off the bone.

axial: break in the 2nd cervical (neck) vertebra.

Barton's: break at the distal end of the palmar side of the radius (larger forearm bone), with dislocation of the distal radioulnar joint (between the two forearm bones).

basilar neck (BAY-sil-ur): break in the femur (thighbone) at the junction of the neck and the shaft.

Bennett's: two-piece intra-articular (joint) break at the base of the metacarpal bone of the thumb.

bimalleolar (bi-mal-EE-oh-lur): break in both the tibial (shinbone) and fibular (lower leg bone) prominences of the ankle.

birth: occurs as the baby passes through the birth canal.

bony mallet: same as MALLET FRACTURE (below).

boxer's: break in the neck of the 5th metacarpus of the hand (knuckle), frequently caused by a punching blow.

bucket-handle: contiguous break in the periphery of the metaphyseal portion (flared end) of a long bone in a child. Thought to result from violent shaking of the child during abuse-related violence. See also CORNER FRACTURE.

bumper: break in the tibial shaft caused by a car bumper hitting the leg below the knee.

burst: break in a vertebra from excess pressure in a vertical direction.

butterfly: fragmented break through a long bone; fragmented bone is triangular in shape and resembles a butterfly. Part of a comminuted fracture.

cartwheel: break in the distal femur (thighbone) or proximal tibia (shinbone) in children. Named when children rode in carts and caught their legs in spoked wheels.

Chance: break through a vertebra caused by combination of excessive flexion and distraction (pulling apart) as when a passenger in a car crash is wearing only the lap portion of a safety belt.

chip: a small bone fragment is pulled away (or chipped off the edge) from the main body of the bone.

clay-shoveler's: a break involving the spinous process (back portion) of a lower cervical (neck) or upper thoracic (chest) vertebra; results from intense traction on the spinous process by the interspinous ligament.

closed, simple: the bones do not pierce the skin.

Colles' (KAHL-ees): break in the distal end of the radius (larger forearm bone) in which the apex of the fracture points to the front, and the distal fragment is displaced to the back.

comminuted: bone is broken into more than two pieces.

complete: runs completely across the bone creating at least two separate fragments.

compound: the bone ends protrude through the skin.

compression: from crushing the bone (compressed toward its center).

condylar: break in the rounded flare at the end of a long bone.

cortical: involves the cortex (hard bone at a bone's periphery).

cotton: trimalleolar break in articular (joint) surface of the tibia (shinbone); involves medial and lateral malleoli, and posterior distal tip of the tibia.

crush: 1. results from a crushing force, usually causing the bone to collapse into itself; 2. a collapsed vertebra.

Darrach-Hughston-Milch: same as GALEAZZI'S FRACTURE (below).

dens: involves the toothlike projection (dens process) of the 2nd cervical vertebra.

depressed: part of the bone is driven into surrounding bone or soft tissue; also refers to sunken position of a fragment in an articular (joint) fracture.

diaphyseal (di-uh-FIZ-ee-ul): break through the shaft of a long bone.

die-punch: an intra-articular (joint) fracture in which a central part of the joint surface has been propelled into the bone. Most commonly applied to certain distal radius (forearm bone) and proximal tibia (shinbone) fractures.

displaced: a bony fragment shifts from its natural position.

dome, **talar dome**: break on the rounded surface (top) of the talus (top foot bone).

Dupuytren's (du-pwe-TRAHNZ): break in the iliac (wing bone) of pelvis.

eminence, **tibial eminence**: avulsion fracture (sudden muscle contraction that pulls its attachment from the bone) of the proximal tibia (shinbone) at the insertion of the anterior cruciate ligament.

epibasal: a break at the base of the thumb or 5th (little finger) metacarpal bone, just above the joint surface.

epicondylar (ep-ee-KAHN-dih-lur): break at the edge of the flare of a long bone.

epiphyseal, **epiphyseal slip** (ep-uh-FIZ-ee-ul): a break through the epiphysis (segment at end of a long bone containing the growth center).

Essex-Lopresti: break in the calcaneus (heelbone) that involves the subtalar joint (between calcaneus and talus).

extracapsular: occurs outside the capsule (fibrous lining of a joint) and does not involve the joint surface.

fatigue, **stress**: break caused by prolonged repetitive activity such as running or marching.

femoral neck: type of hip fracture; occurs across the femoral neck.

fetal: sustained by the fetus in utero; usually associated with bone formation abnormalities such as osteogenesis imperfecta.

fissured: extends along the length of a bone rather than across it.

Galeazzi's: break in the distal third of the radius (larger forearm bone); associated with dislocation of the distal radioulnar joint (between the two forearm bones).

Gosselin's: V-shaped break at end of tibia (shinbone) near the ankle.

greenstick: same as TORUS FRACTURE (below).

Hahn-Steinthal: vertical break in the distal (lower) humerus (upper armbone) separating the capitellum (rounded end) from the rest of the bone.

hairline: non-displaced; appears on x-ray as a crack in the bone.

hangman's, **traumatic spondylolisthesis of the axis**: break in the 2nd cervical (neck) vertebra involving the neural ring of the vertebra and separating the back of the vertebra from the body.

head-splitting: break in the head of the femur (thighbone) or humerus (upper armbone), splitting it into two or more pieces.

hip: break in the upper part of the femur (thighbone); includes femoral neck fracture, intertrochanteric, peritrochanteric and subtrochanteric femur fractures, and greater trochanteric fractures of the femur.

Hoffa: vertical break in a condyle (rounded end) of the femur (thighbone), separating the back portion from the rest of the femur.

ice skater's: a stress fracture seen in the lower part of the fibula (lower leg bone) of children between ages 2–8.

impacted: fracture fragments are driven into each other by the force of the injury.

incomplete: a crack that does not proceed from one side of the bone through the other side.

intercondylar: the fracture line runs between the condyles (rounded ends of long bones), splitting them apart.

intertrochanteric (in-tur-troh-kan-TEHR-ik): break along the line between the greater and lesser trochanters (prominences) of the femur (thighbone). Type of hip fracture.

intra-articular: runs into and involves the joint surface of a bone.

intracapsular: a break within the joint capsule.

intrauterine: same as FETAL (above).

Jefferson: a burst fracture of the 1st cervical (neck) vertebra.

Jones: break in 5th metatarsal (base of toe) involving the upper metaphyseal part (flare) of that bone; has a higher-than-usual rate of nonunions.

juvenile Tillaux: same as TILLAUX FRACTURE (below).

Kocher-Lorenz: involves the capitellum of the humerus (rounded projection at lower end of arm bone) where the articular cartilage and a sliver of the attached subchondral bone (below articular cartilage) is fractured off the rest of the humerus. See also BRYAN AND MORREY CLASSIFICATION.

linear: same as FISSURED FRACTURE (above).

Lisfranc (LISS-frank): same as TARSOMETATARSAL FRACTURE (below).

little league shoulder: stress fracture of the proximal humerus (upper growth plate of armbone) caused by repetititive throwing injury.

Maisonneuve (may-zoh-NOOV): break in the medial malleolus associated with fracture of the proximal fibula (smaller bone of lower leg).

malunited: break that has healed in an inappropriate position.

Malgaigne (mal-GAYN): break at the front of the pelvic ring associated with a dislocation or fracture/dislocation on the opposite side.

mallet: a break in the most distal bone of a finger; the attachment of the extensor tendon of the finger is pulled off the bone, resulting in downward deformity of the tip of the finger.

march: a stress fracture of the 3rd metatarsal caused by prolonged repetitive activity, such as running or marching.

Monteggia: break in thc ulna (smaller forearm bone) with dislocation of the radial head (larger forearm bone). See also BADO CLASSIFICATION.

neoplastic (nee-oh-PLAS-tik): same as PATHOLOGIC FRACTURE (below).

neurogenic, Charcot's joint: a break through an area of bone affected by neurologic disease and caused by the repetitive overstressing of the bone secondary to poor pain perception.

nightstick: break in the midshaft ulna (smaller forearm bone) resulting from a direct blow.

nondisplaced: break without change in the position of the fragments.

oblique: occurs at an oblique angle to the long axis of the bone.

occult: a break that is hidden or not easily identified.

open: same as COMPOUND FRACTURE (above).

osteochondral (ahs-tee-oh-KAHN-drul): break in the articular (joint) surface of a joint involving both cartilage and bone.

overlapping: fragments overlap, which shortens the length of the bone.

parry: same as MONTEGGIA FRACTURE (above).

pathologic: a break through an area of a bone weakened by tumor, infection, injury or surgery.

periarticular: a break that occurs next to and around a joint.

peritrochanteric: type of hip fracture; break in upper part of the femur loosely involving the line connecting the greater and lesser trochanters, but running beyond this area as well.

physeal: same as SALTER FRACTURE (below).

Piedmont: same as GALEAZZI'S FRACTURE (above).

pilon, pylon: break in lower part of the tibia (shinbone) and the articular (joint) surface of the lower tibia at the level of the ankle; caused by a strong upward push across the ankle. See also RÜEDÌ AND ALGOWER CLASSIFICATION.

Plafond (pluh-FAHND): break in the distal end of the tibia (shinbone) involving the articular (joint) surface of the ankle.

plateau: involves the flat part of a bone; usually refers to intra-articular (joint) fractures involving the top of the tibia (shinbone) or proximal part of a phalanx (finger- or toebone).

posterior arch: break in the back half of the arch (circular part of a vertebra surrounding the spine).

Pott's: break in both the medial and lateral malleoli (tips of lower leg bones), causing lateral displacement of the ankle.

pylon: same PILON FRACTURE (above).

reverse Barton's: break through the articular (joint) surface of the distal radius (larger forearm bone) with fracture line positioned toward back of wrist.

reverse Bennett's: two-part, intra-articular (joint) fracture of the base of the 5th metacarpal. Named for its resemblance to the two-part fracture of the base of the metacarpal of the thumb (Bennett's fracture).

reverse Colles': break in the distal end of the radius (larger forearm bone) near its lower joint surface with a displacement toward the palm.

Rolando: three-piece, intra-articular (joint) break at the base of the metacarpal of the thumb; can be shaped like a Y (Rolando Y fracture) or a T (Rolando T fracture).

Salter, Salter-Harris: a break through the growth plate of a child. See also SALTER-HARRIS CLASSIFICATION.

segmental: break in a long bone in which there is an isolated central piece is not connected to either the proximal or distal fragments.

Shepherd: break in posterior process (projection) of talus (top foot bone).

simple, closed: the bones do not pierce the skin.

single column: 1. break in the lower part of the humerus (upper armbone) involving medial or lateral column (circular flares at sides of lower humerus); 2. break in the vertebra involving only one of the three columns described by Denis. See also DENIS CLASSIFICATION OF VERTEBRAL FRACTURES.

Skillern's: break in the lower end of the radius (larger forearm bone) with greenstick fracture of the ulna (smaller forearm bone).

Smith: same as REVERSE COLLES' FRACTURE (above).

spiral, torsion: spiral-shaped break associated with a twisting type of injury.

splinter: lay term for comminuted fracture, bone broken into multiple pieces, giving a splintered appearance.

spontaneous: occurs without specific trauma; usually pathological.

Steida: an avulsion type of break around the knee, with small pieces of bone along the side of the knee joint. Associated with a tear in the anterior cruciate ligament.

stellate (STEL-ayt): star-shaped break caused by direct trauma.

stress: same as FATIGUE FRACTURE (above).

subcapital: below the femoral head at uppermost level of the femoral neck. Type of hip fracture.

subtrochanteric: below the lesser trochanter of the femur (thighbone). Type of hip fracture.

supracondylar: above the condyles of the distal femur (thighbone) or distal humerus (upper armbone).

surgical neck: break in the proximal humerus (upper armbone) below the physeal plate.

talar dome: same as DOME FRACTURE (above).

tarsometatarsal (TMT), Lisfranc: through the base of the metatarsal bones; usually associated with dislocation of the tarso-metatarsal joint.

t-condylar: extends between the two condyles and splits medially and laterally; looks like the letter T on x-ray.

tibial eminence: same as EMINENCE FRACTURE (above).

Tillaux (tee-YOH): break in the anterior, lateral articular surface of the distal tibia (shinbone) in an adolescent when the growth plate is closing.

torsion: same as SPIRAL FRACTURE (above).

torus, greenstick: nondisplaced break, generally at distal end of the radius (larger forearm bone) or tibia (shinbone) in a small child; appears as a rounded bump on the bone.

transcervical: break through the midportion of the femoral neck. Type of hip fracture.

transcolumn: a break in the distal portion of the humerus (upper armbone) crossing transversely across the supracondylar region.

transcondylar: break in the distal humerus (upper armbone) or distal femur (thighbone) extending through the condyles.

transitional: ankle fracture that occurs during the final 18 months of distal (lower) tibial physeal (growth plate) closure. See also JUVENILE TILLAUX FRACTURE, TRIPLANE FRACTURE.

transverse: crosses the cortices perpendicular to long axis of the bone.

trimalleolar (tri-muh-LEE-oh-lur): break in ankle that involves the medial, lateral and posterior malleoli (tips of lower leg bones) of the tibia (shinbone).

triplane: break in the tibia (shinbone) about the lower growth plate; occurs exclusively in the adolescent.

trophic: associated with weakened bones.

tuft: break in the tuft portion (widened end) of the distal phalanx of a finger or toe.

undisplaced: break without change in the position of the fragments.

ununited: break in a bone that has not healed.

wagon wheel: same as CARTWHEEL FRACTURE (above).

Wagstaff: displaced break of the medial malleolus (inner bump of ankle).

wedge: collapse of the front of a vertebra.

willow: same as GREENSTICK FRACTURE (above).

Y: break usually between the condyles (articular surface), spreading medially and laterally; appears on x-ray as the letter Y.

fracture diastasis (di-uh-STAY-sus). *Pathologic condition*. Separation of the fracture fragments.

fracture-dislocation. *Pathologic condition*. Broken bone with dislocation of the joint.

fragilitas osseum congenita (fruh-JIL-uh-tus AHS-ee-um kun-JEN-ih-tuh), **brittle bones**, **osteitis fragilitans**, **osteogenesis imperfecta** /or/ **imperfecta tarta**. *Pathologic condition*. Multiple system connective tissue disorder characterized by fragile bones that fracture easily. Involves the skeleton, eyes, ears, teeth, and vascular tissue.

frame. *Orthopedic appliance*. A structure for holding patients in certain positions.

Bradford: metal frame with attached movable canvas strips.

McConnel: used for holding a patient reclining on his/her back against a backrest, with the knees slightly bent (Fowler's position).

Schlyme (shlime): similar to MCCONNEL.

Montreal: baseboard with slots designed to fit prefabricated pegs. Used for holding a patient on his/her side during surgery.

Jackson: type of radiolucent table.

free bone graft. *Biologic implant.* Bone segment transferred from another area without attachment to the donor site. See also ALLOGRAFT, AUTOGRAFT.

free tendon graft. *Biologic implant.* Tendon segment transferred from another area without attachment to the donor site.

freeze-dried bone graft. *Biologic implant.* Bone graft (from a cadaver) that is washed in solvent to remove the fat, then dried and frozen for later use.

Freiberg's infraction. *Pathologic condition.* Multiple recurrent fractures and associated reparative attempts involving the 2nd metatarsal of the foot; results in pain and deformity of the head of the 2nd metatarsal bone. Usually seen in the second decade of life and usually treated without surgery.

Frejka pillow splint (FRAY-kah), **pillow orthosis**. *Orthopedic appliance.* Cloth pillow used as a brace in congenital dislocation of the hip. Pillow is placed in a harness between the legs, to abduct the legs and keep the hip reduced.

frenic. Incorrect spelling of PHRENIC.

friable. *Description.* Refers to tissue that does not hold together normally, but falls apart easily.

Friedreich's ataxia. *Pathologic condition.* Progressive upper motor neuron disorder that affects the arms and legs, leading to contractures, paralysis, and eventual death. Hereditary.

Frölich's adiposogenital dystrophy. See FRÖLICH'S SYNDROME.

Frölich's appearance. See FRÖLICH'S SYNDROME.

Froment's sign (froh-MAHZ). *Diagnostic sign.* Distal phalanx of the thumb is pressed against the index finger; a weak grasp indicates ulnar nerve palsy.

Frölich's syndrome /or/ **adiposogenital dystrophy** /or/ **appearance** /or/ **syndrome** (FRA-liks), **dystrophia adiposogenitalis**, **Launois-Cleret syndrome**. *Pathologic condition.* Obesity and delayed secondary sexual characteristics, sometimes seen with a pituitary tumor; occasionally associated with slipped capital femoral epiphysis.

frostbite, chillblain, pernio. *Pathologic condition.* Redness, itching, burning sensation of skin exposed to extreme cold; most frequently affects tops of the fingers and toes. Death of tissues can occur if circulation is not maintained.

frozen shoulder, adhesive capsulitis. *Pathologic condition.* A shoulder that is stiff and painful to move. Patient refuses to move the arm, leading to fibrosis (scar tissue) and markedly reduced motion that is difficult to regain.

Frykman classification (FRIK-mun). *Fracture classification.* Identifies different types of distal radius fractures.

full-thickness skin graft (FTSG). *Biological implant, surgical procedure.* Skin removed from an individual to be transferred from one location to another; transplanted skin that takes the full thickness of the dermis without extending into the subcutaneous tissue. See also SPLIT-THICKNESS SKIN GRAFT.

full weight bearing (FWB). *Function.* Carrying the full weight of the body on a leg or legs.

funny bone. *Anatomy.* Popular term for area where the medial epicondyle of the humerus is crossed by the ulnar nerve (at the elbow). Not actually a bone.

fusion arthrodesis, artificial ankylosis. *Surgical procedure.* Fusion of a joint by removing the cartilage and compressing joint surfaces, allowing the bones on either side of the joint to heal together into one bone; eliminates motion.

  intra-articular f. (in-truh-ahr-TIK-yu-lur). *Pathologic condition.* occurs completely within the joint capsule.

G

Gaenslen test. (GENZ-len). *Clinical test*. With patient lying on his/her side and holding the lower leg curled up against the chest, the examiner extends the upper leg at the hip while holding the pelvis steady. Pain in the upper leg denotes abnormalities of the hip, sacroiliac joint, or the L4 nerve root.

gait. *Function*. Process of walking; consists of swing phase (leg moving forward) and stance phase (weight bearing).

> **g. training**. *Treatment*. Teaching a patient how to walk or to use assistive devices such as crutches, or to train the patient to wean off such devices.

Galant's sign, lateral trunk incurvature reflex. *Clinical sign*. Spontaneous bending of an infant toward one side as a blunt object is gently drawn along that side of its trunk. Absence of movement indicates nervous system abnormality.

Galeazzi's fracture (gal-ee-AHT-seez), **Darrach-Hughston-Milch fracture, Piedmont fracture**. *Pathologic condition*. Break in the distal 3rd of the radius (larger forearm bone); associated with dislocation of the distal radio-ulnar joint (between the two forearm bones).

Galeazzi sign (gal-ee-AHT-see), **Allis test**. *Clinical sign*. For determining hip dislocation or limb length discrepancy in an infant. Patient lies on back, both knees bent and feet on the table; knee is noticeably lower on the side with a dislocation or shortening. See also REVERSE ALLIS TEST.

Galeazzi technique (gal-ee-AHT-see). *Surgical procedure*. To prevent a recurrence of lateral dislocation of the patella (kneecap); the semitendinosus tendon is passed through the patella and sutured back upon itself.

gallium scan (GAL-ee-um). *Radiologic test*. Radioisotope is injected into the blood stream in an effort to localize possible infected areas of bone and soft tissue.

gamekeeper's thumb. *Pathologic condition*. Rupture of the ulnar collateral ligament of the metacarpophalangeal joint of the thumb.

gampsodactyly (gamp-soh-DAK-tih-lee), **cavus foot, claw foot, pes cavus**. *Pathologic condition*. Abnormally high-arched foot, usually with clawing of toes. Associated with some forms of neurologic abnormality such as polio or Charcot-Marie-Tooth disease.

ganglion (GANG-lee-un). *Anatomy*. Collection of nerve bodies. Usually represents a center where electrical impulses from numerous cells converge and are transmitted to a second group of nerve cells.

> **g. cyst**. *Pathologic condition*. Fluid-filled sac protruding from the synovial sheath (lining) of a tendon or capsule of a joint, frequently on the back of the wrist.

ganglionectomy (gang-lee-un-EK-tuh-mee). *Surgical procedure*. Excising (cutting out) a ganglion.

gangliosidosis (gang-lee-oh-sih-DOH-sis). *Pathologic condition*. Lipid storage disease characterized by abnormal accumulation of complex sugars, particularly within the nervous tissue, resulting from a series of enzyme abnormalities. Consequences include progressive psychomotor deterioration, death in early childhood. Example: familial amaurotic idiocy, Sandhoff disease. Hereditary.

gangrene (gang-GREEN). *Pathologic condition*. Necrosis (tissue death) from absence or loss of blood supply.

> **gas g.**: gangrenous tissue that has been infected by an anaerobic

(not requiring oxygen) bacteria that forms gas; the gas gives a crackling feeling when the skin is pressed (crepitus).

Garceau procedure (gahr-SO). *Surgical procedure*. Lateral transfer of the tibialis anterior tendon for realignment of a clubfoot.

Garden classification. *Fracture classification*. Describes femoral neck fracture patterns based on the degree of displacement.

Gardner-Wells tongs. *Orthopedic equipment*. Sharp pins with attached arch, for driving into the skull's outer table, to place traction on the skull and neck.

gargoylism (GAR-goyl-izm). *Pathologic condition*. Term used to describe the facial changes encountered in dysostosis multiplex (Hurler's syndrome).

Garré disease (gah-RAY), **sclerosing osteitis**. *Pathologic condition*. Areas of bone become thickened and distended, but do not form abscesses. Cause unknown; may represent a low-grade, chronic osteomyelitis (bone infection).

gas gangrene. See GANGRENE.

gastrocnemius (gas-trahk-NEE-mee-us). *Anatomy*. Large muscle on the back of the leg that bends the knee and ankle; attaches proximally to the distal end of the femur (thighbone) and distally to the heel.

gastrocnemius release, Compere Vulpius procedure. *Surgical procedure*. Lengthening the Achilles tendon by partially releasing it at the level where the gastrocnemius muscle converges onto the tendon (musculotendinous juncture).

gastrocsoleus (gas-trahk-SOH-lee-us), **triceps surae**. *Anatomy*. Muscle grouping of the gastrocnemius and soleus.

Gaucher's disease (gau-SHAYZ). *Pathologic condition*. Enzyme deficiency (a lipid storage disease) that leads to an accumulation of certain fats in the spleen and liver; grouped by severity into infantile, juvenile, and adult types. Major orthopedic implication is the development of avascular necrosis.

gauntlet cast. *Orthopedic appliance*. Forearm cast that incorporates part of the hand. So named because of its resemblance to a knight's glove.

gel cast. *Orthopedic appliance*. Semi-solid cast with gel incorporated in the gauze; used to prevent swelling and to treat skin ulcerations. See also UNNA BOOT.

gemellus (jem-EL-us). *Anatomy*. One of two muscles in the back of the hip (gemellus inferior and gemellus superior) that rotate the thighbone (femur) externally. Plural: gemelli.

genicular arteries (jen-IK-yu-lur). *Anatomy*. Series of arteries that branches off the popliteal artery at the level of the knee to encircle the joint. Includes the medial (inner) and lateral (outer) superior genicular arteries, the medial and lateral inferior genicular arteries, and a middle genicular artery that comes off the femoral artery on the inner side of the thigh.

genicular vessels (jen-IK-yu-lur). *Anatomy*. Small, irregular blood vessels that supply the bone around the knee joint.

genu (JEN-yu), **knee**. *Anatomy*. Hinge-like joint between the femur (thighbone) and the tibia (shinbone); place of articulation between the thigh and leg.

> **g. recurvatum** (ree-KUR-vuh-tum), **back-knee**. *Pathologic condition*. Hyperextended (backward-bending) knee joints that occur when standing or walking; caused by excessively flexible knee ligaments, giving the leg a backward curvature. See also EHLERS-DANLOS SYNDROME, MARFAN'S SYNDROME.

> **g. valgum** (VAL-gum), **g. valgus, tibia valga**. *Abnormal condition*. Knock-knees; ankles remain widely separated while standing with knees touching.

> **g. varum** (VEHR-um), **g. varus, bandylegs, tibia vara**. *Abnormal condition*. Bowlegs; legs whose knees point outward, remaining separated when standing with the ankles together; results in a bowlike appearance.

Gerdy's tubercle (TU-bur-kul). *Anatomy*. Prominence on the outer side of the tibia; attachment for the iliotibial band of the femur (thigh).

giant cell tumor. *Pathologic condition*. Bone tumor composed of characteristic large cells; may be malignant.

giant osteoid osteoma, osteoblastoma (AHS-tee-oyd ahs-tee-OH-muh). *Pathologic condition*. Benign tumor with osteoblasts in areas of osteoid and calcific tissues; usually in the spine of a young person.

gibbous (GIB-us). *Description*. Pertains to one who is humpbacked or has a gibbus.

gibbus (GIB-us). *Abnormal condition*. Change in spine alignment that results in extreme kyphosis (bending-forward deformity) or a sharp dorsal bump. Frequent in tuberculosis of the spine.

Gibson approach. *Surgical technique*. Approach to the hip from back and side, for exposure of the femoral head and trochanteric area.

gigantism. *Pathologic condition*. Condition characterized by abnormal enlargement of the body as a whole or any of its parts. May be associated with Klippel-Trenauny-Weber syndrome or tumors of the pituitary gland.

Gigli saw (JEEL-yee). *Surgical tool*. Type of flexible saw; a wire with cutting edges.

Gilbert prosthesis. *Orthopedic appliance*. Metal replacement for the proximal femur (thighbone).

Gilchrist's disease, blastomycosis. *Pathologic condition*. Infectious fungal disease of the skin and mucus membranes; originates in the lungs, can spread to bone and soft tissues.

Gill procedure. *Surgical procedure*. Excision of the posterior arch for decompression of the nerve roots in a patient with spondylolisthesis (slipping of one vertebra on another).

ginglymus (JING-luh-mus), **hinged joint**. *Anatomy*. A joint between bones that permits motion in only one plane. Example: knee, elbow. Plural: ginglymi.

Girdlestone procedure, resection arthroplasty of the hip. *Surgical procedure*. The complete removal of the head and neck of the femur (thighbone), leaving the patient without a functional hip joint. Used in the treatment of serious infection and in some forms of cancer.

Girdlestone-Taylor procedure. *Surgical procedure*. For correction of hammertoes. Transferring the flexor tendon from the top of the proximal phalanx of the toe to the extensor tendon.

glenohumeral joint (glen-oh-HYU-mur-ul). *Anatomy*. Joint between top of the humerus (upper armbone) and side of the scapula (shoulderblade).

glenoid cavity, glenoid fossa (GLEN-oyd). *Anatomy*. Shallow curved surface on the upper, outer scapula (shoulderblade) and its cartilaginous and fibrous rim, where the humerus articulates with the shoulder girdle.

glenoid fossa (GLEN-oyd FAH-suh). *Anatomy*. See GLENOID CAVITY.

glenoid labrum ligament (GLEN-oyd LAY-brum). *Anatomy*. Connective tissue band along the front of the glenoid fossa. Frequently torn when a shoulder is dislocated.

glenoplasty (GLEN-oh-plas-tee). *Surgical procedure*. Transferring bone to the glenoid to deepen the cup, to prevent dislocation of the shoulder.

gliding joint, arthrodia. *Anatomy*. Type of joint allowing only for a slight sliding motion between two bones, as in the vertebrae. See also DIARTHROSIS.

globoid cell leukodystrophy, diffuse infantile familial sclerosis, Krabbe's disease. *Pathologic condition*. Infantile condition characterized by rapid deterioration of the central nervous system (leukodystrophy). Death usually occurs by age 2. Hereditary; most likely autosomal recessive.

Glomus tumor. *Pathologic condition*. Small, benign vascular growth at the end of a finger or toe. Extremely tender.

glucosamine (glu-KOHS-uh-meen). *Biological substance*. Complex carbohydrate found in joint cartilage; used in the treatment of osteoarthritis.

gluteal lines (GLU-tee-ul). *Anatomy*. Creases between the buttocks and thighs. May be unequal in congenital dislocation of the hip.

gluteus maximus (GLU-tee-us). *Anatomy*. Large buttocks muscle that extends the hip; attached from the iliac crest to the back of the thigh.

gluteus medius (GLU-tee-us MEE-dee-us). *Anatomy*. Buttocks muscle along the outer side of the hip that abducts the hip; attaches from the iliac crest to the greater trochanter.

gluteus minimus (GLU-tee-us) *Anatomy*. Small muscle the abducts and internally rotates the hip; attaches from the outer wing of the ilium to the front of the greater trochanter.

glycoprotein (gli-koh-PRO-teen). *Biological substance*. Category of chemicals made up of a protein to which a sugar is attached.

Goldstein fusion. *Surgical procedure*. Technique for spinal fusion in scoliosis.

Goldstein procedure. *Surgical procedure*. Resection arthroplasty of the hip: the upper end of the femur (thighbone) is excised and the patient continues without a hip joint.

Goldthwait test. *Clinical test*. To differentiate between the back and the sacroiliac joint as the source of pain. With patient lying on his/her back, the examiner's fingers are placed at and between the spinous processes of the lumbar vertebrae. The hip is bent with the knee extended. If pain occurs before there is relative motion between the spinous processes, it is from the sacroiliac joint; if afterward it is referable to the back.

golfer's elbow, medial epicondylitis. *Pathologic condition*. Inflammation of the small bony protuberance at the elbow joint, attachment of flexor muscles of the forearm. From overuse or trauma; pain may accompany muscle contraction.

gomphosis. *Anatomy*. Joint where a bone inserts into a cone-shaped socket. Seen in the joints of the teeth against the jaw. One of three types of fibrous joints. See also SYMPHYSIS, SUTURES.

Gordon approach. *Surgical procedure*. An approach to the proximal end of the ulna (smaller forearm bone); used in reduction of Monteggia fractures.

Gordon reflex. *Clinical sign*. Spontaneous raising of the big toe as lateral pressure is placed on the calf muscles. Indicates central nervous system disease.

Gordon-Taylor technique. *Surgical technique*. Method of amputating the lower extremity at the level of the hip.

Gordon technique, Bröstrom technique for dye injection into the ankle. *Injection technique*. Used for dye injection into the ankle, such as injecting radiographic contrast material into an ankle joint to evaluate an ankle sprain.

Gosselin's fracture. *Pathologic condition*. V-shaped break at the end of the tibia (shinbone) near the ankle.

gouge. *Surgical instrument*. Long-handled tool with a curved cutting face.

gout. *Pathologic condition*. Metabolic disease in which elevation in blood uric acid level causes precipation of uric acid crystals resulting in episodes of acute arthritis affecting the base of the great toe and occasionally other joints.

gouty arthritis. *Pathologic condition*. Joint inflammation caused by uric acid crystals; associated with hyperuricemia (elevated blood uric acid levels).

gouty nodes. *Pathologic condition*. Small nodules of inflammatory tissue surrounding uric acid crystals under the skin.

Gower sign. *Clinical sign*. Using the arms to push the legs and body to an erect position; characteristic of lower extremity weakness in Duchenne's muscular dystrophy. Also may be found in some forms of congenital myopathy and in spinal muscular atrophy.

gracilis (GRAH-sil-us). *Anatomy*. Muscle on the inside of the leg that adducts (moves toward center of body) the hip; attaches from the pubis (a pelvic bone) to the proximal tibia (shinbone).

graft. 1. *Surgical procedure.* Transfer of tissue from one area or one person to another. 2. *Biological implant.* Tissue (e.g., bone, skin) removed from an individual to be transferred from one location to another; may be taken from the same individual or from another. See also ALLOGRAFT, AUTO-GRAFT, DONOR TISSUE, HOMOGRAFT, XENOGRAFT.

> **autogenous g.** (ah-TAH-juh-nus): transfer of tissue to a new site on the same individual.

> **composite g.**: contains more than one kind of tissue, e.g., muscle, nerve, fat, bone.

> **cortical g.**: composed of the hard cortex (outer surface) of the donor bone.

> **dowel g.**: segment of bone removed with a round cutter; resembles a dowel.

> **fibular strut g.** (FIB-yu-lur): segment of fibula transferred to another area, generally to the femoral neck for avascular necrosis of the femur. May be transferred alive (vascular) or nonliving (avascular).

> **free bone g.**: segment of bone transferred from another area without attachment connecting it to the donor site.

> **full thickness g.**: segment of skin involving the full breadth of the dermis transplanted to cover an open wound.

> **hemicylindrical g.** (hem-ee-sil-IN-drih-kal); taken from a long bone or pelvis, shaped as half a cylinder. Used to fill bony defects in long bones.

> **inlay g.**: placement of a segment of bone into a recipient bone that has been prepared by cutting a slot in it, or by creating a prefitted cavity.

> **intercalary g.**: insertion of tissue (bone, nerve, artery or vein) to span a missing bone segment.

> **intraosseous** (in-truh-AHS-ee-us): a bone graft within bone.

> **island pedicle g.**: transfer of a small area of skin ("island") with its attached nerve and blood vessels from one area to another.

> **onlay g.**: cortical bone placed on the outside of an area to be grafted.

> **osteochondral g.**: transfer of a bone segment with attached cartilage into the articular surface of a defective joint, to create a smooth surface.

> **osteoperiosteal g.** (ahs-tee-oh-pehr-ee-AHS-tee-ul): local transfer of a bone segment with periosteum and blood supply to induce bone healing.

> **sliding inlay g.**: bone segment slid down from an adjacent bone to replace a segment of bone removed from half the joint.

> **split-thickness skin g. (STSG)**.: a strip of skin encompassing only the most superficial layers of the dermis, used for covering an open wound.

> **strut g.**: bone graft used as a strut between two areas of bone; most frequently between two ends of a spinal curve in a kyphotic or scoliotic deformity.

> **Wolf's skin g**: a free, full thickness skin graft.

granulation. *Function.* Healing in which injured tissue is replaced by scar tissue.

greater multangular, trapezium. *Anatomy.* Four-sided bone in the wrist at the base of the thumb.

greater saphenous vein (suh-FEE-nus). *Anatomy.* Large vein on the inside of the leg; drains the superficial aspects of the leg.

greater sciatic notch (si-AT-ik). *Anatomy.* Opening in the pelvis that the sciatic nerve passes through. Comprised of the ischium and sacral bony surfaces.

greater trochanter (TROH-kan-tur). *Anatomy.* Large prominence on the outer side of the proximal femur (thighbone); attachment for the gluteus medius and gluteus minimus muscles.

greater tuberosity (tu-bur-AH-sih-tee). *Anatomy.* Large prominence on the proximal part of the humerus (upper armbone); attachment for shoulder muscles.

Green and Banks technique. *Surgical procedure*. Transfer of the flexor carpi ulnaris tendon (tendon belonging to one of the muscles that bends the wrist) to the upper, outer side of the wrist, in cerebral palsy patients.

Green procedure. *Surgical procedure*. The upper part of scapula (shoulderblade) is removed along with some abnormal tissue and pulled down to a more normal position, reattaching muscles that were dissected from the inner border, to hold it in the new position. Performed in cases of Sprengel's deformity.

greenstick fracture, willow fracture. *Pathologic condition*. Break that involves splintering of a long bone; occurs in young children.

Grevlich & Pyle atlas. *Reference.* Tables and radiologic pictures of the wrist and hand from infancy to completion of growth, for estimating bone age.

Grevlich and Pyle method. *Measurement.* Standard for assessment of a child's skeletal development based on wrist and hand x-rays.

Grice and Green procedure. See GRICE PROCEDURE.

Grice procedure, Grice and Green procedure. *Surgical procedure*. Insertion of bone taken from the pelvis, heel or shinbone into the subtalar joint; used in the treatment of congenital vertical talus.

grinding test, Apley's grind test. *Clinical test*. With patient lying face down, the knee is flexed 90° and a downward, twisting force is exerted on the leg, compressing the knee cartilage. Pain in the knee indicates tearing of the meniscus in the knee joint.

groin flap, iliofemoral flap. *Surgical technique.* Large flap of skin and subcutaneous tissue removed from the groin and reattached with its veins and arteries to another site, to cover a large wound.

Gross-Kemph nail. *Surgical implant.* Intermedullary rod used for fixation of fractures of the femur (thighbone).

growth arrest. *Pathologic condition.* Interruption of growth after injury or infection at the epyphyseal plate. May lead to overall shortening or angular deformity of the bone.

growth factors. *Biologic substances.* Complex molecules produced in the body that stimulate tissue growth and repair.

growth plate, epiphyseal plate /or/ **cartilage, physis**. *Anatomy.* In a long bone, the layer of cartilage between the epiphysis (growth center) and the metaphysis, where growth in length occurs.

Guepar prosthesis. *Orthopedic implant.* Artificial replacement of the joint surfaces of the knee. Refers to any of a group of implants designed by the French Canadian organization G.U.E.P.A.R.

Guillain-Barre syndrome (gee-AHN bar-AY), **acute idiopathic polyneuritis**. *Pathologic condition.* Viral syndrome that affects the peripheral nervous system; rapid onset, results in progressive paralysis.

guillotine amputation (GEE-oh-teen). *Surgical procedure.* Removal of an extremity, performed transversely, cutting the muscle, skin and bone at the same level. The wound is left open.

gun stock deformity, cubitus varus. *Pathologic condition.* Smaller-than-normal angle formed by the upper armbone (humerus) and the forearm; the elbow joint deviates toward the midline.

Gustilo classification. *Fracture classification.* Describes differing severities of soft tissue damage associated with open (compound) fractures. Originally described for open fractures of the tibia, it is now commonly applied to most open long bone fractures.

Guyon canal (gee-YOHN). *Anatomy.* Tunnel surrounded by bone and ligament at the ulnar side of the wrist and palm, through which the ulnar nerve and artery pass from the forearm into the hand.

H

habitual dislocation. *Pathologic condition*. Joint dislocation that recurs, most frequently in the kneecap or shoulder. Has a volitional component.

Haglund deformity. *Abnormal condition*. Abnormal prominence (bump) on the back of the calcaneus (heelbone).

Hagie pin. *Surgical implant*. Threaded pin used for fixation of clavicle fractures.

Hahn-Steinthal fracture. *Pathologic condition*. A vertical break in the lower portion of the humerus (upper armbone) separating the capitellum (rounded lower end of humerus) from the rest of the bone.

hairline fracture. *Pathologic condition*. Non-displaced break that appears on x-ray as a crack in the bone.

hallux (HAL-uks). *Anatomy*. The big toe.

> **h. adductus**, **hallux varus** (ad-DUK-tus). *Abnormal condition*. Big toe that is deviated toward the midline of the body.

> **h. dolorosa** (dahl-ur-OH-suh). *Abnormal condition*. Painful big toe.

> **h. extensus** (eks-TEN-sus). *Abnormal condition*. Deformed big toe that is raised and does not lie flat on the horizontal surface.

> **h. flexus** (FLEKS-us). *Abnormal condition*. Big toe that is bent down at the metatarsophalangeal joint and cannot be raised to a neutral position.

> **h. malleus** (muh-LEE-us). *Abnormal condition*. Hammertoe of the big toe; the interphalangeal joint is markedly flexed, forcing the patient to walk on the end of the toe.

> **h. rigidus** (RIJ-ih-dus). *Abnormal condition*. Stiff big toe (at the metatarsophalangeal joint).

> **h. valgus** (VAL-gus), **bunion**. *Pathologic condition*. Painful protrusion of the 1st metatarsophalangeal joint (main joint of big toe) at the inner side of the foot. Toe is deviated outward.

> **h. varus** (VEHR-us). Same as HALLUX ADDUCTUS (above)

halo. *Orthopedic appliance*. Ring placed around the skull to maintain alignment or stability of the neck; held in place with four pins screwed into the skull.

> **h. body cast**: metal struts attached to a halo about the head and to a body cast, to maintain the neck in a specific position.

halo traction. *Treatment*. Technique for distracting the neck by attaching a ringed apparatus to the skull via pins, and pulling on the ring with weights. Keeps an unstable segment of the cervical spine (neck portion) from dislocating, thus protecting the spinal cord and preventing neurological damage.

hamartoma (ham-ahr-TOH-muh). *Pathologic condition*. Normal tissue in an abnormal location or organ.

> **cartilaginous h.**: benign tumorlike lesion resulting from abnormal tissue growth of cartilage. Usually seen in the chest wall.

> **fibrous h**: fibrous malformation, generally found in upper arm or shoulder of children under age 2.

hamate (HAM-ayt). *Anatomy*. Small bone in wrist; innermost bone in the 2nd row of carpal (wrist) bones. Has a hook at the distal end of its palmar surface.

> **hook of the h.**: part of the hamate near the area traversed by the ulnar nerve. Resembles a hook.

hammer toe. *Abnormal condition*. Deformity of a toe consisting of flexion at the proximal interphalangeal joint and extension at the metatarsophalangeal joint. May be flexible or rigid. Usually caused by improperly fitting shoes. In the great toe (hallux malleus), the extended joint is the metatar-sophalangeal joint and the flexed joint is the interphalangeal joint.

hamstrings. *Anatomy*. Group of muscles on the back of the thigh that bend the knee and extend the hip; consists of the semitendonosus, semimem-branosus and biceps femoris.

handgrip dynamometer. *Diagnostic equipment*. Grip used for testing strength; a series of gauges indicate amount of pressure elicited by a grasp or squeeze.

handlebar palsy. *Pathologic condition*. Pressure along the median nerve. Caused by grasping bicycle handlebars with upper body weight on the hands; usually disappears shortly after relief of pressure.

Hand-Schüller-Christian disease. *Pathologic condition*. Multifocal, more agressive form of Langerhans' cell histiocytosis; involves the bone and the hypothalamus or pituitary stalk. Characterized by exophthalmos (eye bulging), skull defects, and diabetes insipidus (characterized by produc-tion of excessive amounts of urine). Usually occurs before age 10.

hanging arm cast. *Orthopedic appliance*. Extends from upper arm to the hand, holding the elbow in a flexed position; used in nonsurgical treat-ment of humerus (upper armbone) fractures. The arm hangs freely within the cast so that its weight helps the humerus to realign itself.

hanging hip procedure. *Surgical procedure*. Muscles crossing hip joint are cut to eliminate the force normally placed against the joint, relieving pain.

hangman's fracture, traumatic spondylolisthesis of the axis. *Pathologic condition*. Break in the 2nd cervical (neck) vertebra involving the neural ring of the vertebra and separating the back of the vertebra from the body.

Hansen-Street nail. *Surgical implant*. Diamond-shaped nail that cuts its own path. Used to stabilize femur (thighbone) fractures.

hard corn, heloma durum. *Abnormal condition*. Callus formed on or about a bony prominence or joint, caused by pressure.

Harmon deltoid transfer. *Surgical procedure*. Transferring origin of deltoid muscle to front of shoulder, to improve function of a paralyzed shoulder.

Harmon hip reconstruction. *Surgical procedure*. Reconstruction of the proxi-mal femur (thighbone), usually in a child who has lost bony substance to infection. In the procedure, the remaining portion of the proximal femur is reshaped so that it may serve as a femoral head for the hip joint.

Harrington rod. *Surgical implant*. Solid steel rod attached to back of the spine. Used in surgical treatment of scoliosis and fixation of certain spinal fractures.

Harris approach. *Surgical technique*. An approach to the outer side of the hip for total joint replacement.

Harris hip score. *Measurement tool*. For grading outcome of reconstruction procedures, to determine quality of surgical result. Takes into account vari-ables such as x-ray appearance, physical findings, and subjective pain.

Harris line. A line seen on x-ray in long bones of a growing child following temporary growth arrest that occurs on a metabolic basis or after injury.

Hauser procedure. *Surgical procedure*. Moving the tibial tubercle from the proximal tibia (shinbone) medially and distally, to keep the patella (kneecap) from dislocating.

Haversian canals (huh-VUR-zjun). *Anatomy*. Microscopic canals within bone that blood vessels branch through, to circulate nutrients.

Hawkins classification. *Fracture classification*. Identifies three severity lev-els of talar neck fractures. Canale modification adds a fourth.

head-splitting fracture. *Pathologic condition*. Break of the head of the femur (thighbone) or humerus (upper armbone), splitting it into two or more pieces.

healing. *Physiologic process*. The method through which the body repairs a wound or injury.

    h. by primary intent: occurs when the wound edges are in direct contact (or when a wound is sutured together).

    h. by secondary intent: occurs when wound edges are not in direct contact.

Heberden nodes (HEE-bur-dun). *Abnormal condition*. Small protrusions of bone at the ends of finger joints; sign of arthritic changes.

heel. *Anatomy*. The hind part of the foot, below the ankle.

    h. bone. *Anatomy*. Popular term for CALCANEUS.

    h. cord, Achilles tendon, tendoachilles. *Anatomy*. Strong connective tissue band that joins the triceps surae (calf muscles) to the calcaneus (heelbone); comprised of the tendons of gastrocnemius and soleus muscles.

        h. pad. *Anatomy*. Firm pad of fat on bottom of foot beneath heelbone.

        syndrome. *Pathologic condition*. Pain and irritation about the heel caused by a heel pad that insufficiently protects the calcaneus (heelbone).

    h. spur. *Pathologic condition*. Bony protrusion from the calcaneus (heelbone). Most common at bottom of the heel where the plantar fascia attaches, can also occur at back of heel at the attachment of the tendoachilles.

    h. valgus (VAL-gus). *Clinical finding*. With patient standing and viewed from the back, the heel is angled away from the midline of the body.

    h. varus (VEHR-us) *Clinical finding*. With patient standing and viewed from the back, the heel is angled toward the midline of the body. Mild heel varus is normal, but when excessive, the finding can be pathologic.

Helbing sign. *Clinical sign*. Lateral displacement of the Achilles tendon in relation to the heel. Sign of heel valgus.

heloma durum (hee-LOH-muh), **hard corn**. *Abnormal condition*. Callus formed on or about a bony prominence or joint, caused by pressure.

heloma molle (hee-LOH-muh MOH-lay), **soft corn**. *Abnormal condition*. Pressure area between the toes that results in the formation of a painful callosity. Usually macerated and softened from moisture between the toes.

hemangioendothelioma (hee-MAN-jee-oh-en-doh-thee-lee-OH-muh). *Pathologic condition*. Rare tumor comprised of blood vessels. Sometimes malignant.

hemangioma (hee-man-jee-OH-muh). *Pathologic condition*. Benign tumor comprised of multiple small blood vessels.

    cavernous h.: large vascular tumor composed of large diameter, thin-walled vessels.

    sclerosing h.: type of slow-growing, benign, fibrous skin nodule of cellular tissue; usually affects lower extremities.

hemangiopericytoma (hee-MAN-jee-oh-pehr-uh-si-TOH-muh). *Pathologic condition*. Rare malignant tumor arising from pericytes of Zimmerman (type of blood vessel cell). Aggressiveness of the tumor varies.

hemangiosarcoma (hee-MAN-jee-oh-sahr-KOH-muh), **angiosarcoma**. *Pathologic condition*. Rare, malignant tumor arising from the cells of the inner wall of blood vessels; occurs most often in skin, soft tissue, breast or liver.

hemiarthroplasty (hem-ee-AHR-throh-plas-tee). *Surgical procedure*. Replacing the femoral head (in the hip) or proximal humerus (in the shoulder).

hemarthrosis (hee-mahr-THROH-sis). *Pathologic condition*. Blood in the joint.

hematoma (hee-muh-TOH-muh). *Pathologic condition*. Collection of blood in the soft tissues.

hematomyelia (hee-mat-oh-mi-EEL-ee-uh). *Pathologic condition*. Collection of blood in the spinal cord.

hemicylindrical graft (hem-ee-sil-IN-drih-kal). *Surgical procedure/biologic* *implant*. Bone graft taken from a long bone or pelvis, shaped as half a cylinder. Used to fill bony defects in long bones.

hemihypertrophy (hem-ee-hi-PUR-troh-fee). *Congenital abnormality*. Having one-half of the body larger than the other.

hemilaminectomy (hem-ee-lam-in-EK-toh-mee). *Surgical procedure*. Removing a portion of the lamina from one side of the spine to expose the underlying dura and nerve roots and/or to relieve pressure on a nerve. See also LAMINECTOMY.

hemimelia (hem-ee-MEE-lee-uh). *Congenital abnormality*. Shortening or incomplete formation of lower segments of an extremity (in upper extremities, the forearm; in lower extremities, the area between knee and ankle).

> **fibular h.**: absence of part or all of the fibula; associated with short femur (thighbone) and absence of the lateral two or three metatarsals (bones in foot).

> **paraxial. h.** (pehr-AKS-ee-ul): absence or partial absence of the pre- or postaxial part (medial or lateral) of mid-portion of a limb (forearm or lower leg).

> > **incomplete**: absence or partial absence of a limb segment.

> > **intercalary complete** (in-TUR-kuh-lehr-ee): limb having a missing central segment while the distal portion is attached, e.g., missing forearm with hand attached to elbow.

hemimelica, dysplasia epiphysealis, epiphyseal osteochondroma, tarso-epiphyseal aclasia, Trevor disease. *Congenital abnormality*. Abnormal development of osteochondromas, usually involving multiple bones in one limb. Three variations: localized (involves one epiphysis); classic (involves more than one bone in a single limb); and generalized (involves multiple bones in more than one limb).

hemipelvectomy (hem-ee-pel-VEK-toh-mee), **hindquarter amputation**, **ilioabdominal amputation**. *Surgical procedure*. Removal of the leg, including the iliac wing.

hemiplegia (hem-ee-PLEE-jee-uh). *Pathologic condition*. Paralysis of one side of the body; may occur at birth or from a stroke or accident.

hemivertebra (hem-ee-VUR-tih-bruh). *Congenital abnormality*. Partial vertebra. Abnormality in formation of the vertebral column; leads to angular changes in the spine.

> **balanced h.**: refers to relationship between two hemivertebrae in a segment of the spine, in which each hemivertebra is missing the opposite half of the bone; the sum effect is to balance each other so that the overall alignment of the spine is preserved.

Henderson arthrodesis (ahr-thro-DEE-sis). *Surgical procedure*. For hip fusion, a large bone segment is taken from the lateral wing of the ilium and placed between the trochanteric area and the ilium of the hip.

hereditary cerebral leukodystrophy (lu-ko-DIS-tro-fee), **Merzbacher Pelizaeus disease.** *Pathologic condition*. Deterioration of the white matter of the central nervous system marked by progressive sclerosis of the frontal lobes of the brain. Hereditary.

hereditary motor sensory neuropathy (HMSN). *Pathologic condition*. Syndrome characterized by progressive degeneration of peripheral nerves. As disease progresses, walking becomes difficult and patient develops certain characteristic deformities of extremities (claw hands, cavovarus feet) as well as muscle weakness and changes in sensation and reflexes. Types:

> **I. Charcot-Marie-Tooth disease (hypertrophic form)** (shar-KOH), **autosomal dominant type, Roussy-Lévy syndrome**: there is demyelinization of the peripheral nerves, with absence of deep tendon reflexes.

II. Charcot-Marie-Tooth disease (neuronal form) (shar-KOH), **variable inheritance type**: reflexes and conduction velocities for peripheral nerves remain normal. Generally slower in progression and milder than type I.

III. Déjérine-Sotta disease (day-zhur-EEN), **autosomal recessive type**: develops in infancy and is highly progressive.

IV. Refsum disease: patient has excessive phytanic acid. Onset in adulthood.

V. neuropathy with spastic paraplesia: distal weakness begins during teen years. Equinus foot deformity develops and difficulty with gait.

VI. optic atrophy with peroneal muscle atrophy: patient develops optic nerve atrophy.

VII. retinitis pigmentosa: patient develops retinitis pigmentosa with distal muscle weakness and atrophy.

hereditary multiple exostosis (eks-ahs-TOH-sis). *Abnormal condition.* Large bony protuberances around the joints; hereditary. Slight chance of becoming malignant.

Herndon and Heyman procedure. *Surgical procedure.* Opening the joints of the tarsometatarsal region and realigning the foot, to correct metatarsus adductus (forefoot adduction).

herniated disc, herniated intervetebral disc /or/ **nucleus pulposus, ruptured** /or/ **slipped disc.** *Pathologic condition.* Extrusion of the cartilaginous tissue in the center of a disc (nucleus pulposus), which can place pressure on a nerve and result in leg or arm pain, numbness, tingling or weakness.

herpetic whitlow. *Pathologic condition.* Herpes infection of a finger, seen in healthcare workers who work around patients' mouths (such as dentists).

heterograft (HET-ur-oh-graft), **xenograft.** *Biological implant.* Tissue transferred from one species to another.

heterotopic bone formation, heterotopic ossification, myositis ossificans. *Pathologic condition.* A disease of muscle in which bone is created within a muscle. Most often associated with trauma, prolonged comas, high calcium concentrations in the blood, and certain surgeries. Leads to stiffness in the joint around the muscle.

hex screw, hexagonal screw. *Surgical instrument.* Screw with a head designed to fit a hexagon-shaped screwdriver.

Hibbs arthrodesis (ahr-thro-DEE-sus). *Surgical procedure.* Hip fusion in which the femoral head is left undisturbed within the acetabulum (hip socket) and a strip of bone is slid down from the pelvis to the proximal part of the femur (thighbone).

Hilgenreiner's epiphyseal angle. *Radiologic measurement.* On an x-ray of a pediatric pelvis, anterior-to-posterior (front-to-back) view, the angle between Hilgenreiner's horizontal line and a line paralleling the proximal femoral physis (growth plate). Normal angle is less than 25°. Greater angles indicate coxa vara (decreased neck shaft angle of the near end of the thighbone.

Hilgenreiner's horizontal line, Hilgenreiner's line, horizontal Y line. *Radiologic measurement.* On an anterior-to-posterior (front-to-back) x-ray view of a pediatric pelvis, the line connecting the upper edge of both triradiate cartilages (growth plate making up inner wall of acetabulum). Method of determining the true horizontal plane of the pelvis.

Hill-Sachs lesion. *Abnormal condition.* Bony defect in the posterior lateral aspect of the humeral head; occurs in recurrent dislocation of the shoulder.

hindfoot. *Anatomy.* The back of the foot; contains the calcaneus (heelbone) and talus (top footbone, immediately below the tibia).

hindquarter amputation, hemipelvectomy, ilioabdominal amputation. *Surgical procedure.* Removal of the leg, including the iliac wing.

hinged joint, ginglymus. *Anatomy*. A joint between bones that permits motion in only one plane. Example: knee, elbow.

hip, hip joint. *Anatomy*. The articulation between the femur (thighbone) and the pelvis at the acetabulum (hip socket). Term also used to denote the area of the body immediately surrounding the joint.

> **h. arthroplasty**. *Surgical procedure*. Hip replacement substituting the hip's natural ball and socket for one made of plastic and metal. Can be total or partial.
>
>> **cemented**: uses artificial parts designed to be cemented into position.
>>
>> **cementless, uncemented**: uses artificial parts with a porous rough surface that allows the bone to heal directly to it without cement.
>>
>> **Charnley**: components designed by Sir John Charnley; for cementing into the bone.
>>
>> **hybrid**: the stem is cemented into position and the acetabulum is press-fit into position (inserted without cement).
>>
>> **partial**: see HEMIARTHROPLASTY.
>>
>> **total**: substitution of both hip joints.
>
> **h. disarticulation (HD)**. *Surgical procedure*. Amputation at the hip joint, including the femoral head.
>
>> **suspension**. *Orthopedic appliance*. Prosthesis suspended by straps, used after hip disarticulation (amputation).
>
> **h. dysplasia** (dis-PLAY-zjuh). *Pathologic condition*. Abnormal shape of the acetabulum (hip socket). Usually the result of a congenital condition, but a normal acetabulum can sometimes grow into an abnormally shaped socket.
>
> **h. flexion contracture**. *Abnormal condition*. Contracture of the flexors of hip, preventing the leg from extending completely when the pelvis is lying flat.
>
> **h. fracture**. *Pathologic condition*. Fracture of the upper part of the femur (thighbone).
>
> **h. hemiarthroplasty**. *Surgical procedure*. Substituting a fractured or diseased femoral head (hip joint) with one made of plastic and metal, while retaining the natural socket.
>
> **h. joint**. *Anatomy*. The articulation between the femur (thighbone) and the pelvis at the acetabulum (hip socket).
>
> **h. pointer**. *Abnormal condition*. Lay term for a contusion in the front of the hip. Seen in football players after being hit and tackled.
>
> **h. reduction**. *Treatment*. Manipulating the femoral head back into the acetabulum (hip socket).
>
>> **closed**: accomplished without opening the joint.
>>
>> **open**: opening the joint capsule.
>
> **h. replacement**: see ARTHROPLASTY (above).
>
> **h. spica**. *Orthopedic appliance*. Body cast for immobilizing the hip joints and/or the thigh. Extends from the nipple line to the lower extremities. Usually has a bar between the legs to keep the hips and legs immobilized.

hip-knee-ankle-foot orthosis (HKAFO). *Orthopedic appliance*. Plastic splint that maintains the hip, knee, ankle and foot in proper alignment; used for paraysis or weakness. May have multiple joints.

His-Haas procedure. *Surgical procedure*. For paralysis of scapular muscles; transfer of the teres major tendon from the humerus (upper armbone) to the 5th and 6th ribs, to hold the scapula (shoulderblade) in correct position.

histiocyte (HISS-tee-oh-site). *Anatomy*. Large mononuclear cell found in connective tissue that helps protect against infection and noxious substances.

histiocytoma (hiss-tee-oh-si-TOH-muh). *Pathologic condition*. A tumor made of histiocytes in a fibrous tissue background.

malignant h.: malignant tumor derived from primitive cells; most frequent in the femur (thighbone) and tibia (shinbone).

histiocytosis X (hiss-tee-oh-si-TOH-sus), **Langerhans' cell histiocytosis (LCH)**. *Pathologic condition*. Group of disorders characterized by proliferation of uniquely shaped Langerhans' cells. Classified on the basis of distribution of affected tissues (listed under LANGERHANS' CELL HISTIOCYTOSIS).

Hodgen splint. *Orthopedic appliance*. Two rods with straps extending between them, on which an extremity is supported.

   Pearson attachment: for fractures of the femur (thighbone); enables the knee to be flexed at varying degrees.

Hoffa fracture. *Pathologic condition*. Vertical break in a femoral condyle (rounded end of thighbone) separating the back of the condyle from the rest of the femur. Best seen on a lateral (side) projection of the knee.

Hoffer procedure. *Surgical procedure*. A split anterior tibia (shinbone) tendon transfer used for treating a varus foot. Half the tendon is moved laterally, creating a yoke that holds the foot up in a neutral position.

Hoffman external skeletal fixation device. *Surgical implant*. Frame attached externally to pins placed through a long bone; holds fracture or osteotomy fragments in alignment.

Hohmann retractor. *Surgical instrument*. Steel device with a hook, for keeping soft tissues out of the surgical field.

Homan sign. *Clinical sign*. The ankle is slowly and gently dorsiflexed; pain at the back of the knee or calf may indicate thrombosis (clot formation) in the deep veins of the leg.

homograft, allograft. *Surgical implant*. Tissue transferred to a member of the same species, e.g., human to human. May be from another individual or a cadaver. See also AUTOGRAFT.

hook of the hamate. *Anatomy*. Part of a wrist bone (hamate) near the area traversed by the ulnar nerve. Resembles a hook.

horizontal Y line, **Hilgenreiner's horizontal line**. *Radiologic measurement*. On a front-to-back x-ray view of a pediatric pelvis, the line connecting the upper edge of both triradiate cartilages (growth plate making up inner wall of acetabulum). Method of determining true horizontal plane of the pelvis.

horn cell (anterior), motor neuron. *Anatomy*. Cell located in the front side of the spinal cord; innervates muscles.

housemaid's knee, prepatellar bursitis. *Pathologic condition*. Inflammation of the bursa in front of the patella (kneecap) after minor or direct trauma. May or may not be infected.

Hubbard tank. *Orthopedic appliance*. Large tank of water that allows control of superficial temperature, range of motion and pain relief; used for rehabilitation.

Hughston jerk test, **pivot-shift test**. *Clinical test*. With knee slightly bent, the leg is bent and extended back and forth while medial or lateral pressure is applied. A snapping sensation indicates knee instability and/or rupture of the anterior cruciate ligament.

Hughston procedure. *Surgical procedure*. Technique for knee ligament repair, reconstruction, or patellar (kneecap) dislocation.

humeral head. *Anatomy*. Upper end of the humerus (upper arm bone); articulates with the glenoid cavity of the scapula (shoulderblade).

humerus (HYU-mur-us) *Anatomy*. The upper armbone, between the forearm and the shoulder.

humpback. *Pathologic condition*. Kyphosis of the spine. Presence of excessive forward curvature of the spine, creating a prominence in the upper back.

   h. deformity of the scaphoid: characteristic appearance of a broken scaphoid bone that has angulated.

Hunter's canal, subsartorial canal. *Anatomy*. Channel in lower leg through which the femoral artery travels; the sartorius muscle forms its roof.

Hunter's syndrome. *Pathologic condition*. Disorder of carbohydrate metabolism. Similar to Hurler's but less severe; death usually by age 20. Hereditary.

Huntington graft. *Surgical procedure*. Moving the fibula (smaller bone in lower leg), with its arterial attachment, medially to bridge a defect (from trauma or infection) in the tibia (shinbone).

Huntington's chorea. *Pathologic condition*. Progressive deterioration of central nervous system characterized by uncontrollable irregular movements of the limbs, trunk and face brought on by attempts at voluntary movement. Accompanied by mental deterioration independent of the movement disorder. Begins between ages 35–40 (occasionally in childhood). Hereditary.

Hurler's syndrome, dysostosis multiplex. *Pathologic condition*. Syndrome characterized by scoliosis, contractures of the joints, progressive coarsening of facial features, corneal clouding, and enlargement of spleen and liver. Usually diagnosed by age 2, with death before age 10 from heart and lung deterioration. Hereditary. See also GARGOYLISM.

hyaline cartilage (HI-uh-leen KAHR-tuh-lidj). *Anatomy*. Smooth, resilient, connective tissue (cartilage) on the ends of long bones that are part of the joint, such as at the shoulder, elbow or knee. See also ELASTIC CARTILAGE, FIBROCARTILAGE.

hyaluronic acid (hi-uh-lu-RAHN-ik). *Biologic substance*. A mucopolysaccharide; forms a gelatinous material in tissue spaces throughout the body. Used as injection in the treatment of osteoarthritis. See also VISCOSUPPLEMENTATION.

hyaluronidase (hi-el-yu-RAHN-ih-dayz). *Biologic substance*. Enzyme added to local anesthetics to hasten and spread their effect, to permit infiltration of fluids given through the skin and to speed the resorption of edema (fluid) or blood from an injured area.

hybrid total hip replacement. *Surgical procedure*. Technique in which the proximal femur prosthesis (the stem) is cemented into position and the acetabulum is press-fit into position (inserted without cement).

hybrid total knee replacement. *Surgical procedure*. Technique in which the tibial prosthesis is cemented into position and the femur is not.

hydracadence, hydraulic knee. *Orthopedic appliance*. Mechanical knee joint sometimes used in artificial legs; a piston makes knee movement smoother and improves gait.

hydrarthrosis (hi-drahr-THROH-sus). *Abnormal condition*. Fluid in a joint.

hydraulic knee. See HYDRACADENCE.

hydrocephalus (hi-droh-SEF-uh-lus). *Pathologic condition*. Excess accumulation of fluid in the brain. Caused by decreased resorption of cerebrospinal fluid or obstruction of its outflow. May result in brain herniation. See also ARNOLD CHIARI SYNDROME.

hydrocortisone. *Drug*. Cortisone derivative. For treating inflammatory and allergic diseases. Long-term systemic use can result in serious side effects, e.g., osteoporosis, immunosuppression.

hydroxyapatite (HA) (hi-droxy-AP-uh-tite). *Biologic substance*. Lattice-like crystal composed of calcium and phosphorous; provides a bone's rigid structure.

hypalgesia (hi-pul-JEE-zjuh). *Abnormal condition*. Decreased ability to recognize or feel pain.

hyperalgesia (hi-pur-al-JEE-zjuh). *Abnormal condition*. Excessive pain or hypersensitivity to pain.

hyperesthesia (hi-pur-es-THEE-zjuh). *Abnormal condition*. Acute sensitivity to touch, pain or other stimulation.

hyperextension. *Function.* Capacity of a joint to be stretched beyond its normal range.

    h. orthosis. *Orthopedic appliance.* Brace used for extending the spine after a compression fracture.

hyperostosis. *Abnormal condition.* Abnormal thickening of bone.

hyperparathyroidism. *Pathologic condition.* The presence of excess parathyroid hormone in the body, resulting in disturbance of calcium metabolism with increase in serum calcium and decrease in phosphorus, loss of calcium from bone, and renal damage with frequent kidney-stone formation.

hyperplasia (hi-pur-PLAY-zjuh). *Anatomic defect.* Increased number of one type of cell; associated with increased frequency of cell division.

hyperreflexia. *Abnormal condition.* Exaggerated or excessive reflex response.

hypertonia (hi-pur-TOH-nee-uh). *Abnormal condition.* Greater-than-normal muscle tone, associated with spasticity.

hypertrophic arthritis (hi-pur-TROH-fik). *Pathologic condition.* Osteoarthritis accompanied by large spurs or bony spikes at the periphery of the joint.

hypertrophic exostosis. *Abnormal condition.* Large spurs at the edges of joints, in certain types of degenerative arthritis.

hypertrophic interstitial neuritis, Déjérine-Sotta disease /or/ **syndrome, familial interstitial hypertrophic neuritis, hypertrophic interstitial neuritis.** *Pathologic condition.* Type III hereditary motor sensory neuropathy, a syndrome characterized by progressive degeneration of the peripheral nerves. Weakness in the hands and feet are associated with localized swelling of the peripheral nerves and sensory changes in the extremities; results in hand and foot deformities. Hereditary; detected in late infancy. See also CHARCOT- MARIE-TOOTH disease.

hypertrophy (hi-PUR-truh-fee). *Abnormal condition.* Enlargement of an area of the body, such as a muscle or nerve, or an organ.

hypesthesia, (hi-pes-THEE-zjuh), **hypoesthesia.** *Description.* Decreased sensation in response to heat, cold or pain.

hyponychium (hi-poh-NIK-ee-um), **base of the nail.** *Anatomy.* The epithelium (lining) of the nail bed beneath a finger- or toenail.

hypoplasia (hi-poh-PLAY-zjuh). *Abnormal condition.* Incomplete development of a tissue or organ.

hypoplastic. *Description.* A tissue or organ having incomplete development.

hypothenar eminence (hi-poh-THEE-nahr). *Anatomy.* Prominence on the ulnar/ palmar portion of the hand; comprised of the short flexors of the little finger.

hypotonia (hi-poh-TOH-nee-uh). *Abnormal condition.* Lower-than-normal muscle tone.

    congenital h.: neuromuscular disorder in young children that causes lower-than-normal levels of muscle tone. See also AMYTONIA CONGENITA.

hypotonic cerebral palsy, flaccid cerebral palsy. *Pathologic condition.* Form of cerebral palsy in which the damage to the nervous system results in a very loose muscle group with little or no tone.

I

iatrogenic (i-at-rih-JEN-ik). *Pathologic description.* Refers to an adverse condition that occurs as the result of treatment.

ibuprofen (i-byu-PRO-fen). *Drug.* NSAID for treating pain and inflammation. Also reduces fever. Trade names: Motrin, Advil, Nuprin.

ice skater's fracture. *Pathologic condition.* Stress fracture in the distal (lower) fibula of children between ages 2–8.

IDET (intradiscal electrothermal therapy). *Surgical treatment.* MInimally invasive method for treating back pain from a damaged or diseased disc; a wire is passed into the disc and heated, shrinking the disc and deadening the nerves that are causing pain.

idiopathic (id-ee-oh-PATH-ik). *Description.* Without known cause.

Ilfeld splint. *Orthopedic appliance.* A splint used in the treatment of congenital dislocation of the hip. Maintains the hips in abduction.

iliac (IL-ee-ak). *Anatomy.* Referring or pertaining to the ilium (large bone forming the lateral wall of the pelvis).

> **i. bone, ilium**: a part of the pelvic bone that is above the hip joint.
> **i. crest**: upper rim of the pelvis, to which abdominal muscles attach.
> **i. horns**: bony prominences that arise from the back of the ilium.
> **i. spine**: bony projections on the ilium wing to which muscles attach.
>> **anterior/inferior (AIIS)**: front, lower edge of the ilac wing.
>> **anterior/superior (ASIS)**: front, upper edge of iliac wing.
>
> **i. vessels**: large blood vessels that make up the distal division of the aorta; divides into the internal and external iliac arteries.
> **i. wing**: the portion of the pelvis that is attached to the sacrum.

iliacus (il-ee-AK-us). *Anatomy.* Muscle that runs along inner surface of the iliac wing to upper part of the femur (thighbone), attaching to the lesser trochanter of the femur via the iliopsoas tendon. Assists in bending the hip.

ilioabdominal amputation (il-ee-o-ab-DAHM-in-ul), **hemipelvectomy, hindquarter amputation**. *Surgical procedure.* Removal of the leg, including the iliac wing.

iliofemoral flap (il-ee-oh-FEM-ur-ul), **groin flap**. *Surgical technique.* Large flap of skin and subcutaneous tissue removed from the groin and reattached with its veins and arteries to another site, to cover a large wound.

iliofemoral ligament (il-ee-oh-FEM-ur-ul), **Y ligament, Bigelow's ligament, Bertin ligament**. *Anatomy.* Connective tissue band at front of hip connecting the anterior/inferior iliac spine to the femur between the neck and trochanters. Reinforces and stabilizes the hip joint. *See also* PUBOFEMORAL LIGAMENT.

iliohypogastric nerve (il-ee-oh-hi-po-GAS-trik). *Anatomy.* Nerve that provides sensation to the buttocks via its anterior and lateral cutaneous branches.

iliolingual nerve (il-ee-oh-LING-wul). *Anatomy.* Nerve that provides sensation to the upper groin.

iliolumbar artery (il-ee-oh-LUM-bahr). *Anatomy.* Blood vessel that travels along the ilium, supplying the deep structures along the inner pelvic wall.

iliolumbar vein (il-ee-oh-LUM-bahr). *Anatomy.* Blood vessel that travels with the iliolumbar arteries and drains the inner pelvic wall.

iliopectineal bursa (il-ee-oh-pek-TIN-ee-ul BUR-suh). *Anatomy.* Fluid-filled sac over the front rim of the pelvis where the iliopsoas muscle and tendon move during contraction.

iliopectineal bursitis (il-ee-oh-pek-TIN-ee-ul bur-SI-tus). *Pathologic condition*. Inflammation of the iliopectineal bursa.

iliopectineal eminence (il-ee-oh-pek-TIN-ee-ul). *Anatomy*. A ridge medial to the anterior/inferior iliac spine, over which the iliacus and psoas major muscles pass; marks the union of the ilium and the pubis.

iliopectineal line (il-ee-oh-pek-TIN-ee-ul). *Anatomy*. A thickening in the superior ramus of the pubus. Used as an anatomic landmark.

iliopsoas (il-ee-oh-SOH-us). *Anatomy*. Confluence of two muscles, the iliacus and psoas major, that bend the hip; attached from the front of the lumbar vertebrae to the lesser trochanter of the femur (thighbone).

    Sharrard i. transfer. *Surgical procedure*. Moving the iliopsoas from an intrapelvic position, through the iliac wing, to a lateral position on the greater trochanter, to act as an abductor instead of flexor of the hip. Used in paralytic patients.

iliotibial band (il-ee-oh-TIB-ee-ul). *Anatomy*. Large connective tissue band (the tendon of the tensor fascia lata) that inserts into the tibia (shinbone); abducts and flexes the hip.

ilium (IL-ee-um), **iliac bone**. *Anatomy*. Large bone forming the side wall of the pelvis.

Ilizarov external fixator (il-ih-ZEHR-ov). *Orthopedic implant*. External fixator device (holds fracture fragments from outside body); multiple thin wires are placed through the different bony fragments and attached to a circular frame.

Ilizarov technique. *Treatment*. For corrrection of angular or length deformity or to stabilize a fracture of an arm or leg. Uses multiple pins that attach to rings around the extremity.

imbrication (im-brih-KAY-shun). *Surgical procedure*. Overlapping tissue to shorten its length and/or increase its strength.

impacted fracture. *Pathologic condition*. Fracture in which the fragments are driven into each other by the force of the injury.

impingement syndrome, **shoulder impingement syndrome**. *Pathologic condition*. Pressure of the humerus (upper armbone) against the acromium (projection of the scapula) when the arm is elevated, leading to painful irritation of the tissues between the humerus or its head and the acromium.

implant. *Surgical material*. A graft or material (plate, prothesis, etc.) placed into a part of the body.

incise (in-SIZE). *Surgical technique*. To cut into, without removal. See also EXCISE.

incision (in-SIH-zjun). *Surgical procedure*. A cut or wound created as part of a surgical procedure.

    i. and drainage (I & D): cutting into tissue or a cavity (as an abscess) and draining the contents.

inclusion cyst. *Pathologic condition*. Abnormal formation of material under the skin or within a tissue.

incomplete fracture. *Pathologic condition*. Break that does not proceed from one side of the bone through the other side.

incurvature reflex (lateral trunk), **Galant's sign**. *Clinical sign*. Spontaneous bending of an infant to one side as a blunt object is gently drawn along that side of its trunk. Absence of movement indicates nervous system abnormality.

Indocin. *Drug*. A trade name of indomethacin, NSAID for treating pain and inflammation.

indomethacin (in-doh-METH-uh-sin). *Drug*. NSAID for treating pain and inflammation. Trade name: Indocin.

induration (in-dur-AY-shun). *Pathologic condition*. Hardening of tissue, usually associated with infection and swelling.

infantile cortical hyperostosis, **Caffey's disease** /or/ **syndrome**, **Caffey-Silverman syndrome**. *Pathologic condition.* Swelling of soft tissue around a bone (most commonly jaw and forearm), accompanied by fever, irritability, elevation in white count and sedimentation rate, and cortical bone thickening. Usually seen in children. Difficult to differentiate from a bone infection.

infantile fibromatosis (fi-broh-muh-TOH-sus), **congenital generalized fibromatosis**. *Congenital abnormality.* Multiple benign fibromas (fibrous connective tissue) in the soft tissues of many areas of the body. Usually presents in childhood and may result in progressive limb and spine abnormalities.

infantile spinal muscular atrophy, **Werdnig-Hoffmann paralysis**. *Congenital abnormality.* Destruction of the anterior cells of the spinal cord; eventually leads to death.

infarct (IN-fahrkt). *Pathologic condition.* Loss of circulation to a specific area of the body, leading to tissue death.

infarction (in-FAHRK-shun). *Pathologic condition.* Death of a tissue.

inferior. *Location.* Refers to a structure that situates lower (farther from the head) than another. See also SUPERIOR.

    i. gemellus (guh-MEL-us). *Anatomy.* Small muscle on the back of the hip that rotates the hip externally. See also SUPERIOR GEMELLUS.

    i. genicular artery (lateral). *Anatomy.* A branch off the popliteal artery at the knee; supplies the top of the lateral tibial articular surface and bone.

    i. gluteal artery (GLU-tee-ul). *Anatomy.* Blood vessel that supplies the buttocks muscles. Exits the pelvis below the piriformis muscle to supply the gluteus medius and gluteus minimus muscles.

    i. gluteal vessels (GLU-tee-ul). *Anatomy.* Large blood vessels that supply the buttocks muscles. Exit the pelvis through the sciatic notch. See also SUPERIOR GLUTEAL VESSELS.

    i. pubic ramus (PYU-bik RAY-mus). *Anatomy.* Part of pubic bone forming the inferior bridge of the obturator foramen. See also SUPERIOR PUBIC RAMUS.

inflatable splint. *Orthopedic appliance.* Plastic splint that becomes rigid when filled with air; used to immobilize fractured bones.

inflatable tourniquet. *Orthopedic appliance.* Air-filled band placed about an extremity to cut off its circulation. Advantage over elastic tourniquet: ability to set its exact pressure, which serves as safeguard from too-tight application.

infraction. *Pathologic condition.* Incomplete break in a bone without displacement of the fragments.

    Freiberg's i.: multiple recurrent fractures and associated reparative attempts involving 2nd metatarsal of the foot, resulting in pain and deformity of the head. Usually seen in second decade of life and treated without surgery.

infrapatellar (in-fruh-puh-TEL-ur). *Location.* Refers to the area below the patella (kneecap) and under the patellar tendon.

    i. fat pad. *Anatomy.* Fatty pad below the kneecap (patella), behind the patellar tendon.

infraspinatus (in-fruh-spin-AT-us). *Anatomy.* Large muscle that stabilizes the shoulder; part of the rotator cuff. Responsible for externally rotating the humerus (upper armbone) at the shoulder. Attaches to back of the scapula (shoulderblade) and spine of the scapula.

ingrown toenail. *Abnormal condition.* Toenail that becomes covered by soft tissue, resulting in inflammation, infection and pain. Causes include tight shoes, improper nail trimming, injuries, fungal infections, abnormalities in foot structure, or recurrent trauma to the area.

    O'Donoghue procedure for i. (o-DAHN-uh-hyu). *Surgical procedure.*

Removal of the lateral (outer) fourth of the nail plate and underlying matrix.

inlay graft. *Surgical procedure*. Placement of a bone segment into a recipient bone that has been prepared by cutting a slot in it, or by creating a prefitted cavity. See also ONLAY GRAFT.

innominate (in-AHM-in-ut), **os coxae**. *Anatomy*. Bone formed by the ilium, ischium and pubis that, in the adult, consolidate into one structure that contains and makes up the pelvis.

> **i. osteotomy**. *Surgical procedure*. Cutting through the innominate bone to realign the acetabulum. Used in treatment of developmental dysplasia of the hip in older children.

>> **double**: cutting through the pelvic bones in the area of the ilium and ischium or between the ilium and pubis to direct the acetabulum in a more favorable direction. Used in treatment of hip dysplasia.

Insall-Burnstein posterior stabilized prosthesis, IB knee, IB prosthesis. *Surgical implant*. Used for knee replacement: the patient's posterior cruciate ligament is preserved and the tibial component is composed of only one piece.

Insall-Burnstein posterior stabilized prosthesis II, IB II knee, IB prosthesis II. *Surgical implant*. Implant replacing the IB knee. Allows a greater variety of instrumentation for facilitating ease of insertion and implant modularity.

Insall-Salvati method for determining patella alta. *Radiologic measurement*. Method for determining the appropriate position of the patella relative to the knee. On lateral view of the knee, the length of the patellar tendon should be approximately equal to the length of the patella and not differ by more than 20%.

Insall's anterior approach, Insall's patellar splitting approach. *Surgical technique*. Involves splitting the tendinous sleeve in front of the patella and peeling it from the bone. At the medial border of the patella, the synovium is split, allowing access to the knee joint underneath.

Insall's patellar splitting approach. See INSALL'S ANTERIOR APPROACH.

Insall's quadriceps snip. *Surgical technique*. For quadriceps contracture in total knee replacement surgery: the quadriceps tendon is separated from the muscle, allowing for full flexion of the knee during the surgery. At the conclusion, the tendon is repaired and effectively lengthened.

Insall's technique for anterior cruciate ligament reconstruction. *Surgical procedure*. For reconstructing a torn anterior cruciate ligament: the lower end of the iliotibial band is detached from its insertion on the tibia, passed through a tunnel drilled at the lower end of the femur (thighbone), and attached at the front end of the upper tibia with a screw.

Insall's technique for patellar realignment, Insall's technique for proximal realignment of the patella. *Surgical procedure*. For realigning the patella (kneecap) to prevent recurring dislocations: involves shifting location where the quadriceps tendon inserts onto the top of the kneecap.

insertion (of a muscle). *Location*. The place onto which a muscle attaches. See also ORIGIN.

in situ (in-SI-tu). *Description*. In place, as a fracture that is fixed without reduction (manipulation) or a cancer that has not invaded any surrounding tissue.

instrumentation. Surgical tools used in support of surgery or a procedure.

intercalary (in-TUR-kuh-lehr-ee). *Anatomic description*. Occurring between two bone segments.

> **i. complete pariaxial hemimelia** (pehr-ee-AX-ee-ul hem-ee-MEE-lee-uh). *Abnormal condition*. Absence of inner or outer halves of the mid-portion of a limb: the forearm (area between elbow and wrist) or lower leg (area between knee and ankle).

i. graft. *Biologic implant*. Tissue (bone, nerve, artery or vein) inserted in such a way as to span a missing segment.

intercondylar (in-tur-KAHN-dul-ur). *Anatomic description*. Between the condyles (rounded ends of a long bone).

    i. fracture. *Pathologic condition*. Break in a bone in which the fracture line runs between the condyles, splitting them apart.

    i. notch. *Anatomy*. The space between two condyles.

intercostal (in-tur-KAHS-tul). *Anatomic description*. Between the ribs.

    i. muscles. *Anatomy*. Muscles between adjacent ribs.

    i. space. *Anatomy*. Space between the ribs.

    i. vessels. *Anatomy*. Blood vessels between the ribs at the lower level of each rib.

interdigital neuroma (nu-ROH-muh), **Morton's neuroma**. *Pathologic condition*. Area of painful enlargement of a nerve between the toes. See also MORTON'S TOE.

intermittent cervical traction. *Treatment*. Traction applied intermittently to the head, relieving pressure on the neck.

intermittent claudication (klah-dih-KAY-shun), **Charcot's syndrome**, **myasthenia angiosclerotica**, **vascular claudication**. *Pathologic condition*. Pain and limping caused by insufficient blood supply to the leg muscles when blood vessels are constricted or obliterated, such as in diabetes or arteriosclerosis.

intermuscular (in-tur-MUS-kyu-lur). *Anatomic description*. Between muscles.

internal derangement. *Abnormal condition*. Abnormality or damage within a joint. Term commonly used when an anatomic problem is suspected (e.g., torn ligament, loose body) but there is no definitive diagnosis.

internal fixation. *Surgical procedure*. Joining two segments of bone with rods, plates or screws, to stabilize the bone and promote healing or fusion. Also refers to the materials used. *See also* EXTERNAL FIXATION.

internal iliac vessels (IL-ee-ak). *Anatomy*. Large blood vessels that are branches of the aorta as it makes its way down the abdominal cavity.

internal obturator (AHB-tu-ray-tur). *Anatomy*. Muscle that stabilizes and rotates the femur (thighbone). Originates at the edge of the obturator foramen; attaches to the back of the proximal femur.

internal rotation. *Function*. Turning inward or toward the midline of the body.

internal rotation gait. *Abnormal function*. Walking with the feet pointing toward the midline of the body instead of forward.

internal rotators. *Anatomic description*. Muscles that rotate an extremity toward the midline of the body.

internal tibial torsion (ITT). *Abnormal condition*. Abnormal shape to the tibia (shinbone) in that it is twisted about its long axis so that its distal portion is rotated toward the midline of the body.

interossei muscles (in-tur-AHS-ee-eye). *Anatomy*. Two layers of small muscles in the hand or foot that move the fingers or toes.

    dorsal: four small muscles on the back of the hand or top of the foot that flex (bend) and abduct (spread) the fingers or toes at the knuckles.

    palmar: three small muscles on the palm side of the hand or bottom of the foot that flex (bend) and adduct (bring together) the fingers or toes at the knuckles.

interosseous ligament (in-tur-AHS-ee-us). *Anatomy*. Connective tissue band joining two bones.

interphalangeal (IP) (in-tur-fuh-LAN-jee-ul). *Anatomic location*. Between the bones of the fingers or toes.

i. dislocation. *Pathologic condition*. Dislocation of a finger or toe.

i. joint. *Anatomy*. Joint between the bones of the fingers or toes.

interscapulothoracic amputation (in-tur-skap-yu-loh-thor-ASS-ik), **forequarter amputation**. *Surgical procedure*. Removal of the arm through the shoulder.

interspinous ligament (in-tur-SPI-nus). *Anatomy*. Dense connective tissue band between the spinous processes of the vertebrae.

intertransverse spinal fusion. *Surgical procedure*. Fusion between the transverse processes of two or more vertebrae.

intertrochanteric crest /or/ **line** (in-tur-troh-kan-TEHR-ik). *Anatomy*. Ridge of bone between the greater and lesser trochanters (bony prominences) on the back of the proximal femur (thighbone).

intertrochanteric fracture (in-tur-troh-kan-TEHR-ik). *Pathologic condition*. Type of hip fracture. Break along the line between the greater and lesser trochanters (bony prominences) of the femur (thighbone).

intertrochanteric osteotomy (in-tur-troh-kan-TEHR-ik). *Surgical procedure*. Cutting the femur (thighbone) in the interochanteric area (upper femur between greater and lesser trochanters) in order to change the alignment of the upper part of the femur.

intervertebral (in-tur-vur-TEE-brul). *Location*. Between the vertebrae.

intervertebral disc (in-tur-vur-TEE-brul), **disc**, **vertebral disc**. *Anatomy*. Disc of cartilage between adjacent vertebrae; absorbs shocks and permits movement of the spine. Named after the vertebrae they reside between (e.g., C4, C5 refers to the disc between the 4th and 5th cervical vertebrae). Also: disk.

i. space. *Anatomy*. The space between two vertebrae.

intra-articular (in-truh-ahr-TIK-yu-lur). *Location*. Within the joint capsule.

i. arthrodesis (ahr-throh-DEE-sus). *Surgical procedure*. Fusion of a joint within the capsule.

i. fracture. *Pathologic condition*. Break that runs into and involves the joint surface of a bone.

i. fusion. *Surgical procedure*. Fusion of a joint that occurs completely within the joint capsule.

intracapsular ankylosis (an-kul-OH-sus). *Abnormal condition*. Fusion within the joint capsule, usually following infection or inflammation.

intracapsular fracture. *Pathologic condition*. A break within the joint capsule.

intradiscal electrothermal therapy (IDET). *Surgical treatment*. Minimally invasive method for treating back pain from a damaged disc; a wire is passed into the disc, and heated, which bonds the collagen in the disc to shrink it and also deadens nerves in the disc that are causing pain.

intramedullary (IM) (in-truh-MED-yu-lehr-ee). *Anatomic description*. Within the medullary (marrow) canal (of a bone).

nail. *Orthopedic implant*. Metal rod placed within the center canal (marrow) of a long bone to fasten together the ends of a fracture or osteotomy.

intramuscular (IM). *Location*. Situated or occurring within, or administered into, a muscle.

intraosseous (in-truh-AHS-ee-us). *Anatomic location*. Within bone.

i. graft. *Biologic implant*. A bone graft within bone.

i. lipoma (li-POH-muh). *Pathologic condition*. A fatty tumor within bone.

i. venography (veen-AH-gruh-fee). *Radiologic test*. X-rays taken after a radiopaque dye is injected into a bone and absorbed into its venous system.

intrapelvic obturator neurectomy (in-truh-PEL-vik AHB-tu-ray-tur nur-EK-toh-mee). *Surgical procedure.* In cerebral palsy, cutting the obturator nerve within the pelvis at the pubic area, to diminish spasticity of the adductor muscles.

intraspinal lesion. *Pathologic condition.* Any tumor or abscess within the spine.

intrauterine fracture, fetal fracture. *Pathologic condition.* A break sustained by a fetus in the uterus. Usually associated with bone formation abnormalities such as osteogenesis imperfecta.

intravenous (IV) (in-truh-VEEN-us). *Location.* Situated or occurring within, or administered into, a vein.

> **i. block**, **i. regional anesthesia**, **Bïer block**. *Technique.* Type of regional anesthesia; pain perception is blocked by anesthetic injected into a vein whose circulation has been blocked through application of a tourniquet.

intrinsic muscles. *Anatomy.* Small muscles of the hands and feet that abduct and adduct the fingers and toes. Their origins and insertions are all contained within the hand or foot.

intrinsic palsy. *Pathologic condition.* Paralysis of the intrinsic muscles (in the hands or feet).

invaginating. *Anatomic condition.* Describes a structure that is folded within itself.

invasive test. *Clinical test.* Diagnostic test that requires the body to be penetrated. Example: arteriogram, myelogram.

inversion ankle stress test, talar tilt test. *Clinical test.* The examiner applies maximum inversion to the ankle; excess inversion indicates instability of the ankle's lateral ligaments.

involucrum (in-voh-LU-crum). *Pathologic structure.* New bone that forms around the sequestrum (infected dead bone). Occurs in an area of chronic osteomyelitis (bone infections).

Iowa hip evaluation system. *Classification scheme.* Method of grading severity of a hip condition; includes patient's clinical state, radiographic findings, and range of motion.

ipsilateral. *Location.* Refers to the same side of the body. See also CONTRALATERAL.

irregular bones. *Anatomy.* Type of bone that lacks symmetry; having a peculiar or complex form. Example: calcaneus. See also FLAT BONES, LONG BONES, SHORT BONES.

irrigation. *Treatment.* The administration of fluid (usually saline) to an area with the purpose of cleaning or purifying it.

> **closed suction i.**: with tubes placed in an infected wound and the tissues closed over them, antibiotic irrigation fluid is passed in one tube and pulled out the other by suction, continually washing the wound.

> **pressure i.**: irrigation using a high-pressure pump.

> **pulsatile i.**: using a pulsatile irrigation pump so as to add the effects of pressure pulsations to the irrigation process.

ischemia (is-KEE-mee-uh). *Pathologic condition.* Inadequate blood supply to a body part. See also INFARCT.

ischemic necrosis (is-KEE-mik nuh-KROH-sus). *Pathologic process.* Death of tissue secondary to loss of circulation.

ischial (ISS-kee-ul). *Anatomy.* Refers to the ischium of the pelvis.

> **i. spine**: small prominence of bone protruding from the ischium.

> **i. tuberosity** (tu-bur-AHS-it-ee): large prominence on the end of the ischium; holds weight of a body seated upright. Attachment for hamstring muscles.

ischial weight bearing brace (ISS-kee-ul). *Orthopedic appliance.* A prosthesis or brace fashioned to allow body weight to be borne by the ischial tuberosity.

ischiectomy (is-kee-EK-toh-mee). *Surgical procedure.* Removal of the ischium.

ischiofemoral arthrodesis (is-kee-oh-FEM-ur-uhl ahr-throh-DEE-sus). *Surgical procedure.* Fusing the proximal femur to the ischium from outside the hip joint.

ischium (ISS-kee-um). *Anatomy.* Segment of pelvic bone between the pubis and the back of the ilium.

ischial. Incorrect spelling of ISCHIAL.

ishium. Incorrect spelling of ISCHIUM.

island pedicle graft. *Surgical procedure.* Transfer of a small area of skin ("island") with its attached nerve and blood vessels from one area to another.

isokinetic muscle contraction (i-soh-kin-ET-ik). *Function.* A muscle shortening at a constant speed over a full range of motion. Used in physical therapy as a form of strengthening exercise.

isometric muscle contraction (i-soh-MET-rik). *Function.* A muscle and its joint are maintained in a constant position while the force exerted by the muscle changes. Used in physical therapy as a form of strengthening exercise.

isotonic muscle contraction (i-soh-TAHN-ik). *Function.* A muscle contracts against a constant weight, while the joint and length of the muscle are allowed to change. Used in physical therapy as a strengthening exercise.

IV (intravenous) (in-truh-VEEN-us). *Location.* Situated or occurring within, or administered into, a vein.

ivory bones, Albers-Schönberg disease, chalk bones, marble bones, osteopetrosis, osteosclerosis fragilis. *Pathologic condition.* Rare disorder characterized by extreme density and fragility of the bones and obliteration of the marrow spaces. Symptoms include pathologic fractures, osteomyelitis of the mandible, cranial nerve palsy, enlargement of the spleen and liver, severe anemia, and possible deafness and blindness. Hereditary.

J

Jackson frame. *Orthopedic appliance*. Type of radiolucent table that holds the patient in the desired position.

Jacobson technique. *Treatment*. Method of consciously, progressively relaxing voluntary muscles; used for achieving relaxation.

Jahss osteotomy. *Surgical procedure*. Removing a wedge from the top of the foot at the level of the tarsometatarsal joint and bending the forefoot upward, to correct a cavus (high-arched) deformity.

Japas osteotomy. *Surgical procedure*. For correcting a cavus (abnormally high-arched) foot. The fascia (tight connective tissue band) on the bottom of the foot is cut, a wedge of bone is removed from the midfoot, and the space is closed to bring the foot out of its abnormal position.

javelin thrower's elbow, **baseball elbow**, **little league elbow**. *Abnormal condition*. Repetitive stress injury of the medial condyle of the humerus at the elbow joint.

Jeanne's sign, fingertip pinch test. *Clinical test*. Strength tested by pressing fingertip to thumb. Loss of strength or inability to perform a pinch is indicative of ulnar nerve dysfunction.

Jefferson fracture. *Pathologic condition*. A burst fracture of the 1st cervical (neck) vertebra.

jerk test, lateral pivot-shift test, pivot-shift test of Hughston. *Clinical test*. Test for instability of the knee. With the knee bent to 90°, medial (inward) rotation and valgus (away from midline) stress is applied to the leg as the knee is slowly extended; as the knee passes through 20° or 30° of flexion, shifting forward indicates a tear of the anterior cruciate ligament.

Jersey finger. *Pathologic condition*. Disruption of the flexor digitorum profundus tendon (tendon responsible for bending the tip of the finger).

Jewett nail. *Surgical implant*. A tri-finned, angulated, metal rod used for repairing hip fractures. The proximal segment is screwed into the femoral neck and the other end is inserted into the central femoral shaft.

Jewett orthosis. *Orthopedic appliance*. Back brace for extending the spine; has metal struts in front and back.

Jobst boot, Jobst sleeve. *Orthopedic supply*. Elastic stocking used for reducing swelling of an extremity.

John C. Wilson arthrodesis. *Surgical procedure*. Extra-articular fusion of the hip joint. A large segment of bone from the ilium is inserted into a segment of bone shaved off the greater trochanter.

Johnson modification of Mason classification. *Fracture classification*. Adds a fourth pattern of radial head fractures to the three in the Mason classification.

joint. *Anatomy*. Connection between two bones, with a cartilaginous and/or ligamentous junction that permits motion between the bones.

    amphiarthrotic j. (am-fee-ahr-THRAH-tik): nonmobile. See also JUNCTURAE CARTILAGINAE.

    ball-and-socket j.: comprised of the large round end of a long bone fitting into a hollow part of another bone, to make swinging and rotating movements possible. Example: hips.

    fibrous j.: the bones are in almost direct contact, held together by fibrous connective tissue; three types: syndesmoses, sutures, gomphoses.

    fixed j.: does not move; absorb shock to help prevent bones from breaking. Example: fontanelles of the skull.

hinged j.: moves forward and backward. Example: knee joint.

pivot j.: allows a rotating movement. Example: elbow (also has hinge joint).

synovial j.: freely movable joint with a synovial lining (fluid secreting membrane), e.g., knee, wrist. Also called DIARTHROSIS.

joint capsule. *Anatomy*. Dense fibrous sheath of tissue stretching across and enclosing two articulating surfaces.

joint mice, loose bodies. *Abnormal condition*. Small pieces of cartilage and/ or bone that have broken loose or formed within the joint.

joint reconstruction. *Surgical procedure*. Removal and replacement of all or part of an arthritic joint and rebuilding it, to allow for restoration of function.

joint replacement, arthroplasty. *Surgical procedure*. Joint reconstruction by creation of an artificial joint or by the removal or reshaping of a joint.

Jones fracture. *Pathologic condition*. A break in the 5th metatarsal involving the proximal (upper) metaphyseal portion (flare) of that bone. Associated with a higher-than-usual rate of nonunions.

Judet view (ZJU-day). *Radiologic test*. X-rays of the pelvis taken from different angles to show various surfaces of the ilium, for a better idea of the shape of the acetabulum (hip socket).

jumper's knee. *Pathologic condition*. Irritation of the patellar tendon (extends from kneecap to top of shinbone) caused by overstress of the tendon.

juncturae cartilaginae (junk-TU-ruh kahr-tih-LAH-jin-ee), **amphiarthrosis**, **amphiarthrotic joint, slightly moveable articulations**. *Anatomy*. Type of synarthrosis (nonmobile joint). Called a symphysis if the bones are connected by flattened disks of fibrocartilage (e.g., the symphysis pubis connecting the two pubic bones at the front of the pelvis), or a syndesmosis (if connected by an interosseous ligament).

juvenile aponeurotic fibroma (ay-pahn-yu-RAH-tik fi-BROH-muh). *Pathologic condition*. Benign calcifying tumor within an aponeurosis (fibrous tissue) of children and adolescents; most frequently seen in the hands and feet as a slow-growing and painless nodule.

juvenile arthritis, juvenile rheumatoid arthritis. *Pathologic condition*. Severe form of arthritis occurring in childhood. Muscle and joint involvement, elevated sedimentation rate; occasionally accompanied by a rash and fever.

juvenile kyphosis (ki-FOH-sus), **Scheuermann's disease**. *Pathologic condition*. Abnormality of the vertebrae in the thoracic or thoracolumbar area; characterized by wedging of at least three consecutive vertebrae and irregularities of the growth plate, resulting in a round back appearance (kyphosis). Can be painful.

juvenile osteoporosis (ahs-tee-oh-puh-ROH-sus). *Abnormal condition*. Decrease in bone mass in an adolescent. Rare.

juvenile spondyloarthropathy (spahn-dul-oh-ahr-THRAH-puh-thee). *Congenital abnormality*. Inflammation and degeneration of the spine, affecting children and adolescents. May result in spinal deformity and various joint abnormalities. Many types.

juxta- (JUKS-tuh). *Prefix*. Alongside (juxta-articular: situated close to a joint).

juxta-cortical chondroma. *Pathologic condition*. Benign tumor comprised of hyaline cartilage, situated beneath the periosteum against the bone cortex.

K

Kapel procedure. *Surgical procedure*. Construction of a ligament from the biceps and triceps tendons, for recurrent dislocation of the elbow.

Kaufer technique. *Surgical procedure*. Lateral transfer of part of the tibialis posterior tendon to correct an adducted foot.

Keen sign. *Radiologic sign*. An increase of the distance between the malleoli at the ankle, seen on x-ray. Sign of syndesmotic distruption.

Keller procedure. *Surgical procedure*. Removal of the proximal portion of the proximal phalanx of the big toe, releasing tension on the toe and correcting its alignment, to treat a bunion.

keloid (KEE-loyd). *Abnormal condition*. Benign overgrowth of skin or scar tissue after injury or surgery. Most common in dark skinned races.

keratoma (keh-ruh-TOH-muh). *Abnormal condition*. A callus or tumor of keratin tissue.

Kerlix dressing. *Orthopedic supply*. Trade name for elasticized cotton material used for holding bandages in place.

Kerrison ronguer (ron-ZJUR). *Surgical instrument*. Small instrument for cutting bone in tight places.

ketoprofen (kee-toh-PRO-fen). *Drug*. NSAID for treating pain and inflammation. Trade names: Orudis, Actron, Oruvail.

ketorolac. *Drug*. NSAID for treating pain and inflammation. Trade name: Toradol.

key pinch. *Function*. The specific way the thumb and index finger come together when grasping a small flat object, e.g. a key.

Kidner procedure. *Surgical procedure*. Removal of an accessory bone on the medial side of the foot through a split in the tibialis posterior tendon. See also ACCESSORY NAVICULUM.

Kienböck disease. *Pathologic condition*. Necrosis (tissue death) of the carpal lunate bone (in the wrist) caused by loss of circulation.

kinematics (kin-uh-MAT-iks). *Science*. Deals with motion or movement of parts of the body.

kineplastic amputation (kin-uh-PLAS-tik). *Surgical procedure*. Amputation with preparation of the stump for suspending and activating a prosthesis with straps; most frequently in the arm.

kinetics (kin-ET-iks). *Science*. The study of motion or changes in motion.

kiphosis. Incorrect spelling of KYPHOSIS.

Kirner's deformity. *Abnormal condition*. Deformity of the little finger: the distal phalanx (last bone of finger) is curled downward (toward palm) and radially (toward thumb). Sporadic; no known association or predispositions. Most common in teenage girls.

Kirschner wire, K-wire. *Surgical implant*. Steel wire of varying sizes used for stabilization of fractures or joints; may be threaded or smooth.

Kite clubfoot cast, Kite's method, Kite's technique. *Treatment*. Gentle serial casting of the foot for correction of clubfoot.

Klenzak orthosis. *Orthopedic appliance*. Spring-loaded short leg brace; jointed attachment can be modified to allow for raising or lowering the foot.

Kling dressing. *Orthopedic supply*. Trade name of a cotton bandage applied over a wound to hold dressings in place.

Klippel-Feil syndrome (file). *Abnormal condition*. Fusion of some cervical (neck) vertebrae, with significant decrease in range of motion. Associated with a short neck and low hairline; may be associated with deafness, urinary tract abnormalities, elevation of the shoulderblade, and/or congenital heart disease.

Klippel-Trenaunay-Weber syndrome. *Pathologic condition*. Arteriovenus abnormalities with enlargement of digits or extremities, with changes of the face and/or skull. Unknown etiology.

Klisic technique. *Surgical procedure*. Technique for reduction of congenital hip dislocation in an older child; involves opening the joint, femoral shortening, and osteotomy of the pelvis.

knee, genu. *Anatomy*. Hinge-like joint between the femur (thighbone) and the tibia (shinbone); place of articulation between the thigh and the leg.

knee-ankle-foot orthosis (KAFO). *Orthopedic appliance*. Plastic brace for stabilizing the ankle and knee joint. Fits inside a shoe and extends to the thigh.

kneecap. *Anatomy*. Popular name for the patella, the bone formed within the patellar tendon; serves to position the quadriceps tendon farther from the knee to improve its ability to straighten the joint.

Kniest dysplasia /or/ **syndrome** (neest). *Congenital abnormality*. Form of dwarfism characterized by short limbs, atypical facial appearance, enlarged and stiff joints, contractures of the fingers, scoliosis and deafness. May be due to a disorder in type II collagen.

Knight-Taylor orthosis. *Orthopedic appliance*. Brace that decreases motion of the lumbar spine; used in the treatment of certain back conditions.

knock-knees, genu valgum, tibia valga. *Abnormal condition*. Knees that are angled away from the body and remain widely separated while standing with knees touching.

Knowles pin. *Surgical implant*. Type of threaded pin used for fixation of femoral neck fractures or slipped capital femoral epiphysis.

knuckles, metacarpal heads. *Anatomy*. Prominences produced by the metacarpophalangeal joints in the hand. Serve as location for joining with the phalanges (the 1st, most proximal, of the finger bones).

Kocher clamp (KO-kur). *Surgical instrument*. Clamp having a serrated surface and pointed teeth at the end, used for holding tissue during surgery.

Kocher-Lorenz fracture (KO-kur). *Pathologic condition*. A break involving the capitellum of the humerus (rounded projection at lower end of armbone) where the articular cartilage and a sliver of the attached subchondral bone (below articular cartilage) is fractured off the rest of the humerus. See also BRYAN AND MORREY CLASSIFICATION.

Kocher maneuver (KO-kur). *Surgical procedure*. Traction with external rotation of the arm, followed by traction and internal rotation; for reduction of a dislocated shoulder.

Kohler's disease. *Pathologic condition*. Osteochondrosis or avascular necrosis of the patella (kneecap) or of the navicular bone in the foot.

Koker. Incorrect spelling of KOCHER.

Krabbe's disease, diffuse infantile familial sclerosis, globoid cell leukodystrophy. *Pathologic condition*. Infantile condition characterized by rapid deterioration of the central nervous system (leukodystrophy). Death is usually by age 2. Hereditary; most likely autosomal recessive.

Krause's bone. *Anatomy*. Small bone on a child's growing acetabulum (hip socket) at junction of the pubis, ilium and ischium; later fuses with the acetabulum.

Krukenberg technique. *Surgical procedure*. Construction of a forearm after amputation at the wrist. The two forearm bones (radius and ulna) are separated to enable grasping.

Kugelberg-Welander disease (VEL-an-dur), **spinal muscular atrophy type III.** *Pathologic condition.* Least severe form of spinal muscular atrophy; patient is able to walk, but gait is abnormal. Normal life span is possible, though patient has a higher risk of pulmonary complications.

Küntscher nail. *Surgical implant.* Type of rod designed to be inserted down the medullary (central) canal of a broken femur (thighbone), to stabilize the bone.

K-wire, Kirschner wire. *Surgical implant.* Steel wire of varying sizes used for stabilization of fractures or joints; may be threaded or smooth.

    K-wire skeletal traction. *Treatment.* Pulling an extremity with a Kirschner wire driven transversely though a long bone.

kyphoplasty. *Surgical procedure.* Surgical correction of a kyphotic (humpback) deformity.

kyphoscoliosis (ki-foh-skoh-lee-OH-sus). *Abnormal condition.* Humpback-shaped backward curvature of the thoracic spine.

kyphosis (ki-FOH-sus). *Anatomic condition.* Curvature of the upper thoracic spine in which the concave surface of the curve faces forward; abnormal if excessive. See also DOWAGER'S HUMP, LORDOSIS.

    congenital. *Pathologic condition.* An increase in the thoracic or lumbar arch of the spine secondary to partial absence or fusion of one or more vertebrae anteriorly; growth occurs only in the posterior half of the vertebral column, causing the deformity to progress over time.

    juvenile k., Scheuermann's disease. *Pathologic condition.* Abnormality of the vertebrae in the thoracic or thoracolumbar area; characterized by wedging of at least three consecutive vertebrae and irregularities of the growth plate, resulting in a round back appearance (kyphosis). Can be painful.

L

L. Abbreviation for LUMBAR VERTEBRA; used with specific number (L1–L5).

lacertus fibrosus (luh-SEHR-tus fi-BROH-sus). *Anatomy*. Fibrous continuation of the biceps muscle as it attaches to the radius (larger forearm bone); extends to the fascia of the forearm muscles.

Lachman test. *Clinical test*. With knee extended, anterior stress is applied to the tibia (shinbone). A feeling of instability indicates a possible tear of the anterior cruciate ligament.

lacuna (luh-KU-nuh). *Anatomy*. One of the minute cavities in bone or cartilage occupied by osteocytes.

lag screw. *Surgical implant*. Screw having a smooth segment near the head; when tightened, the two fragments of bone are pulled against one another. A fully threaded screw may also serve as a lag screw if the fragment closest to the head of the screw is overdrilled so as to allow it to glide across the screw.

Lambotte osteotome (lam-BAHT AHS-tee-oh-tome). *Surgical instrument*. Chisel-like device with a flat handle, used to chip away or split fragments of bone.

Lambrinudi procedure (lam-brin-OO-dee). *Surgical procedure*. Triple arthrodesis (joint fusion) combined with selected osteotomies designed to correct a severe calcaneovarus or cavovarus deformity.

lamellar (luh-MEH-lur). *Anatomic description*. Layer-like, resembling a plate.

    l. bone. *Anatomy*. Layered bone; structured in microscopic layers.

lamina (LAM-in-uh). *Anatomy*. The arch at the back of each vertebra that covers the spinal canal and serves as an attachment for the back muscles. Plural: laminae (LAM-in-i).

laminar flow. Air flow through a room having a modified wind tunnel to remove bacteria and dust; creates a nearly sterile atmosphere.

laminectomy (lam-in-EK-toh-mee). *Surgical procedure*. Removal of the lamina (of spine), to relieve pressure on a nerve or allow access to a portion of the spinal cord. See also HEMILAMINECTOMY.

    decompression l.: removing the lamina (posterior elements of the spinal cord) to alleviate pressure on the spinal cord or nerve root.

laminotomy (lam-in-AH-toh-mee). *Surgical procedure*. Cutting a small hole into the lamina (posterior elements of spinal cord) to gain access to a nerve root or disc or to relieve pressure on a nerve.

Landouzy-Déjérine disease, facioscapulohumeral dystrophy. *Pathologic condition*. Mild, common form of muscular dystrophy; results in loss of arm strength, especially around the shoulder, with wasting of the shoulder girdle muscles; also affects muscles of the face, which may lead to inability to generate facial expressions such as smiling.

Landsmeer ligaments, oblique retinacular ligaments. *Anatomy*. Small ligaments in the fingers that stabilize the tendons of the interosseous and lumbrical muscles.

Langensköld osteotomy. *Surgical procedure*. Cutting through the base of the intertrochanteric regions of the femor to correct coxa vara.

Lange position. *Treatment*. Extension, abduction and internal rotation of the legs to maintain reduction of a congenital hip dislocation; position is maintained with a cast.

Langerhans' cell histiocytosis (LCH), histiocytosis X (hiss-tee-oh-si-TOH-sus). *Pathologic condition*. Group of disorders characterized by proliferation of uniquely shaped Langerhans' cells. Classified on the basis of distribution of affected tissues:

disseminated, **Letterer-Siwi disease**: most serious form, characterized by skin lesions resembling seborrheic dermatitis, enlarged liver, spleen and lymph nodes, bleeding tendencies, and progressive anemia. Appears in early childhood.

multifocal: more aggressive; involves the bone and the hypothalamus or pituitary stalk. Called Hand-Schüller-Christian disease when accompanied by skull defects, exophthalmos (eye bulging) and diabetes insipidus.

unifocal, **eosinophilic granuloma**: most common and benign form. Characterized by a solitary lytic (hole-like) bone lesion in the skull or spine. Onset between ages 5–10.

Langerhans' cells. *Anatomy.* Immature dendritic cells containing large granules. See also DENDRITIC CELLS, LANGERHANS' GRANULES.

Langerhans' granules, **Birbeck granules**. *Intracellular structure.* Racket-shaped structures found inside Langerhans' cells; function unknown.

Langer's lines. *Anatomy.* Skin lines that parallel joint creases. Used as guides for incisions to minimize scar formation.

Lapidus procedure. *Surgical procedure.* To correct a bunion at the big toe. Involves fusion of the first metatarsal bone (innermost ray bone) with the medial cuneiform bone (innermost midfoot bone).

Larsen's syndrome. *Congenital abnormality.* Multiple joint dislocations and marked ligament laxity, flattening of the face and widely spaced eyes; may be accompanied by scoliosis and mental retardation. Rare. Hereditary.

Lasègue's sign (lah-SEGZ). *Clinical sign.* With patient lying on the back with hip flexed and knee extended, the ankle is brought into dorsiflexion. Pain at the back of the leg indicates pressure or stretching of the sciatic nerve, which may be caused by a herniated disc.

lateral. *Anatomic description.* Away from the midline. See also MEDIAL.

l. collateral ligament. *Anatomy.* Connective tissue attachment along the side of certain joints that gives stability to the joint. In the knee and toes, also called the fibular collateral ligament, and in the elbow and fingers, also called radial collateral ligaments.

l. column shortening. *Surgical procedure.* Removing a wedge from the outer half of the foot; usually performed through the cuboid and the outer half of the calcaneus (heelbone). Used in the treatment of varus deformity of the hindfoot and/or forefoot.

l. compartment of the leg, **lateral crural compartment**. *Anatomy.* Fascial compartment of the lower leg (one of four compartments) enclosed by tight connective tissue bands forming sheaths containing the peroneal muscles. See also COMPARTMENT SYNDROME, POSTERIOR COMPARTMENT.

l. epicondolytis, tennis elbow. *Pathologic condition.* Inflammation of the extensor tendons where they attach to the lateral epicondyle of the humerus (upper armbone), from repetitive motion in dorsiflexion of the wrist (as when hitting a backhand while playing tennis).

l. epicondyle (ep-ee-KAHN-dile). *Anatomy.* Small prominence on the outer side of some long bones.

l. femoral circumflex artery (FEM-ur-ul). *Anatomy.* Small blood vessel exiting off the femoral artery; supplies part of the femoral head and neck.

l. inferior genicular artery (jen-IK-yu-lur) *Anatomy.* Branch of popliteal artery at the knee; supplies top of the lateral tibial articular surface and bone.

l. malleolus (mal-EE-uh-lus). *Anatomy.* Distal tip of fibula (smaller bone of lower leg) that articulates with the talus (top foot bone) at the ankle joint.

l. meniscus (men-IS-kus). *Anatomy.* Outer cartilaginous disc within the knee joint.

  l. pinch. *Function.* Pinch of the thumb against the radial side of the index finger, instead of to the pulp.

  l. superior genicular artery. *Anatomy.* Branch of the popliteal artery; supplies the outer portion of the knee.

  l. trunk incurvature reflex, Galant's sign. *Clinical sign.* Spontaneous bending of an infant toward one side as a blunt object is gently drawn along that side of its trunk. Absence of movement indicates nervous system abnormality.

lateralizing osteotomy of the calcaneus. *Surgical procedure.* Cutting the bottom half of the heel and sliding it laterally (outwardly). Used in the treatment of varus deformity of the hindfoot.

latissimus dorsi (luh-TISS-uh-mus DOHR-see). *Anatomy.* Large flat muscle on the posterolateral side of the trunk; pulls the humerus toward the body.

Lauge-Hansen classification. *Fracture classification.* Identifies ankle fractures by the type of stress placed on the ankle at time of injury.

Laugier's sign (LOH-zjee-ayz). *Clinical sign.* If the styloid process of the radius (larger forearm bone) is at the same level as that of the ulna (other forearm bone), it is a sign of fracture of the radius, which has been shortened.

Launois-Cleret syndrome (LOHN-wahz klair-AY), **dystrophia adiposogenitalis, Frolich's syndrome** /or/ **appearance.** *Pathologic condition.* Obesity and delayed secondary sexual characteristics, sometimes with a pituitary tumor; occasionally associated with slipped capital femoral epiphysis.

Leadbetter maneuver. *Treatment.* For reduction of a dislocated hip. The hip is brought into flexion and slight internal rotation is applied. Traction is applied in line with the femur and the hip is then abducted and extended.

Leddy and Packer classification. *Fracture classification.* Describes different severities of Jersey fingers (avulsion injuries of flexor digitorum profundus).

Lederhosen's disease, plantar fibromatosis. *Pathologic condition.* Scarring of the palmar fascia resulting in painful nodules along the bottom of the foot.

Lee technique. *Surgical procedure.* Bone transfer from the iliac crest to repair fractures of the tibial articular surface.

leg. *Anatomy.* The lower extremity, between hip and ankle.

  lower l.: the portion of the leg that spans from the knee to the ankle.

leg cylinder cast. *Orthopedic appliance.* Cast that spans the leg from the upper thigh to the flare of the malleoli (tips of lower leg bones), not incorporating the foot, so as to allow for ankle movement. Commonly used in the nonoperative treatment of patella (kneecap) fractures.

leg length discrepancy (LLD). *Pathologic condition.* Inequality of leg length.

Legg-Calvé-Perthes disease, Calvé-Perthes disease, osteochondritis deformans juvenilis /or/ **juvenilis dorsi, Perthes disease.** *Pathologic condition.* Deterioration and flattening of the femoral head due to insufficient blood supply; may result in severe arthritic changes. Idiopathic (no known cause); generally occurs between ages 4–8. See also CATTERALL CLASSIFICATION.

Leinbach screw. *Surgical implant.* Long flexible screw used for repairing fractures of the olecranon or osteotomies of the proximal ulna (smaller forearm bone).

leiomyosarcoma (li-oh-mi-oh-sahr-KOH-muh). *Pathologic conditon.* Rare malignant tumor of smooth muscles. Appears incapsulated but is usually large and will metastasize.

Lenox-Hill orthosis. *Orthopedic appliance.* Brace for protecting an unstable knee. Also used during rehabilitation after ligament repair about the knee.

L'Episcopo Zachary procedure. *Surgical procedure*. Multiple tendon transfer for correcting internal rotation abduction contractures of the shoulder secondary to paralysis.

Leri sign. *Clinical sign*. Inability to flex the elbow when the wrist on the same side is passively flexed. Seen in hemiplegia.

lesser multangular (mul-TANG-yu-lur), **trapezoid**. *Anatomy*. Small bone in the wrist between the trapezium and the capitate, opposite the 2nd metacarpal.

lesser trochanter (TROH-kan-tur). *Anatomy*. Small protrusion of bone on the proximal side of the femur (thighbone); insertion of the iliopsoas tendon.

Letournel classification. *Fracture classification*. Describes different fracture patterns of the acetabulum.

Letterer-Siwe disease (SEE-wee), **disseminated Langerhans' cell histiocytosis**. *Pathologic condition*. Disseminated and most serious form of Langerhans' cell histiocytosis. Characterized by skin lesions resembling seborrheic dermatitis, bleeding tendencies, enlarged liver, spleen and lymph nodes, and progressive anemia. Appears in early childhood.

leukodystrophy (lu-ko-DIS-tro-fee) *Pathologic condition*. Group of hereditary disorders characterized by deterioration of white matter of the central nervous system.

    globoid cell l., **diffuse infantile familial sclerosis**, **Krabbe's disease**: infantile condition characterized by rapid deterioration of the central nervous system. Death usually by age 2. Most likely autosomal recessive.

    hereditary cerebral l., **Merzbacher Pelizaeus disease**: marked by progressive sclerosis of the frontal lobes of the brain.

    metachromatic l., **sulfatide lipidosis**, **sulfatidosis**: lipid storage disease characterized by abnormal accumulation of fat molecules (sulphatide lipids) with a sulphur chain. Progressive deterioration of the central nervous system, with loss of ability to walk, speech difficulty usually about age 1, death by age 10. Autosomal recessive. Most common leukodystrophy in childhood.

levator scapulae (luh-VAY-tur SKAP-yu-li). *Anatomy*. Muscle that raises the scapula (shoulderblade).

Lhermitte sign. *Clinical sign*. Feeling of pain down the spine upon simultaneous bending the neck and hip by examiner; sign of meningeal irritation.

Lichtbeau technique (LIKT-boh). *Surgical procedure*. Cutting the abductor hallucis tendon to allow the foot to turn out; for forefoot abduction or metatarsus adductus.

ligament (LIG-uh-munt), **ligamentum**. *Anatomy*. Band or sheet of connective tissue connecting two or more bones or two parts of the same bone. See also LIGAMENTUM.

    annular l. (AN-yu-lur): surrounds the wrist, elbow or ankle joint or the flexor tendons of the fingers; at the elbow joint, the ring-shaped cartilage that surrounds the radial head (upper end of larger forearm bone), helping to keep it from dislocating.

    anterior cruciate l. (ACL) (KRU-shee-ut): connects the distal lateral femoral condyle (thighbone) to the top of the tibia (shinbone) across the knee joint; prevents the tibia from slipping forward on the femur.

    anterior longitudinal l. (ALL): secures the vertebral bodies to each other.

    Bardinet's l. (bahr-din-AYZ): the back of the ulnar collateral ligament; joins the humerus to the ulna on the inner side of the arm.

    Bertin l.: same as ILIOFEMORAL (below).

    Bigelow's l.: same as ILIOFEMORAL (below).

iliofemoral l.: at front of hip; reinforces and stabilizes the hip joint by connecting the iliac spine to the femur between the neck and trochanters.

medial collateral l.: gives stability to the inner side of a joint.

nuchal l. (NU-kul): maintains alignment of the head and neck. Attaches to the spinous processes of the neck vertebrae. More prominent in quadripeds in which it supports the head in an upright manner.

posterior cruciate l. (PCL) (KRU-shee-ut): joins the femur (thighbone) to the tibia (shinbone) within the knee joint; prevents the tibia from slipping backward on the femur.

posterior longitudinal l.: tight connective tissue band within the spinal canal of a vertebra; lies against the back of the vertebral body.

radial collateral l.: on radial side of the arm, hand or digit; holds two bones together.

sacrospinous l. (say-kroh-SPI-nus): runs from the ischial spine (bony prominence on ischium) to the lower segment of the sacrum.

sacrotuberous l. (say-kroh-TU-bur-us): runs from the sacrum to the tuberosity on the lower side of the ischium.

spring l.: very thick, strong ligament between the calcaneus (heelbone) and navicular of the foot; supports head of the talus (top foot bone).

talocalcaneal l. (tay-loh-kal-KAY-nee-ul): between the talus (top foot bone) and calcaneus (heel), within the tarsal sinus.

talofibular l. (tay-loh-FIB-yu-lur): holds the talus (top foot bone) and fibula (smaller bone of lower leg) in position on the outer side of the foot.

talonavicular l. (tay-loh-nuh-VIK-yu-lur): joins the talus (top foot bone) to the navicular in the front of the foot.

tibial collateral l.: connects the femur (thighbone) to the tibia (shinbone); acts as a stabilizer of the knee, keeping the tibia from rotating outward.

ulnar collateral l.: accessory ligament of the fingers or at the elbow, on the inner side of the arm.

volar carpal l.: crosses the wrist, attaching to the hamate and trapezium and incorporating the tendons in the front of the forearm and wrist.

Wrisberg l.: attaches outer meniscus to the inner, rear femoral condyle.

Y l.: same as ILIOFEMORAL (above).

ligamentum, ligament. *Anatomy.* Band or sheet of connective tissue connecting two or more bones or two parts of the same bone. See also LIGAMENT.

l. flavum (FLAH-vum): attaches from the lamina of each vertebra to the lamina of the vertebra below.

l. mucosum (myu-KOH-sum): small ligament in the knee that holds the fat pad in a relatively stable position.

l. teres (TEHR-eez): attaches the femoral head to the lower inner side of the acetabulum (hip socket).

ligation (li-GAY-shun). *Surgical procedure.* A tying off of an anatomical channel (e.g., a blood vessel).

ligature (LIG-uh-chur). *Surgical supply.* Thread used for tying off vessels, muscles, etc.

limb, extremity. *Anatomy.* An arm or leg.

l. length discrepancy (LLD). *Pathologic condition.* Inequality of limb length. See also PROXIMAL FOCAL FEMORAL DEFICIENCY.

l. salvage. *Surgical procedure.* Attempt to save an extremity with a malignant bone tumor or extensive trauma by surgical means.

Lindholm procedure. *Surgical procedure.* For repair of a rupture of the Achilles tendon: fascial strips from the tendon are sutured onto themselves.

linea aspera (LIN-ee-uh AS-pur-uh). *Anatomy.* Large ridge extending from the lesser trochanter to just above the knee; attachment of some of the hamstring muscles at the back of the femur (thighbone).

linear fracture, fissure fracture. *Pathologic conditon.* A break that extends along the length of a bone rather than across it.

linear scleroderma. *Pathologic condition.* Non-progressive disease in which the skin and subcutaneous tissue become thin and inflexible, giving the appearance of leather. May cause limb deformities.

Lineback screw. Incorrect spelling of LEINBACH SCREW.

lipid. *Biologic substance.* Name given to the fat molecule.

lipid storage disease. *Pathologic condition.* Series of hereditary disorders of fat (lipid) metabolism, the effects and severity of which are determined by the specific enzyme affected. Examples:

> **gangliosidosis** (gang-lee-oh-sih-DOH-sis): characterized by abnormal accumulation of complex sugar, particularly within nerve tissue; consequences include progressive psychomotor deterioration and death in early childhood. Examples: familial amaurotic idiocy, Sandhoff disease.

> **Gaucher's disease** (go-SHAYZ): leads to accumulation of certain fats in the spleen and liver; grouped by severity into infantile, juvenile and adult types; major orthopedic implication is the development of avascular necrosis.

> **Niemann-Pick disease**: severe form of sphingolipidosis type; growth impairment with progressive neurological deterioration, enlargement of the liver and spleen, and cherry red spots or grayish haze in the retina. Death by age 3. A more benign form occurs rarely in adults.

lipofibroma (li-poh-fi-BROH-muh). *Pathologic condition.* Benign, fatty, fibrous tumor of muscle or subcutaneous tissue.

lipoma (li-POH-muh). *Pathologic condition.* Benign fatty tumor, sometimes palpable beneath the skin.

> **intraosseous l.** (in-truh-AHS-ee-us): a fatty tumor within bone.

liposarcoma (li-poh-sahr-KOH-muh). *Pathologic condition.* Malignant fatty tumor.

Lisfranc amputation (LISS-frank). *Surgical procedure.* Removal of the foot through the tarsometatarsal joint.

Lisfranc dislocation (LISS-frank), **Lisfranc fracture-dislocation, tarsometatarsal fracture-dislocation.** *Pathologic condition.* Traumatic dislocation of the foot at the tarsometatarsal joint. Frequently involves fractures of the bones in the immediate area.

Lisfranc joint (LISS-frank), **midtarsal** /or/ **tarsometatarsal joint.** *Anatomy.* Joint complex between the metatarsal and tarsal bones (cuneiforms and cuboid).

Lister's tubercle. *Anatomy.* Small protuberance of bone on the dorsal surface of the distal end of the radius (larger forearm bone).

listhesis (lis-THEE-sis). *Pathologic condition.* The sliding of one surface across another; describes the slippage of one vertebra relative to an adjoining vertebra. See also SPONDYLOLISTHESIS.

little league /or/ **baseball** /or/ **javelin thrower's elbow.** *Abnormal condition.* Repetitive stress injury of the medial condyle of the humerus at the elbow joint.

little league shoulder, proximal humeral apophysitis. *Pathologic condition.* Stress fracture of the proximal humerus (upper growth plate of armbone) caused by repetititive throwing injury.

Littler procedure for policization. *Surgical procedure.* Procedure used for turning a finger into an opposable thumb.

lobster foot, cleft foot. *Congenital anomaly.* Foot separated into two parts (like a lobster claw), possibly with missing parts (e.g., metatarsal bones and toes).

lobster hand, lobster claw, cleft hand, split-hand, main fourchee. *Congenital anomaly.* Hand separated into two parts (like a lobster claw), associated with missing fingers and metacarpal bones.

local anesthetic. *Drug.* Medication that temporarily removes sensation, including pain; affects a part of the body; may be regional (affects an area of body) or topical (applied to surface).

Localio technique. *Surgical procedure.* Resection of the sacrum for a malignant tumor.

localizer cast technique. *Treatment.* Casting treatment for scoliosis. The patient is placed in a bent or stretched position in a frame to correct the curve while the cast is applied. The cast is changed at intervals to accommodate growth.

locking plate. *Orthopedic implant.* Metallic plate for holding fractured bones together; the screw holes are threaded so that the screws thread onto the plate. Increases stability of the fracture repair by preventing the screws from moving.

　　l. compression p.: offset screw holes allow fractured bones to be compressed together.

Lodine. *Drug.* A trade name of etodolac, NSAID for treating pain and inflammation.

long bone. *Anatomy.* Tubular bone with a growth plate at each end from which normal growth occurs. Example: femur.

longitudinal axis. *Anatomic description.* The long axis of an individual, i.e., from head to foot.

long-leg cast (LLC). *Orthopedic appliance.* Cast extending from the upper thigh to the toes.

　　l. walking c. (LLWC)*:* reinforced at the bottom to allow for weightbearing.

long-leg splint (LLS). *Orthopedic appliance.* Splint extending from the foot to the thigh; must extend above the knee.

long thoracic nerves (thor-ASS-ik). *Anatomy.* Nerves that originate from the 5th, 6th and 7th cranial vertebrae and innervate the serratus anterior muscle.

loose bodies, joint mice. *Abnormal condition.* Small pieces of cartilage and/or bone that have broken loose or formed within the joint.

lordosis (lohr-DOH-sus), **swayback.** *Anatomic condition.* Curvature of the spine in which the curve points forward. Normal in the upper neck (cervical spine) and lower back (lumbar spine). Abnormal if excessive. See also KYPHOSIS.

　　cervical l.: the forward-facing curve of the neck.
　　lumbar l.: the forward-facing curve of the lower back.

Lorenz procedure. *Treatment.* Closed reduction of the hip in childhood.

Lottes nail /or/ **pin.** *Surgical implant.* A triflanged intramedullary nail used in fractures of the tibia (shinbone).

Lou Gehrig disease, amyotrophic lateral sclerosis (ALS), Charcot's disease, motor neuron disease. *Pathologic condition.* Progressive degenerative disease of the spinal cord nerves that control motor function (the muscles); leads to gait and motor abnormalities and eventually death.

Lovejoy drill. *Surgical instrument.* Hand-held, hand propelled drill used for creating holes and driving pins.

low contact dynamic compression plate (LCDCP). *Orthopedic implant.* Metallic plate for compressing fractured bone ends together. Its surface is indented between screw holes to minimize contact between the plate and the bone.

Minimizes bone tissue damage from the plate resting against the bone.

lower motor neuron disease. *Pathologic condition*. Nervous system disease occurring at the anterior horn cell of the spinal cord or distally; affects motor nerves to the extremities, leading to weakness or paralysis. Example: polio.

Lowe syndrome, oculocerebrorenal dystrophy. *Congenital abnormality*. Autosomal recessive abnormality resulting in kidney dysfunction and failure, congenital eye disorders such as cataracts and glaucoma, and severe mental retardation. Death often occurs in childhood.

LP. Abbreviation for LUMBAR PUNCTURE.

L-spine. See LUMBAR SPINE.

lucatio erecta (luk-SAY-shee-oh. *Abnormal condition*. Dislocation of the shoulder below the glenoid; causes the arm to remain raised in an extended position.

Ludloff approach. *Surgical procedure*. Medial approach through the adductor area for reduction of a congenital hip or for aspiration of a pediatric hip.

Ludloff sign. *Clinical sign*. 1. Difficulty raising the thigh from the sitting position; occurs after an injury in which the apophysis of the lesser trochanter is traumatically pulled off. 2. Bruising in the inner side of the groin resulting from the same injury.

lumbago (lum-BAY-goh) *Pathologic condition*. Nonspecific term for pain in the mid and lower back.

lumbar (LUM-bahr). *Anatomic description*. Refers to the lower back, between ribs and pelvis.

> **l. agenesis** (ay-JEN-uh-sis). *Congenital abnormality*. Incomplete development of the spine in the lumbar area; usually associated with other abnormalities of the lower extremities and pelvic organs.

> **l. myelogram** (MI-loh-gram). *Radiologic test*. X-ray of the lumbar spine after injection of radiopaque dye.

> **l. plexus** (PLEK-sus), **lumbosacral plexus**. *Anatomy*. Place where nerve roots exiting the lumbar and sacral spine join to make up the sciatic and femoral nerves.

> **l. puncture (LP)**. *Procedure*. Inserting a needle into the dura (covering of spinal cord and brain) in the lumbar area to withdraw cerebrospinal fluid or insert dye or anesthetic drugs.

> **l. segmental arteries**. *Anatomy*. Small arteries branching from the aorta at the lumbar level.

> **l. spine (LS)**, **L-spine**. *Anatomy*. The five vertebral bones that make up the spine between the ribs and the pelvis.

> **l. vertebra**. *Anatomy*. One of the five bones making up the lumbar spine.

lumbarization (lum-bahr-uh-ZAY-shun). *Pathologic condition*. Absence of fusion of the 1st sacral vertebra to the remainder of the sacrum, resulting in an extra lumbar vertebra. See also TRANSITIONAL VERTEBRA.

lumbosacral (LS) (lum-boh-SAY-krul). *Anatomic description*. Region in the spine between the lumbar and sacral areas.

> **l. corset**. O*rthopedic appliance*. Corset that covers the lumbar spine and extends across the sacrum, to support the lumbosacral junction.

> **l. orthosis**. *Orthopedic appliance*. Brace that extends from the lumbar to the sacral spine, immobilizing the lumbosacral region.

> **l. plexus**. See LUMBAR PLEXUS.

lumbrical muscles (LUM-brih-kul). *Anatomy*. Four small muscles on the palmar side of the hand, or plantar side of the foot, that flex (bend) the fingers or toes at the knuckles and, acting with the interossei muscles, extend (straighten) the last two joints of the fingers or toes.

lumen (LU-min). *Geometric description.* Hollow, central portion; may be of an organ or of a surgical instrument.

lunate (LU-nayt). *Anatomy.* Small bone in the wrist between the navicular and the triquetrium in the proximal row of carpal bones. Articulates with the capitate and the radius (larger forearm bone).

lupus (LU-pus), **systemic lupus erythematosus**. *Pathologic condition.* Inflammatory disease that commonly affects joints, especially in the hands, wrists and knees. Involves connective and vascular tissues of many organs; may be associated with severe arthritis, kidney involvement, abnormalities of the retina, and rash on the face. Usually occurs in the 3rd or 4th decade.

Luque instrumentation (LU-kee). *Orthopedic implant.* Rods and wires used for correcting malalignment and stabilize the spine.

luxation, dislocation. *Pathologic condition.* 1. Movement of a part from its normal position. 2. Loss of the normal relationship of one bone to the other at a joint. Types listed under *DISLOCATION*.

Lyme disease. *Pathologic condition.* Tick-born disease characterized by a rash and arthritic-like syndrome; may become chronic if not treated promptly with antibiotics.

lymphadenopathy (lim-fad-en-AHP-uh-thee). *Pathologic condition.* Abnormal enlargement of lymph nodes.

lymphangiography (lim-fan-gee-AH-gruh-fee). *Radiologic test.* Dye is placed into the skin in the distal part of an extremity through or near the lymphatic vessels and nodes; as the nodes take up the dye, they can be visualized on x-ray.

lymphangioma (lim-fan-gee-OH-muh). *Pathologic condition.* Tumor formed of dilated (enlarged) lymphatic vessels.

lymphedema (limf-uh-DEE-muh). *Pathologic condition.* Swelling (especially in subcutaneous tissues) as a result of lymphatic vessel or lymph node obstruction and accumulation of large amounts of lymphatic fluid in affected region.

    acquired l., Miege's disease: permanent pitting edema usually confined to the legs; onset at puberty. Hereditary (autosomal dominant).

    familial l., Milroys disease: permanent edema that causes pitting in the legs; congenital.

lymph nodes. *Anatomy.* Mass of lymphocytes found in various locations along lymph vessels; serve as a filter of tissue fluids. Part of body's immune system; when swollen and tender, may indicate infection in that region of the body.

lymphoma (lim-FOH-muh). *Pathologic condition.* Malignant tumor of lymphoid tissue.

lyophilization of bone (li-oh-fil-ih-ZAY-shun). *Process.* Technique for preparing bone for a graft. The crystalline structure of the bone is isolated by freezing, then evaporating the frozen fluid portion of the bone in a vacuum.

lysis (LI-sis). *Abnormal process.* Destruction of bone or soft tissue.

lytic (LI-tik). *Process.* Refers to any process that destroys tissue or bone.

M

maceration (mass-ur-AY-shun). *Treatment.* Softening by soaking, as in an area of infection or an area maintained in a moist environment, such as in a cast.

MacEwen and Shands osteotomy (mak-YU-en, ahs-tee-AH-tuh-mee). *Surgical procedure.* Cutting obliquely through the subtrochanteric and inter-trochanteric regions of the hip to correct malalignment of the upper femur (thighbone) in more than one plane.

macrodactyly (mac-roh-DAK-tuh-lee). *Congenital abnormality.* Enlarged digits; characteristic of some congenital dysplasias.

Madelung deformity (mah-deh-LOONG) *Congenital abnormality.* An abnormally shaped distal radius (larger forearm bone) leading it to be triangular in shape in association with dorsal subluxation of the ulna (smaller forearm bone) at the wrist; results in limitations in wrist motion and perhaps early degeneration of the wrist.

Maffucci's syndrome (mah-FU-cheez) *Pathologic condition.* Multiple enchondromas (benign cartilage growth) in bone associated with hemangiomas.

Magilligan procedure. *Radiologic test.* On lateral projection (side view) of the femur (thighbone), method for measuring rotation of the femoral shaft around the long axis in relation to the femoral neck (femoral anteversion).

magnetic resonance imaging (MRI). *Diagnostic test.* Type of imaging technique using high intensity magnetic fields; permits examination of soft tissues inside the body that cannot be seen with x-rays. See also CT SCAN.

Magnuson-Stack procedure (MAG-nuh-sun). *Surgical procedure.* Advancement of the capsule and muscles laterally on the humerus (upper armbone), to limit external rotation of the shoulder and prevent recurrent dislocation.

main en griffe (man ahn GREEF), **claw hand**. *Pathologic condition.* Hyperextension of the metacarpophalangeal joints of the fingers, and flexion of the middle and distal phalanges, giving a clawlike appearance. Frequently associated with neurological disorders and ulnar nerve lesions.

main fourchee (man foor-SHAY), **cleft** /or/ **split hand**, **lobster claw** /or/ **hand**. *Congenital anomaly.* Hand separated into two parts (like a lobster claw), with missing fingers and metacarpal bones.

Maisonneuve fracture. *Pathologic condition.* Break of the medial malleolus associated with a fracture of the proximal fibula (smaller bone of lower leg).

maleolus. Incorrect spelling of MALLEOLUS.

Malgaigne fracture (mal-GAYN). *Pathologic condition.* Break at the front of the pelvic ring associated with a dislocation or fracture/dislocation on the opposite side.

malignant fibrous histiocytoma (MFH) (his-tee-oh-si-TOH-muh). *Pathologic condition.* Tumor derived from primitive and fast-growing fibrous cells; most frequently found in the femur (thighbone) and tibia (shinbone). Often fatal.

malleolus (mal-EE-uh-lus). *Anatomy.* Protuberance on both sides of the ankle joint. Plural: malleoli.

    lateral m., **external m.**: distal tip of fibula (smaller bone of lower leg) that articulates with the talus (top foot bone) at the ankle joint.

    medial m., **internal m.**: distal end of the tibia (shinbone) that articulates with the talus (top foot bone) at the ankle joint; stabilizes the inner side of the ankle.

    posterior m.: small bump in the back of the distal tip of the tibia; not visible because it is covered by the Achilles tendon.

mallet finger. *Abnormal condition.* A finger that cannot be actively extended at the distal phalanx; caused by rupture of the extensor tendon, usually from injury. The distal phalanx will assume a slightly flexed or "dropped" position, giving it the appearance of a mallet.

mallet fracture, bony mallet. *Pathologic condition.* Break of the most distal bone of the finger, where the attachment of the extensor tendon of the finger is pulled off the bone, resulting in downward deformity of the tip of the finger.

mallet toe. *Abnormal condition.* Flexion deformity of the distal interphalangeal joint of a toe.

malum coxae senilis (KAHKS-i). *Pathologic condition.* Deformity of the head of the femur (thighbone) caused by avascular necrosis.

malunion. *Pathologic condition.* Break in a bone that has healed in a less than optimum position.

man en griffe. *Incorrect spelling of* MAIN EN GRIFFE.

man fourchee. *Incorrect spelling* MAIN FOURCHEE.

manubrium (muh-NU-bree-um). *Anatomy.* Proximal (upper) portion of sternum.

Maquet procedure (mah-KAY). *Surgical procedure.* Elevating the tibial tubercle to relieve pressure of the patella against the femoral condyle.

marble bones, Albers-Schönberg disease, chalk bones, ivory bones, osteopetrosis, osteosclerosis fragilis. *Pathologic condition.* Rare, hereditary disorder characterized by extreme density and fragility of the bones and obliteration of the marrow spaces. Symptoms include pathologic fractures, osteomyelitis of the mandible, cranial nerve palsy, enlargement of spleen and liver, severe anemia, and possible deafness and blindness.

march fracture. *Pathologic condition.* Stress fracture of the 3rd metatarsal bone caused by prolonged repetitive activity, such as running or marching.

Marfan's syndrome. *Pathologic condition.* Disorder characterized by arachnodactyly (long fingers), loose lens in the eye, scoliosis, kyphosis, loose joints, pectus excavatum, flat feet, high arched palate, long narrow face, and cardiovascular abnormalities including aortic aneurism. Often seen in basketball players. May lead to premature death secondary to aortic rupture.

Marie-Strümpell disease, ankylosing /or/ **rheumatoid spondylitis, Bechterew's disease.** *Pathologic condition.* Autoimmune connective tissue disorder resulting in the gradual fusion of the joints between vertebrae; causes severe limitation of spinal motion, with back and hip pain.

Markell shoes, reverse last shoes. *Orthopedic appliance.* Shoes in which the left and right lasts (patterns) are reversed, i.e., the right shoe on the left foot. Frequently used as treatment for metatarsus adductus in children.

Maroteaux-Lamy syndrome (mah-roh-TOH lah-MEE). *Pathologic condition.* One of the mucopolysacharidoses (type VI). Characteristics include short stature, coarse facial features, increased urinary dermatan sulfate, significant growth retardation. Normal intelligence. Gradual clouding of corneas, hearing loss, joint stiffness, kyphosis, enlargement of spleen and liver may occur. Hereditary.

marrow (bone). *Anatomy.* Soft, spongy tissue filling the cavities of bones, which in youth is filled with blood-forming cells and in older adults with fat.

marsupialization (mahr-su-pee-ul-ih-ZAY-shun). *Surgical procedure.* Opening a lesion and suturing the skin edges around the periphery, creating a pouch, to allow healing to occur from within.

Martin bandage, Esmarch bandage. *Orthopedic supply.* Elastic band used to squeeze the blood out of an extremity.

Martin closed wedge osteotomy. *Surgical procedure*. Removal of a wedge of bone from neck of femur to reduce a slipped capital femoral epiphysis.

Mason classification. *Fracture classification*. Identifies three fracture patterns of the radial head. Johnson modification adds a 4th fracture pattern.

Massie nail. *Surgical implant*. Sliding nail used in femoral hip and neck fractures; as the nail slides within the bone, the fracture areas are allowed to compress.

matrix (MAY-triks). *Anatomy*. The microscopic substance of a tissue or cell.

> **cartilage m.** (KAHR-tuh-lidj): intercellular substance of cartilage, produced by cartilage cells.

> **cellular m**: intracellular material providing structural support to a cell.

Mayer trapezius transfer. *Surgical procedure*. Moving a segment of the trapezius muscle to the humerus (upper armbone), to accommodate for paralysis of the deltoid muscle.

> **Bateman modification**: takes a small piece of scapula with the muscle.

Mayo classification. *Fracture dislocation classification*. Identifies different types of carpal (wrist) dislocations.

McBride procedure. *Surgical procedure*. For a mild bunion: removal of the bony prominence from inner side of the big toe followed by imbrication (tightening) of the medial capsule (lining) of the metatarsophalangeal joint with release of the conjoined adductor tendon from the proximal phalanx to the 1st metatarsal bone. Also involves removal of the sesamoid bones (small bones under far end of 1st metatarsal bone).

> **modified**: involves only the removal of the lateral (outer) sesamoid bone.

McCauley procedure. *Surgical procedure*. Release of muscles, tendons and ligaments via a medial incision, to correct a clubfoot deformity.

McConnel frame. *Orthopedic appliance*. Structure used during surgery, to hold a patient on his/her back against a backrest with knees slightly bent (Fowler's position); attaches to an operating room table.

McCune-Albright disease /or/ **syndrome**, **Albright's disease** /or/ **syndrome**, **Albright-McCune disease** /or/ **syndrome**, **polyostotic fibrous dysplasia**. *Congenital disorder*. Syndrome characterized by multiple skin lesions (cafe-au-lait spots), endocrine abnormalities (especially precocious puberty) and multiple fibrous dysplasia lesions.

McElvenny procedure. *Surgical procedure*. Fusion of the 1st metatarsus bone, the medial cuneiform and the navicium, to correct an abnormally high arch.

McLaughlin technique. *Surgical technique*. 1. For repair of a crescenteric-shaped rotator cuff tear. 2. For addressing upper humeral indentations resulting from recurrent dislocations of the shoulder; involves moving insertion of the subscapularis tendon (one of the rotator cuff tendons) into the defect. 3. For repair of a partial tear of the rotator cuff; involves chiseling out a piece of tendon in order to access the tear.

McMurray osteotomy. *Surgical procedure*. For nonunion of the femoral neck. A cut is made in the area of the lesser trochanter of the femur to realign the proximal femur, so that weightbearing acts to compress the area of the fracture, causing healing.

McMurray sign. *Clinical sign*. Foot is rotated with knee bent and then extended. A clicking sensation indicates a possible tear of the meniscus in the knee.

meclofenamate (mee-kloh-FEN-am-ate). *Drug*. NSAID for treating pain and inflammation. Trade name: Meclomen.

Meclomen. *Drug*. A trade name of meclofenamate, NSAID for treating pain and inflammation.

medial (MEE-dee-ul). *Anatomic description*. Toward the midline. See also LATERAL.

m. femoral circumflex artery (SUR-kum-fleks). *Anatomy*. Branch of the femoral artery below the inguinal ligament; supplies the bottom of the femoral neck and part of the femoral head.

m. calcar (KAL-cahr), **calcar femorale**. *Pathologic condition*. Dense area of bone. Also, a spur or osteophyte (bony outgrowth at the edge of a joint).

m. collateral ligament. *Anatomy*. Connective tissue attachment that gives stability to the inner side of a joint. In the knee and toes, called the tibial collateral ligament, and in the elbow and fingers, called the ulnar collateral ligaments.

m. epicondyle (ep-ee-KAHN-dile). *Anatomy*. Prominence on outer side of some long bones.

m. epicondylitis, golfer's elbow (MEE-dee-ul ep-ee-kahn-duh-LI-tus). *Pathologic condition*. Inflammation of the small bony prominence at the elbow joint. Caused by overuse or trauma; pain may occur with muscle contraction.

m. inferior genicular artery. *Anatomy*. Branch of popliteal artery at the knee joint; supplies inner side of the proximal tibia (shinbone) and associated ligaments.

m. malleolus (mal-EE-oh-lus). *Anatomy*. Prominence on inner side of the distal end of the tibia (shinbone) that articulates with the talus (top foot bone) at the ankle joint; stabilizes the inner side of the ankle.

m. superior genicular artery. *Anatomy*. Branch of the popliteal artery; supplies the distal portion of the inner side of the femur (thighbone).

median nerve. *Anatomy*. Nerve that supplies the front of the thumb, index, long finger, and the radial side of the ring finger, as well as the intrinsic muscles of the thumb (small muscles that move thumb).

Medical Research Council Scale for Muscle Strength. *Classification scheme*. Five-point grading system: grade 0, absence of any contraction; grade 1, some visible sign of muscular contraction (a flicker); grade 2, some movement of the tested portion; grade 3, the ability to move a joint through a full range of motion against gravity; grade 4, active movement of a joint against gravity plus resistance; grade 5, normal muscle strength.

medulla (meh-DUHL-uh) *Anatomy*. The central portion of a bone or organ.

medullary (MED-yu-lehr-ee). *Anatomic description*. Refers to the marrow or soft marrow-like material in the center of a bone (medulla).

m. canal. *Anatomy*. The marrow and fat-filled canal within a long bone.

m. nail /or/ **pin** /or/ **rod**. *Surgical implant*. Nail inserted within the medullary canal of a long bone, to give stability at a fracture or osteotomy site.

mefenamic acid (mee-fee-NAM-ik). *Drug*. NSAID for treating pain and inflammation. Trade name: Ponstel.

Mehta angle, rib vertebral angle difference. *Radiologic test*. Method for predicting whether a curve in infantile idiopathic scoliosis will progress (get larger). The difference between the rib vertebral angles (RVA) of either rib corresponds to the apical vertebra of a scoliotic curve. If the RVA difference is greater than 20°, the curve is likely to progress. See also RIB VERTEBRALL ANGLE.

Meige's disease (mehj). *Pathologic condition*. Type of familial lymphedema (swelling); permanent fluid in the tissues, causing pitting in the legs. Hereditary; onset at puberty. See also MILROY'S DISEASE.

melorheostosis (mel-or-ee-ahs-TOH-sus). *Pathologic condition*. Rare form of hyperostosis (abnormal bone thickening), with unilateral, linear distribution of bone along the long axis, resembling melting wax. Appears in children or young adults; presents with progressive pain and stiffness, limitation of motion or contractures of the fingers. May be associated with linear scleroderma.

meloxicam (mel-AHKS-ih-cam). *Drug.* NSAID for treating pain and inflammation. Trade name: Mobic.

meningocoele (men-IN-goh-seel). *Congenital abnormality.* Form of spina bifida. Absence of posterior elements of the spine, allowing protrusion (as a sac) of the lining of the brain or spinal cord under the skin. Neurological involvement.

meningomyelocoele (men-in-goh-MI-loh-seel), **myelodysplasia**, **myelomeningocoele**. *Congenital abnormality.* Severe form of spina bifida. Congenital absence of the posterior elements of the spine, allowing protrusion (in form of a sac) of the lining of the brain and spinal cord under the skin and exposing the nerve tissues. Complete loss of neurological function below the level of the abnormality.

meniscal (men-ISS-kul). *Anatomic description.* Referring to a meniscus.

    m. tear. *Pathologic condition.* Causes pain, catching of the knee, and swelling of the knee.

meniscectomy (men-iss-KEK-toh-mee). *Surgical procedure.* Removal of a meniscus (semilunar cartilage of knee) and torn meniscus fragments.

meniscus (men-ISS-kus). *Anatomy.* Wedge-shaped cartilage that acts as a buffer between the femur (thighbone) and tibia (shinbone). Plural: menisci.

    lateral m. *Anatomy.* The outer cartilaginous disc within the knee joint.

        discoid. *Pathologic condition.* Solid cartilage within the knee joint between the femur and tibia, covering the whole outer joint surface of the tibia rather than only its periphery; gives the meniscus an abnormal round shape (as opposed to its usual half-moon shape).

    medial m. *Anatomy.* The inner cartilaginous disc within the knee joint.

merchant view. *Radiologic technique.* X-ray of the knee with patient lying face up and knee bent, so the x-ray beam skims front of knee. Used for evaluating conditions of the patella. See also CONGRUENCE ANGLE, SULCUS ANGLE.

Merzbacher Pelizaeus disease (MERTZ-bah-kur pel-itz-AY-os), **hereditary cerebral leukodystrophy**. *Pathologic condition.* Deterioration of the white matter of the central nervous system marked by progressive sclerosis of the frontal lobes of the brain. Hereditary.

metacarpal (met-uh-KAHR-pul). *Anatomy.* Refers to the metacarpus.

    m. bone: any of the five bones in the hand that span from the wrist to the fingers; their far ends form the knuckles. Numbered from 1–5 (e.g., MC1), beginning from the thumb side.

    m. heads, **knuckles**: prominences produced by the metacarpophalangeal joints in the hand. Serve as the location for joining with the phalanges (1st, most proximal, of the finger bones).

metacarpophalangeal joint (met-uh-KAHR-po-fuh-LAN-jee-ul). *Anatomy.* Junction in the hand between the distal end of a metacarpal bone and a proximal phalanx of a finger or thumb.

metacarpus (met-uh-KAHR-pul). *Anatomy.* The area between the wrist and the fingers.

metachromatic leukodystrophy (lu-koh-DIS-troh-fee), **sulfatide lipidosis**, **sulfatidosis**. *Pathologic condition.* Lipid storage disease characterized by abnormal accumulation of fat molecules (sulphatide lipids) with a sulphur chain. Progressive deterioration of central nervous system, with loss of ability to walk, speech difficulty usually about age 1, death by age 10. Autosomal recessive. Most common leukodystrophy in childhood.

metaphyseal (muh-taf-uh-SEE-ul). *Anatomic description.* Refers to the metaphysis (flared end of a long bone).

m. chondrodysplasia (kahn-droh-dis-PLAY-zjuh), **m. dysostosis**. *Congenital abnormality.* Abnormality of bone formation affecting the growth plates; results in a short stature dwarf with a characteristic peculiar face and severe metaphyseal abnormalities. Three types:

> **Jansen type**: autosomal dominant form characterized by severe shortening of the limbs, prominent forehead, small jaw, markedly flared metaphyses, bowing of lower extremities, high blood calcium levels, and mental retardation.

> **McKusick type**, **cartilage hair hypoplasia**: characterized by bowed legs, short, broad hands, stubby fingers, ligamentous laxity, light blond hair. Autosomal recessive transmission; seen frequently in Amish population. Associated with intestinal malabsorption and atlantoaxial instability.

> **Schmid type**: appears at about 2–3 years of age; characterized by a short stature, genu varum, lumbar lordosis, a waddling gait, and coxa vara. Transmitted in an autosomal dominant pattern and appears to be due to a defect in type X collagen formation.

m. dysostosis (di-us-TOH-sus). See METAPHYSEAL CHONDRODYSPLASIA.

m. dysplasia (dis-PLAY-zjuh), **Pyle's disease**. *Abnormal condition.* Abnormality of bone remodeling process: remodeling does not occcur with growth. X-ray changes include abnormally flared metaphyses.

metaphysis (muh-TAF-uh-sus). *Anatomy.* Junction of the diaphysis (shaft) and epiphysis (growth center) of a long bone. Plural: metaphyses.

metastasis (met-ASS-tuh-sus). *Pathologic condition.* Transfer of disease-producing cells or microorganisms from a disease site to another part of the body, producing similar disease in the new location.

metatarsal (met-uh-TAHR-sul). *Anatomy.* Refers to the metatarsus.

m. bones (MT). Any one of the five small long bones that form the base and ball of the foot; numbered 1 to 5 beginning from the medial side.

metatarsalgia (met-uh-tahr-SAL-jee-uh). *Abnormal condition.* Pain in the metatarsus. The term covers a group of foot disorders.

metatarsophalangeal (MTP) joint (met-uh-TAHR-soh-fal-AN-jee-ul). *Anatomy.* Junction in the foot between the distal ends of a metatarsal bone and the proximal phalanx (toes).

metatarsus (met-uh-TAHR-sus). *Anatomy.* The forefoot. The area extending distally from the cuneiforms and cuboid bones; includes the five metatarsal bones and the bones of the toes.

m. adductus. *Abnormal condition.* A forefoot that turns inward (toward the midline).

m. atavicus (uh-TAV-ik-us). *Abnormal condition.* An abnormally short 1st metatarsal; leads to big toe that turns in. May be genetic.

m. primus varus (PREE-mus VEHR-us). *Abnormal condition.* Forefoot characterized by a first ray (1st metatarsal bone) that turns in, away from the longitudinal axis of the foot.

m. varus (VEHR-us). *Abnormal condition.* Metatarsal bones that turn in, away from the longitudinal axis of the foot.

metatropic dwarf (met-uh-TROH-pik). *Congenital anomaly.* Form of dwarfism characterized by increasing severity of deformity with growth.

methylmethacrylate (meth-ul-muh-THAK-roh-layt). *Orthopedic supply.* Cement used for fixing a prosthesis to bone.

methyprednisolone. *Drug.* Cortisone derative. For treating inflammatory and allergic diseases.

Meyerding and Van Demark technique. *Surgical procedure.* Technique for removal of a Baker's cyst (protrusion of knee joint capsule behind the knee).

micromelic dwarf (mi-kroh-MEE-lik). *Abnormal condition.* Form of dwarfism associated with short arms.

microwave diathermy. *Treatment.* Using microwaves to elevate temperature within the tissues.

midaxillary line. *Anatomic description.* Imaginary line (reference point) drawn down the side of the body from the armpit to the iliac crest.

middle third. *Location.* If a bone is divided into thirds (proximal, middle, distal), the middle third is the central part.

midsagittal plane (mid-SAJ-uh-tul). *Anatomic description.* Imaginary line drawn through the body from the head to the pelvis dividing the body into right and left halves. Used as a reference point for descriptive purposes.

midtarsal joint, **tarsometatarsal joint**, **Lisfranc joint**. *Anatomy.* Joint complex between the metatarsal and tarsal bones (the cuneiforms and the cuboid).

Milch classification. *Fracture classification.* Identifies break patterns in pediatric lateral condyle fractures.

milk-alkali syndrome, **Burnett's syndrome**. *Pathologic condition.* Chronic disorder of the kidneys induced by long-term therapy of a peptic ulcer with alkalis and milk. Causes osteoporosis (porous bone).

Miller procedure. *Surgical procedure.* Fusion of the navicular, first cuniform, and base of first metatarsal bone to form an arch, to correct a flatfoot.

Milroy's disease. *Congenital disorder.* Type of familial lymphedema; permanent fluid in tissues causing pitting in legs. Hereditary. See also MEIGE'S DISEASE.

Milwaukee brace. *Orthopedic appliance.* Brace for treating adolescent idiopathic scoliosis in a growing child. Has a pelvic portion (girdle-like), a neck ring, and a frame with pads to push the trunk in various directions to correct curvature.

Minerva jacket. *Orthopedic appliance.* Body cast that includes the trunk and head, with ears and face left open; used for treating spine deformities.

mini-incision surgery (MIS). *Surgical technique.* Surgical procedures performed with specialized techniques and instrumentation that allow particularly small incisions. Can apply to knee replacement or hip replacement.

"ministroke," transient ischemic attack (TIA). *Pathologic condition.* Temporary interruption in the circulation to a portion of the brain, causing dysfunction of the affected section of the brain. Resolves spontaneously.

Mitchell procedure. *Surgical procedure.* To correct a bunion: a cut is made at the distal end of the 1st metatarsal bone so it can be shifted laterally to correct malalignment.

Mobic. *Drug.* A trade name of meloxicam, NSAID for treating pain and inflammation.

modularity, modular implant. *Surgical implant design.* Describes certain endoprostheses in which some of its segments are available in interchangeable sizes so as to allow for the final implant to more closely fit the patient's particular anatomy and shape.

Moe arthrodesis. *Surgical procedure.* Type of spinal fusion.

mold arthroplasty, Smith-Petersen arthroplasty. *Surgical procedure.* Creation of a new joint by interposing inert material (plastic, metal, etc.) between the reshaped ends of bones.

mongolism, Down syndrome, trisomy 21. *Congenital abnormality.* Presence of three #21 chromosomes; associated with mental retardation, hyperelasticity, heart disease, oblique eyelids, flat skull and flattened facial features.

monoarticular (mahn-oh-ahr-TIK-yu-lur). *Anatomy.* Involving one joint.

monobloc implant. *Orthopedic implant design.* Refers to artifical joint components that are made in one piece, with no interchangeable parts. Seen in some models for knee, hip, and shoulder replacements. See also MODULARITY.

mononeuropathy (mohn-oh-nur-AHP-uh-thee). *Pathologic condition.* Damage or disease affecting one nerve. See also PERIPHERAL NEUROPATHY.

monoplanar external fixator, uniplanar external fixator. *Orthopedic implant.* Device used to stabilize fractures and osteotomies; relies on threaded pins placed onto the bone fragments and attached to a linear, external frame.

monoplegia (mahn-oh-PLE-jee-uh). *Abnormal condition.* Paralysis of one limb.

monostotic fibrous dysplasia (mah-noh-STAH-tik, dis-PLAY-zjuh). *Abnormal condition.* Form of fibrous dysplasia: affects only a single bone.

Montacelli classification. *Disease classification.* Identifies (with x-rays) combinations of coxa valga and femoral anteversion in its relationship to acetabular dysplasia and subluxation of the hip.

Montacelli procedure. *Surgical procedure.* Femoral osteotomy to correct angulation and rotation of the proximal femur (thighbone).

Monteggia fracture (mahn-TEJ-yuh), **parry fracture**. *Pathologic condition.* Break in the ulna (smaller forearm bone) with dislocation of the head of the radius (larger forearm bone). See also BADO CLASSIFICATION.

Montreal frame. *Orthopedic appliance.* Base board with slots designed to fit prefabricated pegs. Used for holding a patient on his/her side during surgery.

Morquio's disease/syndrome (MOHR-kee-ohz), **Brailsford-Morquio disease**, **Morquio-Ullrich disease**, **type IV mucopolysaccharidosis**. *Pathologic condition.* One of a series of hereditary chemical disorders called mucopolysaccharidoses. Results in normal-appearing newborns who develop into short trunk dwarfs (final height 50 inches) with progressive hip disease, joint laxity, atlantoaxial instability and cloudy corneas, with normal faces and intellect.

Morquio-Ullrich disease. (MOHR-kee-oh). See MORQUIO'S DISEASE.

mortise view. *Radiologic test.* An internally rotated view of the ankle joint so that the articulation between the talus (top foot bone) and tibia (shinbone) can be visualized from the frontal x-ray projection.

Morton foot. *Anatomic description.* Foot whose 1st metartasal is shorter than the 2nd. May be painful when pressure of forefoot is applied on 2nd metatarsal.

Morton's neuroma, interdigital neuroma. *Pathologic condition.* Area of painful enlargement of a nerve between the toes. See also MORTON'S TOE.

Morton's syndrome. *Pathologic condition.* Shortening of the 1st metatarsal bone with pain between the heads of the other metatarsal bones.

Morton's test. Pressure is placed across the metatarsal heads; sharp pain indicates the presence of Morton's neuroma.

Morton's toe. *Pathologic condition.* Sharp pain felt between the toes and on ball of the foot upon walking; occurs when two metatarsal bones, most frequently the 3rd and 4th, irritate the interdigital nerve. See also MORTON'S NEUROMA.

motor neuron, anterior horn cell. *Anatomy.* Cell located on the front side of the spinal cord; innervates the proximal muscles.

motor neuron disease, amyotrophic lateral sclerosis (ALS), Charcot's disease, Lou Gehrig disease. *Pathologic condition.* Progressive degenerative disease of the spinal cord nerves that control motor function (the muscles); leads to gait and motor abnormalities and eventually death.

Motrin. *Drug.* Trade name of ibuprofen, NSAID for treating pain and inflammation.

mould arthroplasty. See MOLD ARTHROPLASTY.

MRI (magnetic resonance imaging). *Diagnostic test.* Type of imaging technique using high intensity magnets and computers; permits visualization of soft tissues inside the body that cannot be seen with x-rays. See also CT SCAN.

mucopolysaccharidosis (myu-koh-pah-lee-sak-ur-ih-DOH-sus). *Pathologic condition.* Series of hereditary disorders of mucopolysaccharide (complex sugar) metabolism, the effects and severity of which are determined by the specific enzyme affected. Leads to multiple abnormalities including scoliosis, coarse features and mental retardation. The group includes the following syndromes: Hunter's, Hurler's, Morquio's, Sanfilippo, and Scheie's.

mucopurulent (myu-koh-PYUR-yu-lunt). *Description.* Any exudate that has a mucus appearance and appears to be infected.

Müller osteotomy *Surgical procedure.* An intertrochanteric osteotomy of the proximal femur (thighbone) to change the weight-bearing area of the femoral head in the hip joint.

multangular bone (mul-TANG-yu-lur). *Anatomy.* One of the two cubic-shaped bones of the wrist.

> **greater m., trapezium**: four-sided bone in the wrist at base of the thumb.

> **lesser m., trapezoid**: small bone in the wrist, between the trapezium and capitate; opposite the 2nd metacarpal bone.

multiplanar external fixation. *Orthopedic implant.* Device for stabilizing fractures or osteotomies. Pins or wires are applied into bone fragments from different directions around the extremity, then attached to a frame outside the body. See also ILIZAROV EXTERNAL FIXATION, SMALL WIRE EXTERNAL FIXATOR.

multiple epiphseal dysplasia, (eh-pih-FIZ-ee-ul dis-PLAY-zjuh, **dysplasia epiphysealis multiplex**. *Congenital abnormality.* Abnormality at ends of the long bones, causing difficulty in walking, joint deformities and pain, short stubby fingers, and short limb dwarfism. The condition tends to spare the spine. Two types: Fairbank and Ribbing (less severe). Hereditary.

multiple hereditary exostoses (eks-ahs-TOH-seez). *Abnormal condition.* Large bony protuberances around joints. Slight chance of becoming malignant. Hereditary.

multiple myeloma (mi-uh-LO-muh), **myeloma, plasma cell myeloma, plasmacytoma**. *Pathologic condition.* Most common primary neoplasm (malignant new growth) of bone, with lesions most common in the spine, pelvis and skull; may lead to pathological fractures (may appear on x-ray as holes in the bone). Occurs usually after the 5th decade.

Mumford procedure, distal clavicular resection. *Surgical procedure.* Removal of the outer end of the clavicle (collarbone); for treating pain from acromioclavicular arthritis.

muscle. *Anatomy.* Tissue composed of contractile fibers that, by contracting and relaxing, cause motion.

> **extensor m.**: causes the attached part to straighten.

> **flexor m.**: causes the attached part to bend.

> **intrinsic m.**: small muscles of hands and feet that abduct and adduct the fingers and toes.

> **involuntary m.**: same as SMOOTH (below).

> **skeletal m.**: same as STRIATED (below).

> **smooth m.**: type of muscle found in organs that cause the organ to contract and relax; involuntary in its actions and is not attached to bone.

> **striated m.**: serrated (not smooth) type of muscle, under voluntary

control and attached to bone or connective tissue; responsible for moving different body parts, e.g., arms, legs.

voluntary m.: same as STRIATED (above).

muscle strength, Medical Research Council scale. Grade 0, absence of any contraction; grade 1, some visible sign of muscular contraction (a flicker); grade 2, some movement of tested portion; grade 3, ability to move a joint through a full range of motion against gravity; grade 4, active movement of a joint against gravity plus resistance; grade 5, normal muscle strength.

muscular dystrophy, Duchenne's muscular dystrophy /or/ **paralysis, pseudohypertrophic dystrophy**. *Pathologic condition*. Progressive weakness of the voluntary muscles. Onset generally before age 3, with frequent falls, difficulty getting up, and enlargement of the calf muscles. Hereditary, sex-linked (males); females are carriers. Death before age 25.

    Becker's m.: milder form; onset is in the latter half of the first decade of life and patients can live into adulthood.

    facioscapulohumeral m. (fas-ee-oh-skap-yu-loh-HYU-mur-ul), **Landouzy-Déjérine disease**: mild, common form; results in loss of arm strength, especially around the shoulder, with wasting of the shoulder girdle muscles, and loss of ability to smile.

musculocutaneous nerve (mus-kyu-loh-kyu-TAY-nee-us). *Anatomy*. Nerve in the arm, below shoulder; supplies biceps and part of brachialis muscle before exiting the fascia and supplying volar and lateral portions of the forearm skin.

Mustard iliopsoas transfer (il-ee-oh-SOH-us). *Surgical procedure*. Moving the iliopsoas muscle from an intrapelvic position, through the iliac wing, to a lateral position on the greater trochanter, to act as an abductor instead of a flexor of the hip. Used in paralytic patients lacking hip abduction strength. Similar to Sharrard iliopsoas transfer.

myasthenia angiosclerotica, Charcot's syndrome, intermittent claudication, vascular claudication. *condition*. Limping caused by insufficient blood supply to the leg muscles when blood vessels are constricted or obliterated, such as in diabetes or arteriosclerosis.

myasthenia gravis (mi-us-THEE-nee-uh GRAV-us). *Pathologic condition*. Progressive muscular weakness secondary to an abnormality at the myoneural junction.

myelocoele (MI-loh-seel). *Abnormal condition*. In spina bifida, protrusion of the spinal cord through a defect in the posterior elements of the spine. Usually associated with some paralysis of the upper or lower extremities.

myelodysplasia (mi-loh-dis-PLAY-zjuh). See MYELOMENINGOCOELE.

myelogram (MI-lo-gram). *Radiologic test*. X-ray picture taken after injection of radiopaque dye into the dura; for spinal cord evaluation.

    cervical m.: x-ray of the cervical spine (neck area) after injection of dye.

    lumbar m.: x-ray of the lumbar spine after injection of dye.

myelography (mi-LAHG-ruh-fee). *Radiologic test*. X-ray evaluation of the spinal cord by injection of radiopaque dye into the dura, to outline the contents of the spinal canal.

myeloma (mi-uh-LO-muh). See MULTIPLE MYELOMA.

myelomeningocoele (mi-lo-muh-NIN-go-seel), **meningomyelocoele, myelodysplasia**. *Congenital abnormality*. Form of spine bifida. Congenital absence of the posterior elements of the spine, allowing protrusion (in form of a sac) of the lining of the brain and spinal cord under the skin and exposing nerve tissues. Complete loss of neurological function below level of the abnormality.

myelopathy (mi-LAH-puh-thee). *Abnormal condition.* Abnormality of the spinal cord secondary to extrinsic pressure (e.g., a herniated disc) or associated with radiation damage or diabetic myelopathy.

myo- (MI-oh). *Prefix.* Muscle (myofibril: muscle fiber).

myoelectric prosthesis (mi-oh-ee-LEK-trik). *Orthopedic appliance.* Artificial limb with surface electrodes that attach batteries to remnants of the stump muscles. Contracting the muscles allows electric activity to activate the batteries and enable the limb to function. Most commonly used in the upper extremity to reproduce hand function.

myofibril (mi-oh-FI-brul). *Anatomy.* Muscle fiber.

myofibrosis (mi-oh-fi-BROH-sus). *Abnormal condition.* Scarring within a muscle.

myolysis (mi-oh-LI-sus). *Abnormal function.* Breakdown of muscle.

myoma (mi-OH-muh). *Pathologic condition.* Benign tumor of muscle tissue. Various types.

myoneural (mi-oh-NUR-ul). *Anatomic description.* Refers to the junction between nerve endings and muscle fibers.

myopathy (mi-AH-puh-thee). *Pathologic condition.* General term for an abnormal condition or disease of muscle tissue.

myositis (mi-oh-SI-tus). *Pathologic condition.* Inflammation of muscle.

myositis ossificans (oh-SIF-ih-kans), **heterotopic bone formation, heterotopic ossification**. *Pathologic condition. A* disease of muscle in which bone is created within the muscle. Most often associated with trauma, prolonged comas, high calcium concentrations in the blood, and certain surgeries. Leads to stiffness in the joint around the muscle.

    m. ossificans progressiva (proh-gres-EE-vuh): muscle disease in which there is progressive deposition of calcified material. Often fatal.

myotonia congenita (benign) (mi-oh-TOH-nee-uh kun-JEN-uh-tuh), **amyotonia congenita, Oppenheim's syndrome**. *Abnormal condition.* Rare disorder affecting newborns, characterized by muscle weakness and decreased muscle tone. Normal lab data and imaging studies; apparent normal alertness. Usually improves spontaneously. See also FLOPPY BABY SYNDROME.

myotonic dystrophy (mi-uh-TAHN-ik DIS-troh-fee), **dystrophic myotonia, Steinert's disease**. *Pathologic condition.* Muscle weakness in the face, neck and distal extremities. Patients usually present with weakness of the hands and difficulty walking or tendency to fall. Many die young from pulmonary-cardiac failure; they are especially at risk during anesthesia. Hereditary.

myxoid chondrosarcoma (MIKS-oyd kon-dro-sahr-KOH-muh), **chondromyxosarcoma**. *Pathologic condition.* Malignant cartilaginous tumor containing mucus elements.

myxoma (miks-OH-muh). *Pathologic condition.* Benign tumor of connective tissue; under the microscope, starlike cells are imbedded in a soft matrix having a mucoid appearance.

N

nabumetone. *Drug*. NSAID for treating pain and inflammation. Trade name: Relafen.

Nalfon. *Drug*. Trade name of fenoprofen, NSAID for treating pain and inflammation.

Naffziger syndrome, Scalenus anticus syndrome. *Pathologic condition*. Compression of the brachial plexus and the artery between an enlarged scalenus anticus muscle and the 1st thoracic rib. Pain and cramping may occur in the arm when the arms are held upright. Treatment consists of cutting the scalenus muscle.

nail, rod. *Surgical implant*. Metallic rod used to attach the fragments of broken bones. See also PIN.

    intramedullary n: placed within the center canal (marrow) of a long bone to fasten together the ends of a fracture or osteotomy.

nail fold. *Anatomy*. The rounded surface of skin along the sides of each fingernail and toenail.

nail-patella syndrome (puh-TEL-uh), **onycho-osteodysplasia**. *Pathologic condition*. Growth disturbances of the bones and the fingernails, toenails and toes. The patella may have an abnormal shape, leading to dislocation. May include webbing of the elbow, preventing full extension, and occasionally, scoliosis. Renal disease is significant. Hereditary (autosomal dominant).

naphthylalkalones. *Drug*. Class of NSAIDs (nonsteroidal anti-inflammatory drugs).

Naprelan. *Drug*. A trade name of naproxen, NSAID for treating pain and inflammation.

Naprosyn. *Drug*. A trade name of naproxen, NSAID for treating pain and inflammation.

naproxen (nuh-PRAHKS-en). *Drug*. NSAID for treating pain and inflammation. Also reduces fever. Trade name: Aleve.

navicular (nuh-VIK-yu-lur). *Anatomy*. Bone in the wrist and foot; so named for its boat-like appearance. In the wrist the bone is also called the scaphoid.

    accessory n. bone. *Pathologic condition*. Small secondary center of ossification in the tendon of the tibialis posterior as it inserts on the tarsal navicular. Its presence may lead to pain and tenderness. Sometimes thought to represent a normal variant.

    carpal n., scaphoid. *Anatomy*. One of eight bones that make up the wrist; largest bone in the first row of carpal bones, at the end of the radius.

    tarsal n. *Anatomy*. Bone in the foot, between the talus (top foot bone) and the 1st cunieform on the medial side.

neck righting reflex. *Clinical sign*. In infancy, spontaneous adjustment of body position in response to a change in head position. Absence of reflex indicates severe delay in development.

neck shaft angle. *Measurement*. Angle formed by the femoral (thighbone) neck and shaft, normally 130–140°.

necrosis (nuh-KROH-sus). *Pathologic condition*. Death of tissue.

    avascular n., aseptic n.: loss of circulation to a body part or area, leading to bone or tissue death.

needle. *Surgical device*. Elongated, pointed device used to traverse tissue, usually to pass suture material through tissue when repairing a wound. An alphanumeric system is used to described size and shape.

    cutting n.: tip is sharpened so that it cuts through tissue as it is passed.

    Keith n.: type of straight needle.

Mayo n.: type of curved needle with an eyelet on its backside to allow for a suture to be manually loaded onto it.

tapered n.: tip is blunted so that it burrows through tissue as it is passed.

needle biopsy. *Surgical procedure*. Removal of tissue with a needle for microscopic evaluation.

Neer classification. *Fracture classification*. Identifies different fracture patterns across the proximal humerus based on degree of comminution (fragmentation) and displacement.

Neer prosthesis. *Orthopedic appliance*. Artificial replacement for the proximal humerus (upper armbone) at the shoulder.

Neest (dysplasia, syndrome). Incorrect spelling of KNIEST.

negative Babinski. *Diagnostic sign*. Normal, involuntary lowering of the big toe and closing together of the other toes as the sole of the foot is firmly stroked.

Nélaton's dislocation (NAY-luh-tonz). *Abnormal condition*. Dislocation of the talus (top foot bone) from severe injury that has disrupted the ligaments between the tibia and fibula and displaced the talus within the joint.

Nélaton's line (NAY-luh-tonz). *Clinical sign*. Imaginary line from the anterior superior iliac spine to the ischial tuberosity; when the greater trochanter does not fall on this line, it indicates a possible dislocation of the hip or fracture of the femoral neck.

neonate. A newly born infant, usually less than 1 or 2 days old.

neoplasm (NEE-oh-plaz-um), **tumor**. *Pathologic condition*. New, abnormal growth; may be benign or malignant.

neoplastic fracture (nee-oh-PLAS-tik). *Pathologic condition*. Break in an area of bone weakened by a tumor.

nerve. *Anatomy*. Bundle of neurons that transmits electrochemical impulses from the central nervous system to body tissues.

　　n. cable graft, **nerve** /or/ **cable graft**. *Surgical technique*. Transfer of a portion of a peripheral, expendable sensory nerve to repair a defect in an important nerve. A segment is removed from the nerve and sutured into defect.

　　n. conduction test. *Electrophysiologic test*. Measure of the speed and quality of a nerve impulse as it travels through a nerve. Abnormally slow or weak signals indicate a nerve injury or disease.

　　n. conduction velocity (NCV). *Physiologic finding*. The speed an impulse travels along a nerve; abnormal velocities may be indicative of peripheral nerve damage. See also ELECTROMYOGRAM, NERVE CONDUCTION TEST.

　　n. graft. See NERVE CABLE GRAFT (above).

　　n. tract. *Anatomy*. Bundle of nerve fibers that travel together along the brain or spinal cord. In general, those along the front of the spinal cord are responsible for motor activity, and those at the back are responsible for sensation.

nervous system. *Anatomy*. Compilation of organs and tissues whose purpose is to control and coordinate the functions and movements of the body.

　　autonomic, visceral efferent: maintains the resting function and state of readiness of the body and organ systems. Composed of two, generally antagonistic subsystems: sympathetic and parasympathetic nervous systems.

　　sympathetic: part of the autonomic system that provides quick energy and response.

　　parasympathetic: part of the autonomic system that maintains resting body function and restores energy reserves.

Neufeld nail (NU-feld). *Surgical implant*. Nail used for repair of introchanteric fractures of the proximal femur (thighbone).

neumatic. Incorrect spelling of PNEUMATIC.

neural arch, vertebral arch. *Anatomy.* The bony arch at the back of a vertebra that surrounds the spinal cord.

neuralgia (nu-RAL-juh). *Pathologic condition.* A throbbing or stabbing pain in the distribution of a nerve.

neuralgic amyotrophy. *Pathologic condition.* Atrophy of a muscle due to dysfunction of its nerve.

neuraxon, axon. *Anatomy.* The long tail of a nerve cell; conducts nerve impulses away from the cell.

neurectomy (nu-REK-toh-mee). *Surgical procedure.* Cutting a segment from a nerve, to eliminate function. Used in cerebral palsy patients to decrease the spasticity of a muscle.

neuritis (nu-RI-tus). *Pathologic condition.* Inflammation of a nerve; leads to neuralgia.

neurofibril. *Intracellular anatomy.* Small structure within a nerve cell giving it its structural integrity and support.

neurofibroma (nu-roh-fi-BRO-muh). *Pathologic condition.* Abnormality or tumor of Schwann cells in a nerve, enlarging the nerve. Can result in severe disability.

neurofibromatosis (NF) (nu-roh-fi-bro-muh-TOH-sus). *Pathologic condition.* Hereditary disease characterized by the appearance of neurofibromas (soft tissue tumors). Two types are recognized.

> **type I (NFI), von Recklinghausen's disease**: more common type, syndrome consisting of the appearance of multiple neurofibromas, specific bony abnormalities, abnormally pigmented lesions of the skin (e.g., café-au-lait spots, axillary freckling) leading to gross malformations and dysfunction. Begins in early childhood or (rarely) in infancy.

> **type II (NFII)**: less common form, characterized by the appearance of acoustic neuromas and tumors of the 8th cranial nerve.

neurogenic (nu-ro-JEN-ik). *Anatomic description.* Originating from the nervous system.

> **n. fracture**. *Pathologic condition.* A break through an area of bone weakened by disuse; associated with neurologic disease or caused by repetitive overstressing of the bone secondary to poor pain perception.

neurology (nu-RAH-luh-jee). *Science.* Study of the nervous system and its abnormalities.

neurolysis (nu-roh-LI-sus). *Surgical procedure.* Removal of a scar around a nerve.

neuroma (nu-ROH-muh). Large accumulation of nerve fibers in a localized area, from trauma to a nerve.

neuropathy (nu-RAH-puh-thee). *Pathologic condition.* Any disorder affecting a nerve.

> **peripheral**: damage or disease affecting one or more peripheral nerves. When affecting only one nerve, it is referred to as a mononeuropathy; when affecting many, it is called a polyneuropathy.

neuropraxia (nu-roh-PRAKS-ee-uh). *Pathologic condition.* Traumatic lesion in a nerve that interrupts transmission of electronic impulses.

neurorrhaphy (nu-ROHR-uh-fee). *Surgical procedure.* Repairing a nerve by suturing the segments together.

neurotmesis (nu-raht-MEE-sus). *Abnormal condition.* Complete transection (cut through) of a nerve.

neurovascular (nu-roh-VAS-kyu-lur). *Anatomic description.* Involving both nerves and blood vessels.

Newfeld nail. Incorrect spelling of NEUFELD NAIL.

newmatic. Incorrect spelling of PNEUMATIC.

Nicola procedure. *Surgical procedure.* Repair for recurrent dislocation of the shoulder. The biceps tendon is converted into a restraining ligament for the head of the humerus (upper armbone).

Nicoll graft procedure. *Surgical procedure.* Transfer of cancellous bone to an area where a fractured bone has failed to unite; held in place by plates or wires.

nidus (NI-dus). *Anatomic description.* The focal point of development. May be normal (as the origin of a nerve) or abnormal (as the focus of infection).

Niemann-Pick disease, **sphingomyelolipidosis**. *Pathologic condition.* Severe form of lipid storage disease. There is growth impairment with progressive neurological deterioration, enlargement of the liver and spleen, and cherry red spots or grayish haze in the retina. Death by age 3. A more benign form occurs rarely in adults.

nightstick fracture. *Pathologic condition.* A break in the midshaft ulna (smaller forearm bone) resulting from a direct blow.

90-90 traction. *Treatment.* With the hip and knees bent 90°, a pin is placed in the distal femur for traction; used for fractures in the femur (thighbone).

nodes (gouty). *Pathologic finding.* Small nodules of inflammatory tissue surrounding uric acid crystals under the skin.

nodes, lymph nodes. *Anatomy.* Mass of lymphocytes found in various locations along lymph vessels; serve as a filter of tissue fluids. Part of body's immune system; when swollen and tender, may indicate infection in that region of the body.

nondisplaced fracture. *Pathologic condition.* Break in a bone in which the fracture segments have not moved from their anatomic position.

noninvasive test. *Diagnostic test.* Test that does not invade or permanently alter human tissues, e.g., MRI.

nonossifying (nahn-AHS-ih-fi-ing). *Anatomic description.* In describing tumors, any lesion that does not create bone. In an x-ray, will appear as a bony defect.

nonsuppurative osteomyelitis (nahn-suh-PUR-uh-tiv ahs-tee-oh-mi-uh-LI-tus). *Pathologic condition.* bone infection with no pus produced.

nonunion. *Pathologic condition.* Broken bone or osteotomy site that has failed to heal or unite. See also DELAYED UNION.

non-weightbearing (NWB). *Activity restriction.* Extremity bearing no weight during walking.

NSAID (nonsteroidal anti-inflammatory drug) (EN-sad). *Drug classification.* Class of pain-relieving drugs that acts to suppress inflammation, especially after injury or strain. Relieves inflammation, swelling, stiffness, joint pain. Not based on the steroid or cortisone molecule. Inhibits the actions of both COX-1 and COX-2 enzymes. Includes aspirin (acetylsalicylic acid) and ibuprofen.

> **conventional**: Any NSAID that is not a COX-2 inhibitor.

nuchal ligament (NU-kul). *Anatomy.* Strong ligament that maintains the alignment of the head and neck. Attaches to the spinous processes of the neck vertebrae. More prominent in quadrapeds in which it supports the head in an upright manner.

nucleus pulposus (pul-POH-sus). *Anatomy.* Central portion of a spinal disc; comprised of gelatinous material surrounded by a connective tissue capsule. Acts as a shock absorber in the spine.

numatic. Incorrect spelling of PNEUMATIC.

Nuprin. *Drug.* A trade name of ibuprofen, NSAID for treating pain and inflammation.

O

Ober technique of anterior transfer of the posterior tibialis tendon. *Surgical procedure*. Treatment for an equinus deformity (ankle pointing down) in a patient with weakness of ankle dorsiflexion. The posterior tibialis tendon is detached from its normal insertion and transferred to the dorsum of the foot, toward the front of the ankle, allowing the posterior tibialis muscle to act as a dorsiflexor of the ankle.

Ober test. *Clinical test*. With the patient lying on one side, the thigh is abducted and extended at the hip; if the bent knee fails to touch the opposite knee, an abduction contracture of the hip is indicated.

Ober-Yount procedure. *Surgical procedure*. Technique for correcting an abduction contracture of the hip. Involves the release of the iliotibial band.

oblique fracture. *Pathologic condition*. Break in a bone at an angle to the long axis.

oblique retinacular ligaments, **Landsmeer ligaments**. *Anatomy*. Small ligaments in the fingers that stabilize the tendons of the interosseous and lumbrical muscles.

obstetrical palsy. *Pathologic condition*. Injury to the area of an infant's brachial plexus resulting from trauma sustained by the nerves during the baby's passage through the birth canal.

obturator (AHB-tu-ray-tur). *Anatomy*. Denotes an opening in the bones of the pelvis, just below the acetabulum (hip socket).

    o. artery: branch of internal iliac artery; supplies portions of the iliac wing and extends into the femur (thighbone), sending a branch to the acetabulum.

    o. foramen (for-AY-men): large hole in lower part of the pelvis (bordered by the ischium, pubis and lower part of acetabulum) through which pass the obturator muscles, nerves and blood vessels.

    o. nerve: nerve comprised of branches from the 2nd, 3rd and 4th lumbar cord; supplies inner and lower parts of the hip, inner femur (thighbone), and the adductor magnus, longus and brevis and pectineus gracilis muscles.

occlusion. *Pathologic condition*. Blockage.

occlusive dressing. *Surgical supply*. Dressing that prevents exposure to the air.

occult fracture. *Pathologic condition*. Break that is hidden or not easily identified.

occupational therapy (OT). *Treatment*. The use of assistive, work and play activities to help individuals achieve or maintain daily living and developmental skills lost as a result of an illness or accident, to achieve maximum independence and to enhance quality of life. See also PHYSICAL THERAPY.

O'Connor technique. *Surgical procedure*. Clearing of soft tissue from area of the sinus tarsi (between talus and calcaneus) to relieve pain. Used for treating sinus tarsi syndrome.

oculocerebrorenal dystrophy (OCRL), **Lowe syndrome**. *Congenital abnormality*. Autosomal recessive abnormality resulting in kidney dysfunction and failure, congenital eye disorders such as cataracts and glaucoma, and severe mental retardation. Death often occurs in childhood.

O'Donoghue facetectomy of the patella (oh-DAHN-uh-hyu). *Surgical procedure*. Removal of the medial (inner) or lateral (outer) third of the patella (kneecap), to treat chondromalacia (degeneration of surface cartilage).

O'Donoghue procedure (oh-DAHN-uh-hyu). *Surgical procedure*. Removing the medial (inner) meniscus to repair the anterior cruciate and medial collateral ligaments. No longer performed.

    for ingrown toenail: removal of the outer fourth of the nail plate and underlying matrix.

O'Donoghue's terrible triad (oh-DAHN-uh-hyu) /or/ **unhappy triad**. *Pathologic condition*. Knee injury: a tear of the medial collateral ligament, anterior cruciate ligament (ACL) and medial meniscus. O'Donoghue described as resulting from a tackle injury; since discovered that most ACL tears in football players result from twisting injuries (sudden change in direction).

odontoid (oh-DAHN-toyd). *Anatomy*. Tooth-shaped; refers to the odontoid process of the 2nd cervical vertebra.

    aplasia of the o. *Congenital abnormality*. Partial or complete absence of the odontoid process.

    o. dysplasia (dis-PLAY-zjuh). *Congenital abnormality*. Incomplete formation of the odontoid process; results in instability and possible damage to the spinal cord.

    o. process, dens process. *Anatomy*. Projection of the 2nd cervical vertebra toward the skull; fits within the ring of the 1st cervical vertebra, in front of the spinal cord.

Ogden classification. *Fracture classification*. Identifies fracture patterns of the tibial tubercle (small bump on shinbone, just below knee) in children.

olecranon (oh-LEK-ruh-nahn). *Anatomy*. The tip of the elbow.

    o. bursa: thin, fluid-filled sac that sits over the olecranon process of the elbow, lubricating the overlying skin.

    o. fossa (FAH-suh): indented surface in the distal end of the humerus (upper armbone), where the olecranon process fits when the arm is extended.

    o. process: the elbow; the large process (projection) of the ulna that projects behind the elbow joint, forming the bony prominence of the elbow.

olive pin. *Orthopedic implant*. Wire with a round bump along its length, used in conjunction with small wire external fixators. The bump serves as a point of resistance when it contacts the bone, allowing it to be moved or compressed against another fragment.

Ollier's disease (OH-lee-ayz), **dyschondroplasia**, **enchondromatosis**. *Pathologic condition*. Multiple benign cartilage tumors, usually within the metaphyses of long bones. Called Maffucci's syndrome when associated with multiple hamartomas (benign blood vessel tumors).

onlay graft. *Surgical procedure/biologic implant*. 1. Laying cortical bone on the outside of a bone, to provide it with structural support. 2. The graft itself.

onycho-osteodysplasia, **nail-patella syndrome**. *Pathologic condition*. Growth disturbances of bones and fingernails, toenails and toes. The patella may be abnormally shaped, leading to dislocation. May include webbing of the elbow, preventing full extension, and occasionally scoliosis. Renal disease is significant. Hereditary (autosomal dominant).

open amputation. *Surgical procedure*. The amputation site is left open to allow for drainage, with a dressing covering the soft tissues and bone. See also CLOSED AMPUTATION.

open biopsy. *Surgical procedure*. Removing bodily tissue or fluid for laboratory examination by making an incision in the skin and soft tissues. See also CLOSED BIOPSY.

open dislocation. *Abnormal condition*. Joint dislocation that has ruptured the skin, exposing bone and tissues to the air. See also CLOSED DISLOCATION.

open fracture, **compound fracture**. *Pathologic condition*. Break in which the bone ends protrude through the skin. "Open" is the newer, preferred term.

open hip reduction. *Surgical procedure*. Opening the joint capsule to maneuver the femoral head back into the acetabulum (hip socket). See also CLOSED HIP REDUCTION.

opening wedge osteotomy (ahs-tee-AH-tuh-mee). *Surgical procedure*.

Changing lignment or shape of a bone by cutting it almost all the way across and rotating the cut open (as on a door hinge); the resulting defect is filled with a wedge of bone. See also CLOSING WEDGE OSTEOTOMY.

open reduction. *Surgical procedure.* Directly manipulating a dislocated or fractured bone or joint back to its normal position with surgical intervention. Involves cutting the skin to grasp the affected bony fragments or structures. See also CLOSED REDUCTION.

opponens bar (uh-POH-nunz). *Orthopedic appliance.* Small curved hand brace that holds the thumb away from the palm and index finger in a position for grasping. Used for patients with paralysis.

opponens digiti minimi of the foot (uh-POH-nunz DIJ-uh-tee MIN-uh-mee). *Anatomy.* Farthest part of flexor digiti minimi of the foot, sometimes described as a separate muscle; arises from the base of the 5th metatarsal bone and inserts onto the outer aspect of the proximal phalanx of the little toe.

opponens digiti minimi of the hand (uh-POH-nunz DIJ-uh-tee MIN-uh-mee), **opponens digiti quinti**. *Anatomy.* Small muscle on the ulnar border of the hand that abducts the little finger. Arises from the hook of the hamate and inserts into the entire 5th metacarpal bone.

opponensplasty (uh-POH-nunz-plas-tee). *Surgical procedure.* Transfer of tendons to provide opposition of the thumb to the fingers. Used for treating paralysis of the opponens pollicis muscles.

opponens pollicis (uh-POH-nunz PAHL-uh-sus). *Anatomy.* Muscle that bends the 1st metacarpal, producing opposition to the thumb. Arises from the area of the trapezium in the wrist and lower border of the flexor retinaculum and inserts into the lateral half of the palmar surface of the 1st metacarpal bone.

Oppenheim's syndrome, myotonia congenita (benign), amyotonia congenita. *Abnormal condition.* Rare disorder affecting newborns, characterized by muscle weakness and decreased muscle tone. Normal lab data and imaging studies; apparent normal alertness. Usually improves spontaneously. Term rarely used due to confusion over exact definition. See also FLOPPY BABY SYNDROME.

origin (of a muscle). *Anatomy.* Bony location from which a muscle takes its root. See also INSERTION.

orthopaedics, orthopedics. *Medical specialty.* Deals with the study and treatment of the musculoskeletal system by medical, surgical and/or physical methods.

orthopaedist, orthopedist, orthopaedic surgeon. *Medical specialist.* Physician specializing in the diagnosis and treatment of the musculoskeletal system (disorders affecting bones and their supporting structures) by medical, surgical and/or physical methods.

orthosis (or-THO-sus), **orthotic**. *Orthopedic appliance.* Brace used to correct an abnormality or support a part of the body. Plural: orthoses.

> **ankle foot o. (AFO):** spans the foot and ankle region.
> **dynamic o.:** allows motion, to aid in ambulation.
> **functional o:** designed to allow for as much function as possible of a joint or limb, while providing stability and/or limiting range of motion.
> **hinged knee o. (HKO):** equipped with hinges to allow the knee joint to bend; helps provide stability to the knee.
> **hip knee o. (HKO):** spans from the waist to the foot; helps control motion for all the major joints of the lower extremity.
> **hip knee ankle foot o. (HKAFO):** spans from the waist to the foot; helps control motion for all the major joints of the lower extremity.
> **humeral o.:** spans varying portions of the upper arm, to help stabilize the humerus. Frequently used in the treatment of humeral shaft fractures.

parapodium o. (pehr-uh-POH-dee-um): platform with uprights for fastening legs and pelvis; enables paraplegic patients (primarily children) to stand and possibly move about by rocking while holding onto a walker.

patellar tendon bearing o.: cast or brace that places part of the body's weight on the area around the front of the knee.

standing frame o: holds a small child lacking strength or muscle control in the upright position.

thoracic o: brace supporting the chest and lower spine in the treatment of scoliosis.

thoracolumbosacral o. (thor-uh-koh-lum-boh-SAY-krul): brace that encompasses the thoracic area, lumbar area and sacrum.

Toronto o. /or/ **brace**: maintains legs in abduction, allowing movement of the hips. Used in the treatment of Perthes disease in the '70s and early '80s.

total contact o.: describes a prosthesis used for amputations, that surrounds and touches the remaining limb on all sides.

UCBL o.: plastic form molded to the foot and placed in a shoe to hold the heel in specific alignment, eliminating flat foot appearance. Developed by Univ. of Calif., Berkeley laboratory.

wrist o.: spans the wrist, helping provide stability to the wrist joint. See also COCK-UP SPLINT.

wrist-driven flexor hinge o.: enables quadriplegics (with normal function of C5 and C6 nerve roots) to grasp an object by dorsiflexing the wrist.

orthotic (or-THAH-tik), **orthosis**. *Orthopedic appliance.* Brace used to correct an abnormality or support a part of the body.

orthotics (or-THAH-tiks). *Scientific specialty.* Deals with the making and fitting of various kinds of braces and supports.

orthotist (OR-thuh-tist). *Health care professional.* Person skilled in the making and fitting of various kinds of braces and supports.

Ortolani sign/test. *Clinical test.* The hips are abducted and pressure is applied to the outer side of the thigh in an attempt to force the femoral head into the acetabulum (hip socket). Slipping the femur back into its socket is indication of hip dislocation in a child.

Orudis. *Drug.* Trade name of ketoprofen, NSAID for treating pain and inflammation.

Oruvail. *Drug.* Trade name of ketoprofen, NSAID for treating pain and inflammation.

os (AHS). *Anatomy.* Bone.

o. breve, **short bones**: cubical bones whose sides are roughly equal. Example: lunate. See also FLAT BONES, IRREGULAR BONES, LONG BONES.

o. calcis (KAL-sis), **calcaneus**: the heel or heelbone.

o. coxae (ahs-KAHKS-i), **innominate**: bone formed by the ilium, ischium and pubis that, in the adult, consolidate into one structure that contains and makes up the pelvis.

o. naviculare (nuh-vick-yu-LEHR-uh), **tarsal naviculum**: bone in the foot between the cuneiforms and the talus (top foot bone).

o. trigonum (tri-GO-num): small bone behind the talus in some people. Not universally present.

Osgood-Schlatter disease. *Pathologic condition.* Apophysitis of the tibial tubercle. Syndrome of tenderness and swelling of the patellar tendon and proximal tibial tubercle at the knee, in boys age 11–15.

Osmond-Clarke procedure, **Putti Platt procedure**. *Surgical procedure.* 1. For recurrent dislocation of the shoulder; anterior approach for repairing the joint capsule followed by advancing the subcapularis tendon. 2. Two-stage multiple ligament release for treatment of the vertical talus (rocker bottom foot).

osseous (AH-see-us). *Description.* Pertaining to bone.

ossific (ah-SIF-ik). *Description.* Pertaining to ossification; producing or becoming bone.

ossification (ah-sif-ih-KAY-shun). *Process.* Biologic method through which bone is created.

ostectomy (ahs-TEK-toh-mee). *Surgical procedure.* Surgical removal of bone.

osteitis (ahs-tee-I-tis). *Pathologic condition.* Inflammatory process in bone, similar to that in soft tissue. May be secondary to infection or foreign material.

    o. deformans, Paget's disease: chronic thickening and deformity of a bone resulting from unregulated bone absorption and deposition; can be associated with fractures and malignant degeneration. Occurs after middle age; mild cases may be undetected.

    o. fragilitans: see OSTEOGENESIS IMPERFECTA.

    o. fibrosa cystica (fi-BROH-suh SIS-tih-kuh): bone resorption with replacement by fibrous tissue; caused by hyperparathyroidism.

    o. pubis: inflammation of pubic bone; associated with pregnancy, childbirth, or with placement of bone anchors. Usually resolves spontaneously.

osteoarthritis (ahs-tee-oh-ahr-THRI-tis), **osteoarthrosis, degenerative arthritis, degenerative joint disease**. *Pathologic condition.* Inflammation of a joint. Loss of cartilage in joints secondary to age, obesity or abnormal use or function of a joint. Usually characterized by swelling, pain and restriction of motion.

osteoarthropathy (ahs-tee-oh-ahr-THRAH-puh-thee). *Pathologic condition.* Degeneration of a joint; the finding inherent to osteoarthritis.

osteoarthrosis (ahs-tee-ahr-THROH-sis). See OSTEOARTHRITIS.

osteoblast (AHS-tee-oh-blast). *Anatomy.* Cell that creates bone during growth or after a fracture.

osteoblastoma (ahs-tee-oh-blass-TOH-muh), **giant osteoid osteoma**. *Pathologic condition.* Benign tumor with osteoblasts in the areas of osteoid and calcific tissues, usually in the spine of a young person.

osteochondral fracture (ahs-tee-oh-KAHN-drul). *Pathologic condition.* Break in the articular surface of a joint involving both cartilage and bone.

osteochondral graft (ahs-tee-oh-KAHN-drul). *Surgical procedure.* Transfer of a bone segment with attached cartilage onto the articular surface of a defective joint, to create a smooth surface.

osteochondritis (ahs-tee-oh-kahn-DRI-tus). *Pathologic condition.* Inflammation of the junction between bone and cartilage.

    o. deformans juvenilis /or/ **juvenilis dorsi**, **Legg-Calvé-Perthes** /or/ **Calvé-Perthes** /or/ **Perthes disease**: deterioration and flattening of the femoral head due to insufficient blood supply; may result in severe arthritic changes. Idiopathic (no known cause); generally occurs between ages 4–8. See also CATTERALL CLASSIFICATION.

    o. dissecans (DIS-uh-kanz): separation of part of the joint cartilage with its underlying bone, leaving a loose fragment in the joint; most frequently in the knee, followed by the elbow and the ankle.

    o. ischiopubica (is-kee-oh-PYU-bih-kuh): inflammation of the bone-cartilage junction at the pubis of the pelvis.

osteochondroma (ahs-tee-oh-kahn-DRO-muh), **hypertrophic exostosis** *Pathologic condition.* Large spurs at the edges of joints, in certain types of degenerative arthritis.

osteochandrohmatosis (ahs-tee-oh-kahn-droh-muh-TOH-sus), **chondromatosis.** *Pathologic condition.* Multiple small cartilaginous formations in the synovial membrane that may become detached and fall into the joint as loose bodies (joint mice). Causes pain, swelling and stiffness.

osteochondrosarcoma (ahs-tee-oh-kahn-dro-sahr-KOH-muh). *Pathologic condition.* Malignant tumor of bone and cartilage.

osteochondrosis (ahs-tee-oh-kahn-DROH-sis). *Pathologic condition.* Group of disorders of the ossification centers in children. May be associated with degeneration or avascular necrosis of the epiphyses followed by reossification.

    o. deformans tibia, Blount's disease, Blount-Barber disease: stunting of growth at the inner, upper portion of the tibial (shinbone) growth plate. Produces bowlegs in children.

osteoclasis (ahs-tee-oh-KLAY-sus). *Treatment.* Breaking a bone to realign it.

osteoclast (AHS-tee-oh-klast). *Anatomy.* Multi-nucleated cell that absorbs and removes bony tissue.

osteoclastoma (ahs-tee-oh-klas-TOH-muh). *Pathologic condition.* Giant cell tumor of bone; affects the metaphyses and epiphyses of long bones. Usually benign, sometimes malignant.

osteocyte (AHS-tee-oh-site). *Anatomy.* Basic cell of bone that maintains mature bone. Occupies a lacuna (depression) in the bone while branches extend to make contact with other cells.

osteodystrophy (ahs-tee-oh-DIS-truh-fee). *Pathologic condition.* Abnormality in bone formation. Each is named according to the etiology, e.g., Albright's hereditary osteodystrophy, renal osteodystrophy.

    azotemic o. (ay-zoh-TEE-mik): bone depletion due to excessive calcium loss through the urine, caused by kidney failure.

osteofibrochondrosarcoma (ahs-tee-oh-fi-broh-kahn-droh-sahr-KOH-muh). *Pathologic condition.* Malignant bone tumor having both fibrous, osteoid and cartilage tissue in its mass.

osteofibroma (ahs-tee-oh-fi-BROH-muh). *Pathologic condition.* Benign lesion of bone; majority of tissue is comprised of connective tissue that appears fibrous.

osteogenesis imperfecta (ahs-tee-oh-JEN-uh-sus im-pur-FEK-tuh), **osteogenesis imperfecta tarte, brittle bones, fragilitas osseum congenita, osteitis fragilitans**. *Pathologic condition.* Multiple system connecfive tissue disorder characterized by fragile bones that fracture easily. Involves the skeleton, eyes, ears, teeth, and vascular tissue. Hereditary.

osteogenic sarcoma (ahs-tee-oh-JEN-ik sahr-KOH-muh), **osteosarcoma**. *Pathologic condition.* A malignant tumor of bone.

osteoid (AHS-tee-oyd). *Anatomy.* The base tissue of bone.

    o. osteoma (ahs-tee-OH-muh). *Pathologic condition.* Small benign tumor of bone, whose nidus (central point of origin) has a characteristic appearance on x-ray; usually painful, especially at night.

osteolysis (ahs-tee-oh-LI-sus). *Abnormal function.* Process of bone absorption or destruction.

osteoma (ahs-tee-OH-muh), **exostosis, hyperostosis**. *Pathologic condition.* Bony growth projecting from normal bone, usually near a joint. Benign.

osteomalacia (ahs-tee-oh-muh-LAY-shuh). *Pathologic condition.* A gradual softening and bending of the bones, resulting in pain and deformity. Caused by kidney abnormalities such as renal disease, and vitamin D deficiency. The juvenile form of this condition is known as rickets.

osteomyelitis (ahs-tee-oh-mi-uh-LI-tus). *Pathologic condition.* Infection in bone.

    chronic o.: persistent, ongoing; generally lasts longer than six weeks.

    nonsuppurative o. (nahn-SUH-pur-uh-tiv): no pus is produced.

    suppurative o. (SUH-pur-uh-tiv): bone infection producing pus.

osteon (AHS-tee-ahn). *Anatomy.* Vascular cells in osseous (bone) tissue.

osteonecrosis (ahs-tee-oh-nek-ROH-sus), **aseptic necrosis, avascular necrosis**. *Pathologic condition.* Bone death caused by loss of circulation to the bone, with no accompanying infection.

osteopath, doctor of osteopathic medicine. *Medical specialist.* Physician who practices osteopathy.

osteopathia striata (ahs-tee-oh-PATH-ee-uh stree-AH-tuh), **Voorhoeve's disease**. *Abnormal condition.* Condition characterized by the formation of abnormal lines or striations seen on x-ray in the metaphysis of long bones. There are no definite clinical findings. Rare.

osteopathy (ahs-tee-AH-puh-thee). *Medical specialty.* Discipline having the basic concept that correct alignment or adjustment in the body will allow it to remedy itself against toxic conditions, infections, tumors, etc.

osteopenia (ahs-tee-oh-PEE-nee-uh). *Pathologic condition.* Decrease in the amount of calcification in bone; can be associated with disuse, as after a cast for a fracture or, systemically (affecting the whole body), representing a transitional state of bone thinning as the patient progresses toward the development of osteoporosis. See also OSTEOPOROSIS.

osteoperiosteal graft (ahs-tee-oh-pehr-ee-AHS-tee-ul). 1. *Surgical procedure.* Local transfer of a bone segment with periosteum and blood supply to induce bone healing. 2. *Biologic material.* Segment of bone, adjacent periosteum and vascular tissue used for filling in a bony defect.

osteoperiostitis (ahs-tee-oh-pehr-ee-ahs-TI-tus). *Pathologic condition.* Inflammation of the periosteum (fibrous covering of a long bone).

osteopetrosis (ahs-tee-oh-pet-ROH-sus), **Albers-Schönberg disease, chalk** /or/ **ivory** /or/ **marble bones, osteosclerosis fragilis**. *Pathologic condition.* Rare disorder characterized by extreme density and fragility of the bones, and obliteration of marrow spaces. Symptoms include pathologic fractures, osteomyelitis of the mandible, cranial nerve palsy, enlargement of the spleen and liver, severe anemia, and possible deafness and blindness. Hereditary.

osteophyte (AHS-tee-oh-fite), **spur**. *Pathologic condition.* Outgrowth of bone usually at the edge of a joint or a vertebra; indicates an arthritic or inflammatory process. See also CALCAR.

osteoplasty (AHS-tee-oh-plas-tee). *Surgical procedure.* 1. Repair of bone with a bone graft. 2. Reshaping a bone or bone segment.

osteopoikilosis (ahs-tee-oh-poy-kil-OH-sus). *Abnormal condition.* Areas of dense bony tissue within bone; tend to be discovered accidentally on x-ray. Hereditary.

osteoporosis (ahs-tee-oh-puh-ROH-sus). *Pathologic condition.* Decrease in amount of bone or skeletal tissue; defined by the World Health Organization as a T-score of 2.5 or below. Best diagnosed with a dual energy x-ray absorptiometry (DEXA) scan.

    juvenile o.: decrease in bone mass in an adolescent. Rare.

    postmenopausal o. (type I): related to the high amount of bone absorption that takes place during the first six years immediately following menopause. Affects bone marrow much more than it does cortical bone. Associated with vertebral and distal radius (wrist) fractures.

    senile o. (type II): affects elderly men and women (age 70 and above); affects both bone marrow and cortical bone, with equal absorption. Associated with hip, vertebral and distal (wrist) radius fractures.

osteoradionecrosis (ahs-tee-oh-ray-dee-oh-nuh-KROH-sus). *Pathologic condition.* Death of bone caused by radiation, frequently in bone surrounding a radiated tumor.

osteosarcoma (ahs-tee-oh-sahr-KOH-muh). See OSTEOGENIC SARCOMA.

osteosclerosis (ahs-tee-oh-sklehr-OH-sus). *Abnormal condition.* X-ray finding of bone thickening; most commonly associated with changes in the bone surrounding the cartilage in arthritic joints; also encountered in osteonecrosis.

    o. congenita, achondroplasia achondrodystrophy, chondrodystrophia fetalis, chondrodystrophy, Parrot's disease. *Congenital abnormality.* Abnormality of growth cartilage of the extremities, resulting in a short-limbed dwarf, generally accompanied by an apparent enlargement of the front of the skull. Trunk length is normal. Hereditary.

o. cutis: inappropriate formation of bone in the skin.

o. fragilis. See OSTEOPETROSIS.

osteosis (ahs-tee-OH-sus). *Abnormal condition.* Abnormal bone formation.

osteosynthesis (ahs-tee-oh-SIN-thuh-sus). *Physiologic process.* Mending together of fractured bone pieces; uses internal fixation devices to achieve healing.

osteotome. (AHS-tee-oh-tome). *Surgical instrument.* Chisel-shaped tool used for cutting bone.

osteotomy (ahs-tee-AH-tuh-mee). *Surgical procedure.* Cutting of bone.

Baker and Hill o.: inserting a wedge of bone into the calcaneus (heelbone) to realign a foot that turns out (heel valgus).

Chevron o.: making a V-shaped cut into the 1st metatarsal bone so it can be realigned. Used in treatment of bunions. See also HALLUX VALGUS.

crescentic o.: cutting either end of a long bone in the leg into a semi-circle so that alignment can be correct in all three dimensions.

closing wedge o.: removing a wedge from one side of a long bone and straightening the bone, to realign a malunion or deformity.

Coke and Jahss o.: removing a wedge from the top of the foot at the level of the naviculocuneiform joint and bending the forefoot upward, to correct a cavus deformity.

derotation o.: cutting a long bone into two segments, then rotating one into alignment. Both segments are held in the new position with a plate or fixation device.

dial o.: method of cutting the acetabulum (hip socket) from the pelvis, to allow redirection of the acetabulum.

distraction o.: cutting a bone so it may be pulled apart, to heal in a lengthened position.

dorsal wedge o.: cutting a bone, with a wedge taken from the back so the base is directed to the back.

dorsiflexion o. of the first ray (DOR-suh-flek-shun): cutting a wedge of bone and tissue from the 1st ray of the foot (bones of midfoot and forefoot that support the great toe) inclusive of the 1st tarsometatarsal joint and fusing the joint in an upwardly bent position (dorsiflexion). For treating forefoot pain from excessive weight across the 1st ray.

Dwyer calcaneal o.: cutting the calcaneus (heelbone) to realign the back portion of the foot (hindfoot).

innominate o.: cutting through the innominate bone to realign the acetabulum (hip socket). Most commonly used in the treatment of developmental dysplasia of the hip (congenital hip dislocation) in older children.

double: cutting through pelvic bones in area of the ilium and ischium or between the ilium and pubis, to direct the acetabulum (hip socket) in a more favorable direction. Used in treatment of hip dysplasia.

Salter (see below).

intertrochanteric o. (in-tur-troh-kan-TEHR-ik): cutting the femur (thighbone) in the intertrochanteric area (upper femur between the greater and lesser trochanters).

Jahss o.: removing a wedge from the top of the foot at the level of the tarsometatarsal joints and bending the forefoot upward, to correct a cavus (high-arched) deformity.

Japas o.: for correcting a cavus (abnormally high-arched) foot. The fascia (tight connective tissue band) on the bottom of the foot is cut, a wedge of bone is removed from the midfoot, and the space is closed to bring the foot out of its abnormal position.

Langenskiold /or/ **Langensköld o.**: cutting through the base of the intertrochanteric regions of the femor to correct coxa vara.

lateralizing o. of the calcaneus: cutting the bottom half of the heel and sliding it laterally (outward). Used in treatment of varus deformity of the hindfoot.

opening wedge o.: changing the alignment or shape of a bone by cutting it almost all the way across and rotating the cut open (as on a door hinge); the resulting defect is filled with a wedge of bone. See also CLOSING WEDGE OSTEOTOMY.

Pauwel's Y o.: for coxa vara, to bring the femoral neck and head to a more normal position. Also used to encourage fracture healing in non-unions about the femoral neck.

Pemberton o.: cutting a segment of bone from around the acetabulum (hip socket), to allow the acetabulum to be rotated so as to better cover the head of the femur; for congenital hip dislocation in the immature pelvis.

Platou o.: cutting the proximal femur (thighbone) to correct rotational deformity of the hip; plates and screws are used to maintain position.

Salter innominate o.: cutting through the pelvis in area of the innominate bone and turning a segment of the pelvis to cover the femoral head. For congenital hip dislocation or subluxation.

Schanz: displacing the upper shaft of the femur (thighbone) medially and giving a buttress effect to the lower side of the pelvis, to lessen hip pain.

Sofield: cutting a severely deformed bony segment of an extremity into at least three to four small segments and threading them onto a rod, to realign the extremity. Used in osteogenesis imperfecta to correct marked bowing of the legs or arms.

Southwick: cutting proximal femur (thighbone), to realign the femoral head in the acetabulum (hip socket) in severe slipped capital femoral epiphysis. Precise cut will result in correction of alignment in three planes.

Steele: cutting through the innominate bone above the acetabulum to allow rotation of the acetabulum. For treatment of acetabular dysplasia.

Sutherland o.: double innominate osteotomy of the pelvis; a cut is made above the acetabulum (hip socket) and another lateral to the symphysis pubis; the acetabulum is rotated to cover the femoral head. Useful in hip dysplasia.

tibial o. (TIB-ee-ul): cutting through the tibia to realign it, usually to correct deformities about the knee.

varus derotational o. (VEHR-us): to correct a valgus deformity; cutting the distal segment of a long bone to decrease its angulation with respect to its proximal segment.

Otto disease, **Otto pelvis, protrusio acetabuli**, **arthrokadysis**. *Pathologic condition.* Protrusion of the acetabulum (hip socket) into the pelvis.

Otto pelvis. See OTTO DISEASE.

overhead suspension. *Treatment.* Holding an arm or leg above the head to help control swelling (edema) in tissues.

overlapping fracture. *Pathologic condition.* A break in which fragments overlap, which shortens the length of the bone.

oxaprozin (ahks-uh-PRO-zin). *Drug.* NSAID for treating pain and inflammation. Trade name: Daypro.

P

pachyonychia (pak-ee-oh-NIK-ee-uh). *Abnormal condition.* Thickening of the fingernails or toenails; may be associated with fungal infecfions. Most common in the elderly.

Paget's disease, osteitis deformans. *Pathologic condition.* Chronic thickening and deformity of a bone resulting from unregulated bone absorption and deposition; can be associated with fractures and malignant degeneration. Occurs after middle age; mild cases may be undetected.

palindromic, palindromia. *Description.* Relapsing or recurring of a condition.

    p. rheumatism. *Pathologic condition.* Outdated term for type of arthritis; joint symptoms persist for a few days, then disappear; usually turns out to be early rheumatoid arthritis or other inflammatory process.

palliative (PAL-ee-uh-tiv). *Description.* Refers to any method of decreasing severity or alleviating symptoms without correction of underlying disease.

palm. *Anatomy.* The volar (under) surface of the hand; the front surface of the hand in anatomic position.

palmar (PAHL-mur). *Anatomic description.* Refers to the front of the hand in the anatomic position (side opposite the knuckles).

    p. fascia (FASH-uh). *Anatomy.* Connective tissue underneath the skin of the palm. Gives rigidity to the skin, to avoid slipping or bunching.

    p. fasciectomy (fash-ee-EK-toh-mee). *Surgical procedure.* Removal of the palmar fascia from underneath the skin of the palm.

    p. fasciotomy (fash-ee-AHT-uh-mee). *Surgical procedure.* Cutting of the palmar fascia.

    p. fibromatosis (fi-broh-muh-TOH-sus), **Dupuytren's contracture**. *Pathologic condition.* Loss of motion due to contracture of connective tissues underneath the skin of the palm, caused by a proliferation of fibroblasts (necessary in production of scar tissue). Nodules and cords form, causing loss of motion in the finger joints.

    p. interossei muscles (in-tur-AHS-ee-eye). *Anatomy.* Three small muscles on the palm side of the hand or bottom of the foot that flex (bend) and adduct (bring together) the fingers or toes.

palmaris longus (pahl-MEHR-us). *Anatomy.* Long thin muscle that bends the wrist. Extends from the forearm into the wrist area, where it blends with the palmar fascia. Frequently used in tendon transfer.

palmaris tendon graft. (pahl-MEHR-us). *Surgical procedure.* Transfer of a segment of the palmaris longus tendon to another part of the body, such as in the repair of the collateral ligament of the thumb metacarpal bone.

palmer. Incorrect spelling of PALMAR.

palpate. *Physical exam technique.* Feeling or pressing a body part to gain information (induration, swelling, tenderness, instability, etc.) about possible ailments.

palsy (PAHL-zee). *Pathologic condition.* Loss of nerve function.

    intrinsic p.: paralysis of the intrinsic muscles (in the hands or feet).

    obstetrical p.: birth injury to the area of an infant's brachial plexus.

pammer. Incorrect spelling of PALMAR.

Panner's disease. *Pathologic condition.* Loss of circulation (avascular necrosis) of the capitellum (in elbow) with varying degrees of collapse, pain and arthritis. One of the osteochondroses. Etiology is unknown.

pantalar arthrodesis (pan-TAY-lur ahr-thro-DEE-sus), **pantalar fusion**.

Surgical procedure. Fusion of the talonavicular joint (just below the ankle, between talus and naviculum) and subtalar (between talus and calcaneus) into a solid mass, usually for severe arthritis of the ankle and hindfoot.

pantalar fusion. See PANTALAR ARTHRODESIS.

paracentesis (pehr-uh-sen-TEE-sus). *Treatment.* Insertion of a hollow needle into a cavity to remove or infuse fluid.

paraffin bath. *Treatment.* Kneading with warm paraffin; used after hand surgery or in arthritis to restore range of motion.

paralysis. *Pathologic condition.* Loss of ability to actively move a muscle.

> **p. agitans**. See PARKINSON'S DISEASE.

paraplegia (pehr-uh-PLEE-juh). *Abnormal condition.* Paralysis of the lower extremities. See also QUADRIPLEGIA.

parapodium orthosis (pehr-uh-POH-dee-um ahr-THOH-sus). *Orthopedic appliance.* Platform with uprights for fastening legs and pelvis; enables paraplegic patients (primarily children) to stand and possibly move about by rocking while holding onto a walker.

parasympathetic nervous system. *Anatomy.* Part of the autonomic system that maintains resting body function and restores energy reserves. See also SYMPATHETIC NERVOUS SYSTEM.

paraxial hemimelia (pehr-uh-AKS-ee-ul hem-ee-MEE-lee-uh). *Congenital abnormality.* Absence or partial absence of the pre- or postaxial part (medial or lateral) of the mid-portion of a limb (forearm or lower leg).

> **intercalary**: most distal segment of the limb is spared (hands or feet).
> **terminal**: malformation includes the hands or feet. Example: fibular or tibial hemimelia for lower leg and ulnar or radial hemimelia for the forearm.

parevertebral muscle spasm (pehr-uh-vur-TEE-brul). *Abnormal condition.* Muscle spasm or cramp in area next to the spine but not involving the spine.

parenteral (puh-RENT-uh-rul). *Treatment.* Introduction of medication, etc., via the bloodstream.

> **p. nutrition**: feeding a patient via the veins.
> **total p. nutrition (TPN)**: feeding a patient through major veins so as to support all his/her nutritional needs without requiring any oral input.
> **peripheral p. nutrition (PPN)**: supplementing a patient's nutritional needs through one of the peripheral veins.

paresis (pehr-EE-sus). *Abnormal condition.* Partial loss of muscle function, usually from nerve damage. See also PARALYSIS.

paresthesia (pehr-iz-THEE-zjuh). *Abnormal condition.* Abnormal sensation, (e.g., tingling, burning) usually associated with irritation or injury of a nerve.

Parkinson's disease, paralysis agitans. *Pathologic condition.* Degenerative, gradually progressive disease of the brain; results in abnormal movements and tremors at rest. Movements may be rhythmic or rigid. Can be fatal.

paronychia (pehr-uh-NIK-ee-uh). *Pathologic condition.* Infection of the nail fold.

parosteal sarcoma (pehr-AHS-tee-ul). *Pathologic condition.* Malignant tumor beginning along the periostium, usually behind the knee. Slowly progressive, eventual metastasis; prognosis better than for osteogenic sarcoma.

parrot-beak meniscus tear. *Pathologic condition.* Tear in the meniscus formed by a medial or lateral extension of a radial meniscal tear (extending from the central meniscus toward the periphery). Resulting shape of torn portion resembles a parrot's beak.

Parrot's disease. 1. *Pathologic condition.* Pseudoparalysis in an infant secondary to syphilitic osteochondritis. 2. *Pathologic condition.* Extreme malnutrition; marasmus. 3. *Congenital abnormality.* (Also called ACHONDROPLASIA, ACHONDRODYSTROPHY, CHONDRODYSTROPHIA FETALIS, CHONDRODYSTROPHY,

OSTEOSCLEROSIS CONGENITA.) Abnormality of growth cartilage of the extremities, resulting in a short-limbed dwarf, generally accompanied by an apparent enlargement of the front of the skull. Trunk length is normal. Hereditary.

parry fracture, Monteggia fracture. *Pathologic condition*. Break in the ulna (smaller forearm bone) with dislocation of the radial head (larger forearm bone). See also BADO CLASSIFICATION.

pars. *Anatomy*. Part or portion. In orthopedics, usually describes a part of the back of a vertebra.

    p. interarticularis (ahr-tik-yu-LEHR-us): portion of the back of the spine between and superior and inferior facets of the vertebra.

partial weightbearing (PWB). *Activity restriction*. Refers to ambulation with assistive devices; only a portion of full body weight is placed on an extremity. See also NON-WEIGHTBEARING.

passive exercise. *Treatment*. Physical therapy in which a limb is moved by the therapist or a machine, to restore a joint's range of motion.

passive range of motion. *Function*. The range of motion attained when a limb is moved passively by a therapist or examiner.

patella (puh-TEL-uh), **kneecap**. *Anatomy*. Bone formed within the patellar tendon; serves to position the quadriceps tendon farther from the knee to improve its ability to straighten the joint.

patellar (puh-TEL-ur). *Anatomic description*. Refers to the patella (kneecap).

    p. fat pad. *Anatomy*. Pad of fat inside the knee, just below the patella.

    p. shaving. *Surgical procedure*. Smoothing the back of the patella (kneecap) with a shaver.

    p. tendinitis. *Pathologic condition*. Inflammation of the patellar tendon (between the patella and the tibia).

    p. tendon bearing brace /or/ **cast** /or/ **orthosis**. *Orthopedic appliance*. Appliance that places part of the body's weight on the area around the front of the knee.

    p. tendonitis. Alternate spelling of PATELLAR TENDINITIS.

    p. tendon reflex, quadriceps reflex. *Clinical finding*. Spontaneous quick jerky movement of the knee when the patellar tendon is tapped. One of the deep tendon reflexes.

    p. tendon transfer. *Surgical procedure*. Shifting of insertion (point of attachment) of the patellar tendon, for recurrent dislocation of the patella.

patellectomy (pat-el-EK-toh-mee). *Surgical procedure*. Removal of the patella (kneecap).

pathognomonic (path-ahg-no-MAHN-ik). *Description*. Diagnostic.

pathologic fracture. *Pathologic condition*. A break through an area of a bone weakened by tumor, infection, injury or surgery.

Patrick's test, FAbER sign, figure-4 test. *Clinical sign/test*. With patient lying on his/her back, the thigh and knee are bent, and the foot is placed above the patella (kneecap) of the opposite leg. The knee on the affected side is then depressed. Pain indicates an abnormality of the hip joint or sacroiliac joint.

Pauwel's classification. *Fracture classification*. Describes different types of femoral neck fractures based on the angle of the fracture.

Pauwel's Y osteotomy. *Surgical procedure*. For coxa vara (shallow neck shaft angle of proximal femur), to bring the femoral neck and head to a more normal position. Also used to encourage fracture healing in nonunions about the femoral neck.

Pavlik harness. *Orthopedic appliance*. Used for treating congenital hip dislocation in an infant. The legs are kept in flexion with abduction at the hip and knee; movement is still possible.

Pearson attachment (to Hodgen splint). *Orthopedic appliance*. Allows the knee to be flexed at varying degrees while the leg rests in the splint (two rods with strapping between them); for fractures of the femur (thighbone).

pectoral girdle (PEK-tor-al), **shoulder girdle**. *Anatomy*. The bony arch supporting the arms; consists of the scapula, coracoid process and clavicle (corresponds to the pelvic girdle of the legs).

pectoralis major (pek-tor-AL-us). *Anatomy*. Large muscle in front of chest that moves the arm toward the body; attached to the clavicle and sternum.

pectoralis minor (pek-tor-AL-us). *Anatomy*. Small muscle in the front of the chest that pulls the scapula (shoulderblade) forward.

pectus carinatum (PEK-tus kehr-in-AH-tum). *Congenital abnormality*. The sternum and anterior rib cage pressed outward; gives the appearance of a chicken breast.

pectus excavatum (PEK-tus eks-kuh-VAH-tum), **pectus recurvatum**. *Congenital abnormality*. The sternum and anterior rib cage, pressed inward, forming a cavity in front of the chest.

pectus recurvatum. See PECTUS EXCAVATUM.

pedicle (PED-uh-kul). *Anatomic description*. Skin, bone, blood vessels, etc., that serve as an attachment or support for another part; portion of tissue attached by a stalk.

    p. flap. *Surgical technique*. Flap of transplanted tissue that maintains its circulation with a long pedicle; may include muscle, fascia and even bone that share the same vascular stalk.

    vertebral p. *Anatomy*. The part of a vertebra that extends back from the vertebral body to form the front half of the spinal canal.

pegboard. *Orthopedic appliance*. A board with holes that pegs attach to; used for holding a patient on his/her side during surgery.

Pellegrini-Stieda disease. *Abnormal condition*. Calcification along the collateral ligament of the knee, usually in association with injury or chronic irritation. Visible on x-ray.

pelvic (PEL-vik). *Anatomic description*. Refers to the pelvis.

    p. band suspension. *Orthopedic appliance*. Band fastened around the pelvis, which attaches to another band that holds an artificial limb.

    p. bone *Anatomy*. Popular term used to indicate any of the bones that make up the bony pelvis: the ilium, sacrum, pubis and ischium.

    p. femoral angle (FEM-ur-ul). *Clinical measurement*. Measure of hip flexion contracture in a cerebral palsy patient; with patient standing, the angle formed between the sacrum's upper surface and the longitudinal axis of the femur (thighbone).

    p. flexion contracture. *Abnormal condition*. Contracture of pelvic flexors such that the limb cannot be completely extended when pelvis remains flat.

    p. girdle. *Anatomy*. Bony arch that supports the legs; consists of the pelvis and femur.

    p. ring. *Anatomy*. Weightbearing ring of the bony pelvis that transmits force across the hips to the spine. Comprised of the sacrum, ischium, ilium and pubic bones and attached ligaments.

    p. sling. *Orthopedic appliance*. Sling used in treating pelvic fractures. With patient lying in the sling, the pelvis is forced against itself, thereby closing the ring.

    p. traction. *Treatment*. With a band around the pelvis, traction is applied toward the foot. Used for relieving pain from herniated disc disease.

pelvis (PEL-vis). *Anatomy*. The ring of bone at the base of the trunk formed by the pubis, ilium, ischium and sacrum with their attached ligaments.

Pemberton osteotomy. *Surgical procedure*. For congenital hip dislocation in an immature pelvis. Cutting a segment of bone from around the acetabulum (hip socket), allowing the acetabulum to be rotated so as to better cover the head of the femur.

peracentesis. Incorrect spelling of PARACENTESIS.

peralysis. Incorrect spelling of PARALYSIS.

perenteral. Incorrect spelling of PARENTERAL.

periarticular (pehr-ee-ahr-TIK-yu-lur). *Anatomic description*. Area immediately adjacent to a joint.

    p. fracture. *Pathologic condition*. A break that occurs around a joint.

perichondrium (pehr-i-KAHN-dree-um). *Anatomy*. Ring of tissue around the cartilage of a long bone.

perilunate dislocation (pehr-ee-LU-nayt). *Abnormal condition*. Dislocation of the lunate bone of the wrist; differing degrees of severity. Requires reduction.

periosteal sarcoma (pehr-ee-AHS-tee-ul sahr-KOH-muh). *Pathologic condition*. Malignant tumor of the periosteum (thin tissue that surrounds and supports the bone).

periosteum (pehr-ee-AHS-tee-um). *Anatomy*. Thin soft tissue covering of a long bone. In the adult bone provides blood and nutrients. In the immature bone, contributes to its growth.

periostitis (pehr-ee-ahs-TI-tus). *Pathologic condition*. Inflammation of the periosteum.

peripheral neuropathy (nu-RAH-puh-thee). *Pathologic condition*. Damage or disease affecting one or more peripheral nerves. When affecting only one nerve, it is referred to as a mononeuropathy; when affecting many, it is called a polyneuropathy.

peripheral parenteral nutrition (PPN): supplementing a patient's nutritional needs through one of the peripheral veins.

peripheral vascular system (VAS-kyu-lur). *Anatomy*. Blood vessel system to the arms and legs.

peristernal perichondritis, costochondritis, costosternal syndrome, Tietze's syndrome. *Pathologic condition*. Inflammation, pain, and tenderness of the cartilage connecting the ribs to the sternum (breastbone). The pain is exacerbated with deep breathing.

pernio, chillblain, frostbite. *Pathologic condition*. Redness, itching, burning sensation of skin exposed to extreme cold; most frequently affects tops of fingers and toes. Tissue death can occur if circulation is not maintained.

peroneal (pehr-uh-NEE-ul). *Anatomic description*. Relating to the fibula, or peroneus (smaller bone of lower leg).

    p. atrophy, Charcot-Marie-Tooth disease. *Pathologic condition*. Progressive degeneration of peripheral nerves, making ambulation difficult. Associated with certain foot deformities, weakness, atrophy of muscles, and reflex changes. Hereditary. See also HEREDITARY MOTOR SENSORY NEUROPATHY.

    p. bone, fibula. *Anatomy*. Smaller of the two bones of the lower leg; articulates with talus (top foot bone) below and tibia (shinbone) above.

    p. muscles. *Anatomy*. Attached to the fibula or lateral border of the leg. See also PERONEUS BREVIS, PERONEUS LONGUS, PERONEUS TERTIUS.

    p. nerve. *Anatomy*. Branch of sciatic nerve, which runs down lower leg.

        common: in the upper leg, the sciatic nerve splits into the tibial and the common peroneal (fibular) nerve, which wraps around the lateral fibula and splits into the deep and superficial peroneal nerves. These supply the side and front of the lower leg.

            deep: supplies muscles of the anterior compartment of the lower leg (anterior tibialis, extensor digitorum longus, peroneus tertius, extensor hallucis longus) and provides sensation to the top portion of the first web space of the foot (between 1st and 2nd toes)

superficial: branch of the common peroneal nerve; supplies peroneus brevis and longus muscles and provides sensation to the outer portion of the lower leg and most of the top of the foot.

p. snapping syndrome. *Pathologic condition*. Painful ankle abnormality characterized by the sudden dislocation of the peroneal tendons (running along outer side of ankle) from their groove behind the fibula. See also DUVRIES TECHNIQUE.

p. spastic flatfoot. *Pathologic condition*. Abnormal fusion of hindfoot bones (tarsal coalition), making foot rigid; may be painful.

peroneus (pehr-uh-NEE-us), **fibula, peroneal bone**. *Anatomy*. Smaller of the two bones of the lower leg; articulates with the talus (top foot bone) below, and the tibia (shinbone) above.

p. brevis (BREV-us): small muscle attached to the fibula or lateral border of the leg; everts the foot (brings outer part of foot upward).

p. longus: long muscle on outer side of the fibula that passes behind the fibula to the 1st metatarsal underneath the foot. Assists in plantarflexion (pointing downward) of the foot.

p. tertius (TUR-shee-us): muscle on the front and outer part of the lower legs and ankle that helps to evert the foot (raise foot upward and outward).

Perthes disease (PEHR-teez), **Calvé-Perthes** /or/ **Legg-Calvé-Perthes disease**, **osteochondritis deformans juvenilis** /or/ **juvenilis dorsi**. *Pathologic condition*. Deterioration and flattening of the femoral head due to insufficient blood supply; may result in severe arthritic changes. No known cause; generally occurs between ages 4–8. See also CATTERALL CLASSIFICATION.

pes. *Anatomy*. Foot.

p. anserinus (an-sehr-EE-nus). *Anatomy*. The expansion hamstring muscles (sartorius, gracilis, semitendinosus) as they attach to the upper and inner (medial) border of the tibia (shinbone). So named because the attachment is shaped like a swan's foot.

p. cavus (KAY-vus), **cavus foot, claw foot, gampsodactyly**. *Pathologic condition*. Abnormally high-arched foot; usually with clawing of the toes. Associated with some forms of neurologic abnormality such as polio or Charcot-Marie-Tooth disease.

p. equinovarus (ee-kwi-noh-VEHR-us), **clubfoot, equinovarus deformity, talipes equinovarus**. *Congenital abnormality*. Rigid, inwardly rotated foot that bends down and in; if untreated, rests on outer edge and cannot be placed flat on the walking surface.

p. planovalgus (plan-oh-VAL-gus), **planovalgus deformity, talipes planovalgus**. *Congenital abnormality*. Flat foot deviated to the inner side.

p. planus (PLAN-us), **fallen arch, flatfoot, splayfoot, talipes planus**. *Abnormal condition*. Foot that lacks an arch; foot whose metatarsal arch, which runs from the heel to the ball of the foot, is flattened or collapsed. May be congenital or developed over time.

flexible: foot with whose arch collapses when weight is applied and resumes its arched position when the weight is removed.

rigid: a foot whose metatarsal arch is constantly flat.

petaling. *Technique*. Padding the edges of a cast.

Petrie cast. *Orthopedic appliance*. Bilateral long leg casts held apart by two cross-beams so each hip is held in 45° of abduction and slight internal rotation; used in the nonoperative treatment of Legg-Calvé-Perthes disease.

phalangectomy (fal-un-JEK-toh-mee). *Surgical procedure.* Removal of one of the bones of a finger or toe.

phalanges (fuh-LAN-jees). The bones that form a thumb, finger or toe.

phalanx (FAL-anks). *Anatomy.* Any of the bones forming the fingers, thumbs or toes. Numbered I-V (from the thumb or great toe). Plural: phalanges.

>   **distal**: the last (end) bone in a finger, thumb or toe.

>   **middle**: central bone of finger or toe; not present in thumb or great toe.

>   **proximal**: the first (nearest the body) bone of a finger, toe or thumb.

Phemister acromioclavicular pin fixation. *Surgical procedure.* For treatment of acromioclavicular joint dislocation. After reducing the end of the clavicle into position, two crossing K-wires are placed from lateral to medial across the AC joint. The wires are removed after healing (usually 6–12 weeks).

Phemister approach. *Surgical procedure.* Dissection of the leg along the back and inner sides of the tibia (shinbone), to gain access to the tibia.

Phemister onlay bone graft. *Surgical procedure.* Placement of two onlay strips of bone along the sides of a tibial (shinbone) nonunion, to achieve healing.

Phemister's epiphysiodesis. *Surgical technique.* For fusing a growth plate: a segment of bone is placed into the growth plate in an attempt to halt its growth.

Phemister's strut graft technique. *Surgical procedure.* For treatment of avascular necrosis of the femoral head: a segment of bone is packed up into the avascular area.

phlebitis (fluh-BI-tus). *Pathologic condition.* Inflammation of a vein.

phlebogram (FLEE-buh-gram), **venogram**. *Radiologic test.* Visualization of the venous tree of an extremity or region of the body after injection of dye into a vein. Often used for identifying a blockage of a vein, as a thrombophlebitis, or in the identification of ongoing internal bleeding after a pelvic fracture.

phlebothrombosis (flee-boh-thrahm-BOH-sus). *Pathologic condition.* Obliteration or clotting within a vein. See also THROMBOSIS.

phocomelia. *Congenital abnormality.* Defect in the development of an extremity in that the hands and feet are excessively close to the torso, attached to the torso either directly or by means of a poorly formed bone.

phrenic nerve (FREN-ik). *Anatomy.* Nerve that innervates the diaphragm; consists of branches from 3rd, 4th and 5th cervical roots.

phospholipid. *Biologic substance.* Class of chemicals produced in the body containing a fat molecule attached to phosphorus. Seen especially in neural tissue.

physeal fracture (FIZ-ee-ul), **Salter** /or/ **Salter-Harris fracture**. *Pathologic condition.* Break through the growth plate of a child. See also SALTER-HARRIS CLASSIFICATION.

physeal plate (FIZ-ee-ul). *Anatomy.* See PHYSIS.

physiatrist (fiz-ee-AT-rist). *Medical specialist.* Physician who treats disorders of the nervous and musculoskeletal systems without surgery.

physical therapy (PT), **physiotherapy**. *Treatment.* Treatment of musculoskeletal problems and disease by physical and mechanical means, such as massage, exercise, heat, cold. See also OCCUPATIONAL THERAPY.

physiotherapy (fiz-ee-oh-THEHR-uh-pee). See PHYSICAL THERAPY.

physis (FI-sis), **growth plate**, **epiphyseal** /or/ **physeal plate** /or/ **cartilage**. *Anatomy.* In a long bone, the layer of cartilage between the epiphysis (growth center) and the metaphysis, where growth in length occurs. Plural: physes.

Piedmont fracture, **Darrach-Hughston-Milch fracture**, **Galeazzi's fracture**. *Pathologic condition.* Break in the distal third of the radius (larger forearm bone); associated with dislocation of the distal radioulnar joint (between the two forearm bones).

Pierrot-Murphy procedure. *Surgical procedure.* Moving the tendoachilles forward from its attachment on the back of the heelbone, to weaken the pull of the muscle. Used in cerebral palsy.

piezoelectric effect (PEEZ-oh-ee-lek-trik). *Physical property.* Capacity of certain materials, including bone, to convert a portion of the energy from a mechanical stress (compression) into electrical energy or an electrical charge.

pigeon-toed. *Clinical finding.* An inward turning of the feet. See also TIBIAL TORSION.

pigmented villonodular synovitis PVNS (vil-uh-NAHD-yu-lur si-noh-VI-tus). *Pathologic condition.* Lesion that arises in a joint causing swelling and intermittent pain, and yielding blood-tinged fluid upon aspiration. Microscopically similar to a giant cell tumor of a tendon sheath.

pillow orthosis, Frejka pillow splint. *Orthopedic appliance.* Cloth pillow used as a brace in congenital dislocation of the hip. Pillow is inserted between the legs and held in a harness, to abduct the legs and keep the hip reduced.

pilon. Alternate spelling of PYLON.

pin. *Surgical implant.* Short, thin piece of wire, plastic or metal used for fixation of fractured bone ends.

PIP (proximal interphalangeal) joint. *Anatomy.* Joint between the middle and proximal phalanges of a toe (except for big toe) or finger (except for thumb).

> **arthroplasty**. *Surgical procedure.* Replacement of the PIP joint with a plastic or metal hinged joint.

> **fusion**. *Surgical procedure.* Fusion of the PIP joint of a finger or toe.

Pipkin classification. *Fracture classification.* Describes patterns of femoral head fractures associated with hip dislocations.

pirexia. Incorrect spelling of PYREXIA.

piriformis muscle (peer-uh-FORM-us). *Anatomy.* Small muscle originating inside the pelvis that rotates the thigh laterally; extends to the back of the greater trochanter of the femur (thighbone).

piroxicam (peer-AHK-sih-kam). *Drug.* NSAID for treating pain and inflammation. Trade name: Feldene, Fexicam.

pislform (PIZ-uh-form). *Anatomy.* Small bone in palm of hand, just proximal to the hook of the hamate, that articulates with the triquetrum.

piston sign. *Clinical sign.* In the operating room during hip replacement, the hip is flexed and a pull-push motion exerted on the thigh; a feeling of instability indicates a loose hip.

pivot shift test of Hughston, jerk test, lateral pivot-shift test. *Clinical test.* Test for instability of the knee. With the knee bent to 90°, medial (inward) rotation and valgus (away from midline) stress is applied to the leg as the knee is slowly extended; as the knee passes through 20° or 30° of flexion, shifting forward indicates a tear of the anterior cruciate ligament.

Plafond fracture (pluh-FOND). *Pathologic condition.* Break in the distal end of the tibia (shinbone) involving the articular (joint) surface of the ankle.

planovalgus deformity (play-no-VAL-gus), **pes planovalgus, talipes planovalgus**. *Abnormal condition.* Flat foot whose inner side rests on the ground.

plantar (PLAN-tur). *Anatomic description.* Refers to the bottom of the foot.

> **p. aponeurosis** (ap-ohn-yu-ROH-sus). *Anatomy.* Tight connective tissue band on the sole of the foot that forms part of the arch. Bands spanning the long arch of the foot also act as a bowstring to keep the arch from collapsing.

> **p. fascia**: same as PLANTAR APONEUROSIS (above).

> **p. fasciitis** (fash-e-I-tis). *Pathologic condition.* Inflammation of the plantar fascia (sling of tough tissue along bottom of foot).

p. reflex. *Clinical finding*. Toe movement in response to stroking the bottom of the foot firmly from heel to toe. May be normal or abnormal.

p. wart. *Pathologic condition*. A wart on the bottom of the foot.

plantarflexion. *Function*. Bending the foot or toes downward.

plantaris (plan-TEHR-us). *Anatomy*. Small muscle attached to the heel that points the toes downward.

planter. *Incorrect spelling of* PLANTAR.

planus (PLAN-us). *Description*. Flat.

plasma cell myeloma (mi-uh-LOH-muh), **plasmacytoma, multiple myeloma, myeloma**. *Pathologic condition*. Most common primary neoplasm (malignant new growth) of bone, with lesions most common in the spine, pelvis and skull; may lead to pathological fractures (may appear on x-ray as holes in bone). Occurs usually after the 5th decade.

plasmacytoma (plaz-muh-si-TOH-muh). See PLASMA CELL MYELOMA.

plastazote. *Material*. Soft rubbery substance used for making soft braces and shoe inserts.

plate. *Orthopedic implant*. A thin metal device affixed to bone with screws; used for immobilizing bones or bone fragments to promote healing.

plateau fracture. *Pathologic condition*. Break involving flat portion of a bone. Most often used in reference to intra-articular (joint) fractures involving the top of the tibia (shinbone) or proximal part of a phalanx (finger- or toebone).

Platou osteotomy. *Surgical procedure*. Cutting the proximal femur (thighbone) for correction of rotational deformity of the hip; plates and screws are used to maintain position.

platysma (pluh-TIZ-muh) *Anatomy*. Superficial muscle around the neck that depresses corners of the mouth; responsible for some facial expressions.

plethysmography (pleth-iz-MAH-gruh-fee). *Test*. Determines the amount of blood flow in an extremity by measuring changes in volume.

plexus. *Anatomy*. A network of nerves or vessels.

>**brachial p.** (BRAY-kee-ul): complex of nerves from the 5th, 6th, 7th and 8th cervical and 1st and 2nd thoracic segments of the spinal cord, which interconnect in the region of the neck, shoulder and armpit; innervates part of the chest, shoulders and arms.

>**lumbar p.** (LUM-bahr): place where nerve roots exiting the lumbar and sacral spine join to make up the sciatic and femoral nerves.

>**sacral p.** (SAY-krul): network of nerves that give sensation to the area around the buttocks and rectum, and control of the bladder and sphincters.

plica. (PLI-kuh). *Anatomy*. Folded segment of synovium (joint lining) within a joint, usually the knee joint. May cause pain if enlarged or swollen.

pneumatic knee (nu-MA-tik). *Orthopedic appliance*. Artificial knee joint that uses air or gas to dampen knee motion during ambulation. Diminishes stiffness.

pneumoarthrogram (nu-moh-AHR-throh-gram). *Radiologic test*. X-ray showing outline of the articular surface of a joint, after injection of air into the joint. Because air is thin compared to tissue, it serves as reverse contrast medium.

podiatrist (poh-DI-uh-trist), **chiropodist**. *Medical specialist*. Doctor of podiatric medicine; trained and licensed to diagnose and treat foot problems.

Poland syndrome. *Congenital abnormality*. Absence of a portion of the pectoralis major muscle in the chest; associated with syndactyly of the hand.

polio, poliomyelitis. *Pathologic condition*. Viral inflammation of the nerves of the anterior horns of spinal cord, leading to muscle paralysis in severe cases.

poliomyelitis (poh-lee-oh-mi-uh-LI-tus). *See* POLIO.

pollicization (pahl-uh-sih-ZAY-shun). *Surgical procedure*. Transplanting a digit to replace a thumb.

polyarteritis nodosa (pah-lee-ahr-tur-RI-tus). *Pathologic condition.* Inflammation of many small and medium-size arteries; leads to damage to various organ systems, such as kidneys, heart, intestines.

polyarthritis (pah-lee-ahr-THRI-tus). *Pathologic condition.* Arthritis in more than one joint.

polycentric knee prosthesis. *Orthopedic appliance.* Artificial knee whose center of rotation changes as the leg goes through its full range of motion; gives a more normal range than a simple hinge.

polydactyly (pah-lee-DAK-tuh-lee). *Congenital abnormality.* More than the normal number of digits on the hand and/or foot.

polyethylene. *Material.* Plastic used in making artificial acetabular cups and portions of artificial knees.

    highly cross-linked p.: specially treated during manufacturing to make it more resuistant to wear.

polyostotic fibrous dysplasia (pah-lee-uh-STAH-tik, dis-PLAY-zjuh), **Albright's disease** /or/ **syndrome, Albright-McCune** /or/ **McCune-Albright disease** /or/ **syndrome.** *Congenital disorder.* Syndrome characterized by multiple skin lesions (cafe-au-lait spots), endocrine abnormalities (especially precocious puberty), and multiple fibrous dysplasia lesions.

polypropylene (pahl-ee-PROH-puh-leen). *Material.* Plastic used in making braces.

Ponstel. *Drug.* A trade name of mefenamic acid, NSAID for treating pain and inflammation.

popliteal (pah-pluh-TEE-ul). *Anatomic description.* Refers to the popliteus muscle.

    p. angle. *Clinical finding.* Maneuver for estimating severity of hamstring tightness. Patient lies face up on an exam table. The examiner bends the knee and hip to 90°. While maintaining the hip bent to 90°, the knee is brought to extension. The maximum number of degrees the knee can be straightened is then noted.

    p. artery. *Anatomy.* Large artery that is a continuation of the femoral artery as it crosses the back of the knee (in the popliteal space), becoming the anterior tibial artery, posterior tibial artery, and peroneal artery.

    p. cyst, Baker cyst. *Pathologic condition.* Sac located in the popliteal fossa (back of leg behind knee), filled with synovial fluid leaked from the knee joint.

    p. fossa: same as POPLITEAL SPACE (below).

    p. space, p. fossa. *Anatomy.* Diamond-shaped area along the back of the knee, flanked by four muscles. Large nerves and vessels use the space as a conduit to the lower leg.

popliteus (pah-pluh-TEE-us). *Anatomy.* The area in back of the knee.

    p. muscle: small oblique muscle that rotates the tibia (shinbone) medially on the femur (thighbone). Extends from lateral posterior side of the distal femur across the knee joint, inserting medially on the proximal tibia.

    p. tendon: the tendon of the popliteus muscle. Often visible in the outer side of the knee during arthroscopic surgery.

posterior, dorsal. *Anatomy.* Back of the body or body part in anatomic position; posterior surface of the hand is opposite the palm. Opposite: ANTERIOR.

    p. arch fracture. *Pathologic condition.* Break in the back half of the arch (circular part of a vertebra surrounding the spine).

    p. calcaneal osteotomy. See POSTERIOR OSTEOTOMY OF THE CALCANEUS.

    p. compartment of the leg, p. crural compartment. *Anatomy.* Two of the four fascial compartments enclosed by tight, connective tissue bands forming sheaths containing different muscle groups of the lower leg; contains the gastrocnemius, solius, tibialis posterior, and flexor hallucis muscles. See also ANTERIOR COMPARTMENT, COMPARTMENT SYNDROME.

p. cruciate ligament (PCL) (KRU-shee-ut). *Anatomy.* Connective tissue band joining the femur (thighbone) to the tibia (shinbone) within the knee joint; prevents the tibia from slipping backward on the femur.

rupture/tear: a tearing of the posterior cruciate ligament.

sprain: a stretching of the PCL without actual rupture.

p. crural compartment. See POSTERIOR COMPARTMENT OF THE LEG (above).

p. decompression. *Surgical procedure.* Removal of an area from the back of the spine, to alleviate excessive pressure on the cord.

p. longitudinal ligament. *Anatomy.* Tight connective tissue band within the spinal canal of a vertebra; lies against the back of the vertebral body.

p. malleolus (mal-ee-OH-lus). *Anatomy.* Rear lip of the distal tibia (shinbone) where it articulates with the talus (top footbone). Not visible because it is covered by the Achilles tendon.

p. osteotomy of the calcaneus, p. calcaneal osteotomy. *Surgical procedure.* Cutting bottom half of the heel and sliding it posteriorly. Used in treatment of cavus deformity of hindfoot related to a weak gastrocnemius muscle.

p. scalene muscle (SKAY-leen). *Anatomy.* One of three muscles (scalenus anticus, scalenus medius, scalenus posterior) that flex the neck (includes lateral flexion); attaches from the transverse process of the cervical vertebra to the outer surface of the first two ribs.

p. spinal sclerosis, tabes dorsalis. *Pathologic condition.* Loss of sensation and positioning sense in the legs; effect of syphilis on the spinal cord.

p. superior iliac spine. *Anatomy.* Bony prominence along the back of the pelvis above the attachment of the sacrum to the iliac wing.

p. tibial artery. *Anatomy.* Continuation of popliteal artery behind the knee as it supplies the back of the calf and portions of the bottom of the foot.

p. tibial nerve. *Anatomy.* Continuation of sciatic nerve after it breaks off from the popliteal to supply the rear calf muscles, such as the soleus and gastrocnemius.

p. tibial pulse. *Clinical finding.* Pulsations of the posterior tibial artery behind the medial malleolus at the ankle.

p. tibial tendon (PTT). *Anatomy.* Tendon of posterior tibialis muscle that runs along the back of the tibia (shinbone) under the medial malleolus. Inserts into inner side of the navicular and under, inner side of the foot bones.

posterolateral fusion. *Surgical procedure.* Fusion of the back of the spine, extending laterally to the transverse processes.

Pott's disease. *Pathologic condition.* Tuberculosis of the spine. May lead to collapse of the spine and kyphosis (bending-forward deformity of spine).

Pott's fracture. *Pathologic condition.* Break in both the medial and lateral malleoli (tips of lower leg bones), causing lateral displacement of the ankle.

Prader-Willi syndrome. *Congenital abnormality.* Syndrome of poor muscle tone (a floppy baby), morbid obesity, short height, small hands and feet, mental retardation and small genitals. May develop developmental dysplasia of the hip, knock knees, flat feet, and scoliosis.

prednisone. *Drug.* Cortisone derivative. For treating inflammatory and allergic diseases. Long-term systemic use can result in serious side effects, e.g., osteoporosis, immunosuppression. Prolonged topical use can cause cataract, glaucoma.

prehension (pre-HEN-shun). *Function.* Ability to grasp or grab.

prepatella bursa (pree-puh-TEL-uh). *Anatomy.* Thin, fluid-filled sac in the front of the patella (kneecap), under the subcutaneous tissue; may become enlarged by infection or trauma-induced inflammation.

prepatellar bursitis, "housemaid's knee." *Pathologic condition.* Inflammation of the bursa in front of the patella (kneecap) after minor or direct trauma. May or may not be infected.

press-fit /or/ **uncemented total hip replacement**. *Surgical procedure.* Technique for replacing the hip using prostheses (artificial parts) with a porous rough surface, which allows the bone to heal directly to it without cement.

pressure sore, bed sore, decubitus ulcer. *Pathologic condition.* Break in the skin caused by pressure and immobilization.

Prieser disease. *Pathologic condition.* Necrosis (tissue death) of the navicular bone (at the wrist) following a fracture.

process. *Anatomy.* A prominence or projecting part of a bone.

profunda femoris (pro-FUN-duh fem-OR-us), **deep femoral artery**. *Anatomy.* Branch of the femoral artery that supplies upper and inner thigh regions.

progressive arthroophthalmopathy (ahr-thro-ahf-thal-MAH-puh-thee), **Stickler syndrome**. *Pathologic condition.* Syndrome characterized by joint abnormalities (seen at birth), severe hip and knee problems, with bony enlargements of the knees, ankles and wrists; significant nearsightedness and astigmatism, possible retinal detachment. Patients generally have a normal lifespan and intelligence. Some systemic effects, e.g. high fever, high sed rate, spleen enlargement. Hereditary.

progressive diaphyseal dysplasia (di-uh-FIZ-ee-ul dis-PLAY-zjuh), **Camurati-Engelmann, Engelmann disease, diaphyseal dysplasia**. *Pathologic condition.* Type of dwarfism resulting from an abnormality in growth of the long bones. Characteristics include short, wide long bones and early joint arthritis.

pronate (PRO-nayt). *Function.* Turning the hand in the palm-down position or the foot in the sole-down position. See also SUPINATE.

pronation (pro-NAY-shun). *Function.* In the hand, turning the palm down. In the foot, flattening the arch. See also SUPINATION.

pronator (PRO-nay-tur). *Anatomy.* Muscle that rotates a part toward the midline.

    p. quadratus (qwah-DRAT-us): small muscle at the distal portion of the forearm that pronates the forearm. Crosses between the two forearm bones (radius and ulna) on the palmar surface.

    p. teres (TEHR-eez): small muscle that pronates the forearm. Arises at the medial epicondyle of the humerus (upper armbone), crossing laterally from the front of the elbow to the radius (larger forearm bone). Supplied by the median nerve.

prone. *Anatomic description.* Lying face down.

    p. rectus test. *Clinical test.* With patient lying face down, knees are extended, then bent; rising of buttocks indicates a tight rectus femoris muscle.

prosthesis (prahs-THEE-sus). *Orthopedic implant.* Artificial substitute for an missing part, such as a limb. See also ENDOPROSTHESIS.

    cemented: designed to be cemented onto bone.

    cementless: same as PRESS-FIT (below).

    myoelectric (mi-oh-ee-LEK-trik): artificial limb with surface electrodes that attach batteries to remnants of the stump muscles. Contracting the muscles allows electric activity to activate the batteries and enable the limb to function. Most commonly used in the upper extremity to reproduce hand function.

    press-fit: has a porous surface for impacting into position; bony ingrowth will adhere the prosthesis to the bone.

prosthetics (prahs-THET-iks). *Medical field.* The art and science of designing, making and fitting artificial parts for the body, such as limbs.

prosthetist (PRAHS-thuh-tist). *Health care professional.* Licensed specialist in designing, making, and fitting artificial body parts, such as limbs.

prostrate leg raising test, contralateral straight leg raising test, Fajerzstajn test, sciatic phenomenon, well leg raising test of Fajersztajn. *Clinical test.* With the patient lying on his/her back, a leg is raised with the knee in extension. Pain in the opposite leg indicates irritation of the nerve as it exits the spine. Sign of herniated disc disease.

protrusio acetabuli, arthrokatadysis, Otto disease, Otto pelvis. *Pathologic condition.* Protrusion of the acetabulum (hip socket) into the pelvis. Seen in degenerative conditions such as osteomalacia and rheumatoid arthritis.

proximal (PRAHKS-uh-mul). *Anatomic description.* Toward the cephalad (head) or the center of the body. See also DISTAL.

    p. focal femoral deficiency (PFFD). *Congenital abnormality.* Defect in formation of the femur (thighbone). Characterized by a short femur. In more severe cases, various portions of the pelvis and foot may be affected.

    p. interphalangeal joint (PIP) (in-tur-fal-un-GEE-ul). *Anatomy.* Joint between the middle and proximal phalanges of a toe (except for big toe) or finger (except for thumb). Numbered I - V (from thumb or big toe).

        arthroplasty. *Surgical procedure.* Replacement of the PIP joint with a plastic or metal hinged joint.

            fusion. *Surgical procedure.* Fusion of the PIP joint of a finger or toe.

    p. third. *Location.* If a bone is divided into thirds (proximal, middle, distal), the proximal third is nearest the center of the body.

pseudoarthrosis (su-do-ahr-THRO-sus). *Abnormal condition.* A fracture or osteotomy that has failed to heal or unite, forming a false joint between two separate pieces of bone.

pseudogout, calcium pyrophosphate deposition disease. *Pathologic condition.* Abnormal precipitation of calcium pyrophosphate into crystals that deposit into joints, most commonly the knee, resulting in pain and inflammation. Can sometimes be detected on x-ray. See also CHONDROCALCINOSIS.

pseudohypertrophic dystrophy, Duchenne's muscular dystrophy /or/ **paralysis.** *Pathologic condition.* Progressive weakness of the voluntary muscles. Onset generally before age 3, with frequent falls, difficulty getting up, and enlargement of calf muscles. Hereditary, sex-linked (males; females are carriers). Death before age 25. See also BECKER'S MUSCULAR DYSTROPHY.

pseudohypoparathyroidism (SU-doh-HI-po-pehr-uh-THI-royd-iz-um), **Albright's hereditary osteodystrophy, Seabright Bantam syndrome.** *Pathologic condition.* Syndrome characterized by resistance to the effects of parathyroid hormone; includes small stature, obesity, mental deficiency, delayed teeth formation, short metacarpals with a relatively long index finger, and tendency to develop cataracts. Calcification of the basal ganglia of the brain, hypocalcemia, and hyperphosphatemia may occur. May be hereditary.

Pseudomonas (su-doh-MOH-nus). *Organism.* Aerobic bacteria infrequently seen in orthopedic infections.

psoas muscle (SO-us). *Anatomy.* Muscle that bends the hip. Arises from the lumbar spine, runs distally across the hip and inserts into the lesser trochanter.

psoriatic arthritis. *Pathologic condition.* Form of arthritis (joint inflammation and deterioration) associated with psoriasis.

PT. Abbreviation for PHYSICAL THERAPY.

pubic bone (PYU-bik). See PUBIS.

pubis, pubic bone. *Anatomy*. The front part of the pelvis to the side of the symphysis pubi (where halves of the pelvis join).

Pugh nail. *Othopedic implant*. Sliding or telescoping nail used for fixation of femoral trochanteric or neck fractures.

pulp pinch. *Function*. A pinch using the pad of the finger against the thumb pad. See also SIDE PINCH.

pulse electromagnetic field (PEMF). *Treatment*. A type of electromagnetic field used for inducing bone healing in fractures or osteotomies.

pump bump. *Pathologic condition*. Prominence over the back outer side of the heel. Caused by wearing shoes with heels that press on the heelbone.

punched out lesion. *Radiologic finding*. Abnormality that appears on x-ray as a hole punched out of the bone. Suggests presence of a destructive lesion.

punctate epiphyseal dysplasia, chondrodysplasia, chondystrophia calcificans congenita, chondrodysplasia punctata, congenita punctata. *Congenital abnormality*. Malformation of bones resulting in joint deformations and leading to a form of dwarfism. Characterized by limb deformities, spine abnormalities, varus defomation of hips, difficulty walking, and x-ray appearance of stippled, calcified epiphyses. The stippling is present at birth, but usually disappears by 1 year of age. See also CONRADI-HUNERMANN DISEASE, RHIZOMELIC FORM.

purulent (PYUR-yu-lunt). *Pathologic condition*. Infected. Denotes presence of pus.

Putti-Platt procedure. *Surgical procedure*. 1. For recurrent dislocation of the shoulder; anterior approach for repairing the joint capsule followed by advancing the subcapularis tendon. Also called Osmond-Clarke procedure. 2. Multiple ligament release for treatment of vertical talus (rocker bottom foot).

Pyle's disease, metaphyseal dysplasia. *Abnormal condition*. Abnormality of the remodeling process: bone remodeling does not occcur with growth. X-ray changes include abnormally flared metaphyses.

pylon (PI-lohn). 1. *Orthopedic supply*. Post used as the weightbearing portion of a temporary prosthesis (artificial limb). 2. *Anatomy*. Part of a bone serving as the primary weightbearing post. Commonly used to describe the base of the tibia (shinbone) or the bases of the phalanges of the fingers.

    p. fracture: break in lower part of the tibia (shinbone) and articular (joint) surface of the lower tibia at the level of the ankle; caused by a strong upward push across the ankle. See also RÜEDÏ AND ALGOWER CLASSIFICATION.

pyogen. *Bacterial organism*. Bacterium capable of causing pus.

pyogenic (pi-oh-JEN-ik). *Pathologic condition*. Producing pus.

pyramidal tract. *Anatomy*. Nerve tracts in the front of the spinal cord that are involved in locomotor activity.

pyranocarboxylic acids. *Drug*. Class of NSAIDs (nonsteroidal anti-inflammatory drugs).

pyrexia (pi-REKS-ee-uh) *Pathologic condition*. Fever.

pyrroles. *Drug*. Class of NSAIDs (nonsteroidal anti-inflammatory drugs).

Q

Q angle. *Clinical measurement.* Angle formed by the intersection of a line drawn from the center of the patella to the tibial tubercle, and another from the center of the patella to the anterior superior iliac spine. A high angle indicates a valgus relationship between the knee and thigh and can predispose the patient to patellar subluxation or patellar maltracking (patella riding slightly to outside of normal).

quadratus femoris (kwahd-RAY-tus FEM-ur-us). *Anatomy.* Small muscle on the back of the hip, between the gamelli muscles; externally rotates the hip.

quadratus lumborum (kwahd-RAY-tus lum-BOR-um). *Anatomy.* Muscle that bends the vertebral column; attaches from the last rib to the iliac crest in the back.

quadriceps (KWAH-druh-seps). *Anatomy.* Largest muscle in the body, situated at the front of the thigh; extends (straightens) the knee. Made up of four muscles or heads (vastus intermedius, vastus lateralis, vastus medialis and rectus femoris). Supplied by the femoral nerve.

   q. reflex. *Function/Clinical finding.* Elicited by tapping the patellar tendon, which stimulates the quadriceps muscle to contract.

quadricepsplasty (KWAH-druh-seps-plas-tee). *Surgical procedure.* Elongating the quadriceps to improve knee flexion.

quadrilateral brim (kwah-druh-LAT-ur-ul). *Orthopedic appliance.* Type of surface at the top of an above-knee amputation orthosis designed to accommodate the stump. The socket is oftsen referred to as a quadrilateral socket and the brim is the portion that actually bears the weight of the body.

quadriplegia (kwah-druh-PLEE-juh). *Pathogic condition.* Paralysis of all four limbs.

quadriplegic (kwah-druh-PLEE-jik). An individual who is paralyzed in all four limbs.

quads. *Anatomy.* Slang for quadriceps, the four muscles on the front of the thigh.

rachischisis (rah-KIS-kih-sis). *Pathologic condition.* An opening or a complete separation in the spinal column.

radial (RAY-de-ul). *Anatomic description.* Pertaining to the radius (larger forearm bone).

    r. artery. *Anatomy.* One of the two large arteries of the forearm; extends along the radial border (thumb side) of the forearm into the hand; commonly used for determining an individual's pulse.

    r. clubhand, **clubhand**, **talipomanus**. *Congenital anomaly.* Absence of the radius (larger forearm bone) and thumb, with the wrist deviated toward the thumb side.

    r. collateral ligament. *Anatomy.* Connective tissue band (1) running along the outer side of the elbow connecting the humerus and the ulna; acts as a restraining ligament of the elbow, keeping the ulna from rotating inward; (2) running along the outer side of the interphalangeal and metacarpophalangeal joints of the fingers and thumb.

    r. deviation. *Anatomic description.* Bending of the hand or wrist toward the radial side of the arm.

    r. head. *Anatomy.* Top of the radius (larger forearm bone) on the outer side of the arm: articulates with the capitellum of the humerus (upper armbone) and rotates in a notch on the proximal ulna (smaller forearm bone).

    r. nerve. *Anatomy.* Nerve extending along the radial border of the forearm; powers the muscles that extend the wrist, fingers and thumb, and provides sensation to the back of the wrist.

radicular pain (ruh-DIK-yu-lur). *Pathologic condition.* Pain that radiates down a specific course, nerve or route. Caused by irritation of a nerve that is proximal (closer to center of body and spinal cord) to where pain is perceived.

radiculitis (ruh-dik-yu-LI-tus). *Pathologic condition.* Inflammation of the part of a nerve that lies within the dura of the spine prior to exiting the spinal column.

radiculopathy (ruh-dik-yu-LAH-puh-thee). *Pathologic condition.* Localized disease or irritation of the spinal nerve roots. Usually secondary to a herniated disc, tumor or injury.

radioulnar synostosis (ray-dee-oh-UL-nur sin-ahs-TOH-sus). *Pathologic condition.* Fusion between the two forearm bones (radius and ulna). Occurs in congenital anomalies or is secondary to trauma.

radius (RAY-dee-us). *Anatomy.* Larger of the two forearm bones. See also ULNA.

RA factor. *Lab test.* Finding of a protein that suggests presence of rheumatoid arthritis. The test is imperfect as the rheumatoid factor may be present in normal individuals (false positive) and absent in patients who have rheumatoid arthritis (false negative). See also RA TEST.

Raiter's syndrome. *Pathologic condition.* Consists of urethritis (inflammation of the urethra), iridocyclitis (inflammation of the front of the eye), and arthritis.

rakyskeesis. Incorrect spelling of RACHISCHISIS.

ramus (RAY-mus). *Anatomy.* 1. Division or branch of a nerve or blood vessel. 2. Irregularly shaped bone, e.g., the pubic ramus in the pelvis. Plural: rami.

range of motion (ROM). *Measurement.* Full range that an extremity moves; measured in degrees of a circle.

    active. 1. *Clinical finding.* Range of motion attained when a limb is moved under the patient's own power and without assistance. 2. *Treatment.* Exercise performed by patient, under the guidance of a physical therapist; a joint or limb is moved using the limb's own power or muscles.

active-assist. *Treatment.* Exercises done under guidance of a physical therapist: a joint or limb is moved by the patient and aided by gentle stretches from the therapist.

passive. 1. *Clinical finding.* Range of motion attained when a limb is moved passively by a therapist or examiner. 2. *Treatment.* Exercise performed in which a joint or limb is moved by the therapist.

Ratcliff classification. *Fracture classification.* Describes four patterns of avascular necrosis following proximal femur fractures in children.

RA test. See RHEUMATOID FACTOR.

ray. *Anatomy.* One of five projections of a hand or foot; consists of the metacarpal or metatarsal bone and its associated phalanx. Numbered 1 through 5, thumb to small finger in the hand, and from great toe to little toe in the foot.

r. amputation. *Surgical procedure.* Removing an entire metacarpal and associated finger of a hand, or metatarsal and associated toe of a foot.

Raynaud disease. *Pathologic condition.* Insufficient blood supply at the ends of the fingers caused by excessive blood vessel constriction. Can result in gangrene (death) of one or more fingers.

Raynaud phenomenon (ray-NOHZ) *Pathologic condition.* Excessive constriction of blood vessels to the fingers as a result of cold weather or other stimuli.

razorback deformity. *Pathologic condition.* A sharp prominence of multiple ribs in the back. Seen in severe scoliosis.

reamer (REE-mur). *Surgical tool.* Drilling tool used to shape or widen a hole.

acetabular r: used to prepare the acetabulum (hip socket) for acceptance of an artificial cup.

chamfer r: used for preparing or shaping the side or surface of a bone, most commonly during joint reconstruction.

triple r: drill-like device used to prepare the proximal femur for acceptance of a compression hip screw. So named because it has three different widths along its length.

rectus femoris (REK-tus FEM-rus). *Anatomy.* One of four quadriceps muscles on the front of the thigh that bends the hip and extends the knee. (The others are vastus intermedius, vastus lateralis, vastus medialis.) Arises from the pelvis and inserts distally into the patella (kneecap) and the upper part of the tibia.

recurrent dislocation. *Pathologic condition.* Joint dislocation that has occurred more than once.

recurvatum (ree-KURV-uh-tum). *Abnormal function.* Backward movement of an extremity beyond its normal range.

r. genu: backward movement of the knee beyond its normal range.

reduction. *Surgical procedure.* Manipulating a dislocated or fractured bone or joint back to its normal position.

closed: externally manipulating the bone without cutting the skin.

open: cutting the skin to grasp the affected bony fragments or structures.

open r. and internal fixation: placing screws and/or plates inside or along a fractured bone; designed to remain in the body indefinitely. Refers also to the materials used.

reefing. *Surgical procedure.* Tightening a joint capsule or muscle around a joint to improve function.

referred pain. *Pathologic condition.* Pain that is away from the actual site of injury.

reflex. *Physiology*. Sudden, involuntary reaction in response to a stimulus.

> **muscular r**. *Physiology*. Sudden, involuntary muscular reaction in response to a sudden stretch of a muscle.

> **r. sympathetic dystrophy (RSD)** (DIS-truh-fee), **Sudeck atrophy**. *Pathologic condition*. Nonfunctioning extremity caused by exquisite tenderness or pain from inappropriate firing of pain and sympathetic nerve fibers; usually triggered by an injury. Leads to scarring, loss of hair around the injured part and thinning of skin. Treatment may require psychotherapy, physical therapy, and sympathetic blocks. In general, the longer the injured body part is not used, the more difficult it is to achieve a successful recovery.

Refsum disease. *Pathologic condition*. Type IV hereditary motor sensory neuropathy, a syndrome characterized by the progressive degeneration of the peripheral nerves; patient has excessive phytanic acid. Onset in adulthood.

reimplantation. *Surgical procedure*. Reattaching a body part to its original site, as a digit after traumatic amputation.

reinnervation potentials. *Physiologic property*. Pattern of electrical potentials in muscle whose nerves have been injured and are restoring themselves back into the muscle. As the nerves heal, they are somewhat unstable, leading to extraneous electrical activity about the neuromuscular unit. Used for diagnosis of return of function.

Relafen. *Drug*. A trade name of nabumetone, NSAID for treating pain and inflammation.

remission. 1. Lessening or abatement of the signs and symptoms of a disease. 2. The period when symptoms abate or when no evidence of disease is present. See also EXACERBATION.

renal osteodystrophy (REE-nul ahs-tee-oh-DIS-truh-fee), **renal rickets**. *Pathologic condition*. Osteodystrophy (loss of mineral within bone) from severe renal (kidney) disease leading to abnormalities in calcium-phosphorus balance. In children, can lead to bone and growth deformities.

renal rickets. See RENAL OSTEODYSTROPHY.

resect, excise. *Surgical procedure*. To remove a tissue, tumor or body part.

resection, excision, extirpation. *Surgical procedure*. Cutting out; removal. Partial or complete removal or surgical destruction of bone, muscle, tumor, etc.

> **r. arthroplasty**: excision of a joint; patient is allowed to continue without a joint. Usually employed in the treatment of serious infections involving a joint and/or an artificial joint. See also GIRDLESTONE PROCEDURE.

resorption. *Process*. The removal of bone tissue by the body.

reticular cartilage (KAHR-tuh-lidj). *Anatomy*. Outdated term for fibrocartilage.

retinaculum (ret-in-AK-yu-lum). *Anatomy*. Band of connective tissue used for holding a particular structure, as the patella (knee joint), in position.

retrocalcaneal (ret-roh-kal-KAY-nee-ul). *Anatomic description*. Refers to the area behind the heel where the Achilles tendon inserts.

> **r. exostosis** (eks-ahs-TOH-sus), **posterior heel spur**. *Pathologic condition*. Projection of bone behind the heel that protrudes into the tendoachilles; associated with inflammation in the tendon.

retrolisthesis (ret-roh-lis-THEE-sis), **retrospondylolisthesis**. *Pathologic condition*. Spine abnormality: the vertebrae have moved posteriorly from the normal position. Associated with degenerative arthritis.

retropatellar fat pad (ret-tro-puh-TEL-ur). *Anatomy*. Fat segment behind and below the patella, external to the knee joint capsule.

retroversion. *Anatomic description*. Posterior rotation of a structure relative to another. See also ANTEVERSION.

acetabular r. *Pathologic condition.* Posterior rotation of the hip socket, as in total hip replacement when the cup is placed pointing excessively toward the back of the pelvis.

femoral r. *Pathologic condition.* Posterior rotation of the neck of the thighbone (femur) about the long axis of its shaft, causing feet and legs to turn out.

reverse Allis test. *Clinical test.* For evaluating leg length discrepancy and determining whether the femur (thighbone) or tibia (shinbone) is responsible for the shortening. First, the Allis test is done with patient lying on his/her back, then the patient is rolled onto prone position (face down), with knees and ankles bent to 90°. If one knee sits farther down the table than the other, it indicates that a limb-length discrepancy stems from the femur, and if one ankle sits higher than the other, it indicates the discrepancy is from the tibia.

reverse Barton's fracture. *Pathologic condition.* A break through the articular (joint) surface of the distal radius (larger forearm bone) with the fracture line positioned toward the back of the wrist.

reverse Bennett's fracture. *Pathologic condition.* Two-part, intra-articular (joint) fracture of base of the 5th metacarpal bone. Named for its resemblance to the two-part fracture of the base of metacarpal of thumb (Bennett's fracture).

reverse Colles' fracture, Smith fracture. *Pathologic condition.* Break in the distal end of the radius (larger forearm bone) near its lower joint surface with displacement toward the palm.

reverse last shoes, Markell shoes. *Orthopedic appliance.* Shoes in which the left and right lasts (patterns) are reversed, i.e., right shoe on left foot. Frequently used as treatment for metatarsus adductus in children.

reverse Trendelenburg. *Position.* Patient lies on his/her back with the head of the bed tilted up 45° so that the patient's head sits higher than the pelvis. See also TRENDELENBURG POSITION.

rhabdomyoma (rab-doh-mi-OH-muh). *Pathologic condition.* Benign tumor of striated muscle.

rhabdomyosarcoma (rab-doh-mi-oh-sar-KOH-muh). *Pathologic condition.* Malignant tumor of muscle.

rheumatoid arthritis (RA) (RU-muh-toyd). *Pathologic condition.* Autoimmune disease that affects connective tissue; results in chronic inflammation, swelling and destruction of many joints, especially those of the back, hands and feet. Occurs more often in women. See also ANKYLOSING SPONDYLITIS.

juvenile: group of autoimmune diseases that afflict children; similar to rheumatoid arthritis in adults.

rheumatoid factor (RF), RA test. *Lab test.* Finding of a protein that suggests presence of rheumatoid arthritis. The test is imperfect as the rheumatoid factor may be present in normal individuals (false positive) and absent in patients who have rheumatoid arthritis (false negative).

rheumatoid spondylitis, ankylosing spondylitis, Bechterew's disease, Marie-Strumpell disease. *Pathologic condition.* Autoimmune connective tissue disorder resulting in the gradual fusion of the joints between vertebrae; causes severe limitation of spinal motion, with back and hip pain.

rheumatologist. *Medical specialist.* Physician who specializes in the treatment of arthritis and other rheumatic diseases that may affect joints, muscles, bones, skin and other tissues.

rhizomelia (ri-zoh-MEE-lee-uh). *Pathologic condition.* Shortening of the upper portion of a limb (upper arm or brachium in the upper extremity; thigh in the lower extremity). Seen in some types of dwarfism.

rhizomelic (ri-zoh-MEE-lik). *Pathologic condition.* Having a short proximal (close to body) limb segment.

rhizotomy (ri-ZAH-tuh-mee). *Surgical procedure.* Cutting nerve branches at the point of exit from the spinal cord, to relieve pain or to reduce spasticity of the extremities.

rhomboid major (RAHM-boyd). *Anatomy.* Large muscle in the back that holds the shoulder and adducts it toward the midline; attaches between the spinous processes and the medial border of the scapula (shoulderblade).

rhomboid minor (RAHM-boyd). *Anatomy.* Small muscle in the back below the rhomboid major; holds the shoulder adducted toward the midline.

ribs. *Anatomy.* Twelve pairs of bones attached to the vertebrae in the back and curving gently forward to the sternum in front. Together they form the structure for the chest.

> **floating**: lowest two ribs (11th, 12th), so named because they do not attach at the front to the sternum (breastbone).

rib vertebral angle (RVA). *Radiologic measurement.* The angle in which a rib intersects with its vertebra. The difference between the RVA on either side of the apex vertebra of a curve (the backbone at the center of a scoliosis curve) is the cornerstone for the Mehta angle or the RVAD.

rib vertebral angle difference (RVAD), Mehta angle. *Radiologic test.* Method for predicting whether a curve in infantile idiopathic scoliosis will progress (get larger). The difference between the rib vertebral angles (RVA) of either rib corresponds to the apical vertebra of a scoliotic curve. If the RVA difference is greater than 20°, the curve is likely to progress.

RICE. *Treatment.* Acronym for Rest, Ice, Compression (with an elastic ankle wrap), and Elevation.

rice bodies. *Pathologic condition.* Small fragments or growths of fibrous tissue within a joint that resemble rice grains; result from damage to the synovium of the joint. Seen in rheumatoid arthritis.

rickets. *Pathologic condition.* Disease caused by inadequate vitamin D. The bone is poorly calcified, resulting in weakening and enlargement of the ends. Gives rise to deformities, e.g., bowing of legs, a prominence on ends of ribs. See also OSTEOMALACIA.

> **vitamin D-resistant r.**: results from body's inability to utilize vitamin D. Results in joint enlargement, short stature, and poorly calcified bone, giving rise to deformities, e.g., bowing of the legs. Frequently associated with renal abnormalities.

> **renal r., renal osteodystrophy**: osteodystrophy (loss of mineral within bone) from severe renal (kidney) disease leading to abnormalities in calcium-phosphorus balance. In children, can lead to bone and growth deformities.

Riley Day syndrome, dysautononia, familial dysautonomia. *Pathologic condition.* Abnormality of the autonomic nervous system, causing numerous problems including difficulty controlling body temperature, insensitivity to pain, motor uncoordination, lack of tearing, intolerance to anesthetics. Hereditary.

ring constriction, annular band, amniotic band /or/ **groove**. *Congenital abnormality.* Constricting ring produced by thin band of amniotic membrane that may encircle an arm, leg or digit in utero; may be so deep as to sever blood vessels and nerves. See also STREETER'S DYSPLASIA.

Risser localizer. *Treatment.* Applying a cast with selected points of pressure for correction of scoliosis.

rizomelia. Incorrect spelling of rhizomelia.

rocker-bottom foot. *Congenital abnormality.* Foot deformity characterized by rigidity and rocker-bottom appearance: marked plantar flexion of the talus (top foot bone) and dorsiflexion of the forefoot. May be congenital. See also CONGENITAL VERTICAL TALUS.

rod, nail. *Surgical implant*. Slender metallic implant used for attaching the fragments of broken bones. See also PIN.

roentgen (RENT-gen). Unit of x-ray or gamma radiation.

roentgenogram (RENT-gen-uh-gram). *Radiologic test*. An x-ray. Types listed under X-RAY.

Rolando fracture. *Pathologic condition*. A three-piece, intra-articular (joint) break at the base of the metacarpal bone of the thumb; can be shaped like a Y (Rolando Y fracture) or a T (Rolando T fracture).

Romberg sign/test. *Clinical test/sign*. Imbalance when standing with eyes closed; indicates abnormality of the central nervous system.

rongeur (rahn-ZJUR), **bone nippers**. *Surgical instrument*. Spring-loaded cutting tool for taking small bites from bone.

Kerrison r.: small, narrow instrument for cutting bone in tight places.

rotational flap. *Surgical procedure*. Section of skin cut with its blood supply intact, rotated to cover or fill a skin defect such as after removal of a tumor or scar.

rotator cuff. *Anatomy*. Group of muscles and tendons that hold the humerus (upper armbone) to the shoulder blade and serve to rotate the humerus while keeping it centered in the shoulder socket.

muscles: muscles that abduct and rotate the humerus in the glenoid (on the shoulderblade). Comprised of the teres minor, infraspinatus, supraspinatus, and subscapularis.

rudimentary. *Description*. Refers to incomplete development of a part.

r. rib. *Pathologic condition*. Incompletely formed extra rib; greater clinical significance when in the neck or lung area (cervical or lower part of thoracic vertebrae).

Rüedi and Algöwer classification. *Fracture classification*. Classification of various levels of severity of pylon fractures.

type I: bones minimally displaced; bone fragments largely maintain their anatomic positions.

type II: fractures with more than one fragment involving the joint surface but with minimal or no displacement (from original anatomic positions).

type III: most severe; has shifting of the intraarticular fracture fragments.

ruptured disc, herniated /or/ **slipped disc, nucleus pulposus**. *Pathologic condition*. Extrusion of the cartilaginous tissue in the center of a disc (nucleus pulposus), which can place pressure on a nerve and result in leg or arm pain, numbness, tingling or weakness.

Rush nail/rod/pin. *Orthopedic supply*. Device for fixing fractures of long bones.

Russell-Taylor classification. *Fracture classification*. Identifies different patterns of subtrochanteric femur fractures.

Russell traction. *Treatment*. Traction used for fractures of the femur (thighbone) in children. A sling is placed under the knee and straps apply traction over the tibia (shinbone), resulting in a force that pulls the femur into alignment.

Rust sign. *Clinical finding*. Patient holds his/her head as he/she lies down or gets up. Indicates pain or instability. May be seen in patients who have cancer of the cervical vertebrae, rheumatoid arthritis or severe spondylosis or spinal stenosis.

S

S. Abbreviation for sacral vertebra; used with specific number (S1–L5).

Saber-cut incision. *Surgical technique*. A precise cut to the top and front of the shoulder over the acromioclavicular joint.

sacral (SAY-krul). *Anatomy*. Refers to the sacrum, the caudal segment of the spinal canal that forms part of the pelvis.

    s. agenesis (ay-JEN-uh-sus). *Pathologic condition*. Partial or total absence of the sacrum. Part of the caudal regression syndrome.

    s. ala (AH-luh). *Anatomy*. Prominences on the upper side of the sacrum medial to the iliac crest and lateral to its attachment to the spine.

    s. bone. *Anatomy*. See SACRUM.

    s. inclination. *Radiologic measurement*. On a lateral view of the pelvis taken with patient standing, the angle between a line drawn along the back of the S1 vertebra and a vertical line. An increase in inclination may result from an increase in normal lumbar lordosis and may be associated with spondylolisthesis of the lumbar spine (slipping of a lumbar vertebra).

    s. plexus (PLEK-sus). *Anatomy*. Network of nerves that supplies sensation to the area around the buttocks and rectum, and control of the bladder and sphincters.

sacralization. *Pathologic condition*. Absence of fusion of the 1st sacral vertebra to the rest of the sacrum, resulting in an extra lumbar vertebra. See also TRANSITIONAL VERTEBRA.

sacrectomy (say-KREK-tuh-mee). *Surgical procedure*. Removal of the sacrum.

sacrococcygeal (say-kroh-kahk-SIJ-ee-ul). *Anatomy*. Refers to the sacrum and the small segments of vertebrae that comprise the coccyx (tailbone).

sacrocoxalgia (say-kroh-kahks-AL-juh). *Pathologic condition*. Pain in the sacrum and coccyx.

sacrodynia (say-kroh-DIN-ee-uh). *Pathologic condition*. Pain in the sacrum.

sacroiliac joint (sak-roh-IL-ee-ak). *Anatomy*. Joint created by the junction of the sacrum and iliac wings.

sacroiliac subluxation (sak-roh-IL-ee-ak). *Pathologic condition*. Partial or incomplete dislocation of the sacroiliac joint, resulting in abnormal alignment of the sacrum and ilium.

sacrospinous ligament (say-kroh-SPI-nus). *Anatomy*. Connective tissue band that runs from the ischial spine (bony prominence on ischium) to the lower segment of the sacrum.

sacrotuberous ligament (say-kroh-TU-bur-us). *Anatomy*. Connective tissue band that runs from the sacrum to the tuberosity on the lower side of the ischium.

sacrovertebral angle (say-kroh-vur-TEE-brul). *Measurement*. Angle between the sacrum and the 1st lumbar vertebra.

sacrum (SAY-krum), **sacral bone**. *Anatomy*. Part of spinal column; curved triangular bone (comprised of five fused vertebrae) beneath the lumbar spine and above the coccyx.

Sage rod. *Surgical implant*. Solid intermedullary rod used for internal fixation of fractures.

sagittal plane (SAJ-ih-tul). *Location*. Imaginary plane running from front to back, dividing the body into left and right sides; cutting a body in or through a sagittal plane allows inspection of the body from the anterior/posterior direction (front to back) as seen from the side. See also MIDSAGITTAL PLANE.

sagittal rotation (SAJ-ih-tul) *Anatomic description*. Rotation about the sagittal plane.

Saint Vitus dance. See ST. VITUS DANCE.

Salflex. *Drug*. Trade name of salsalate, NSAID for treating pain and inflammation.

salicylic acids. *Drug*. Class of NSAIDs (nonsteroidal anti-inflammatory drugs).

salsalate. *Drug*. NSAID for treating pain and inflammation. Trade name: Disalcid, Salflex.

Salter classification, Salter-Harris classification. *Fracture classification*. Classification of fractures across the physeal plate (growth plate).

Salter fracture, Salter-Harris fracture. *Pathologic condition*. Break through the physeal plate (growth plate) of a child. See also SALTER-HARRIS CLASSIFICATION.

Salter innominate osteotomy. *Surgical procedure*. Cutting through the pelvis in the area of the innominate bone and turning a segment of the pelvis to cover the femoral head. For congenital hip dislocation or subluxation.

Sanfilippo syndrome. *Pathologic condition*. Series of hereditary disorders of carbohydrate metabolism resulting in multiple organ pathology, such as enlargement of spleen and liver, scoliosis, and contractures of joints. Similar to Hurler's syndrome, with less severe features. Death often by age 20.

saphenous nerve (SAF-eh-nus). *Anatomy*. Branch of the femoral nerve; travels from the pelvis down the inside of the leg, supplying sensation to the inside of the foot, ankle and calf.

saphenous vein (SAF-eh-nus). *Anatomy*. Large vein along the inner side of the calf and leg, draining into the external iliac vein.

sarcoidosis, Boeck's disease /or/ **sarcoid**. *Pathologic condition*. Chronic inflammatory disorder characterized by tiny soft nodules in the skin, lungs, liver, spleen and eyes. Affects almost all systems of the body. Unknown origin.

sarcoma (sahr-KOH-muh). *Pathologic condition*. Malignant tumor of connective tissue, bone, cartilage or striated muscle; spreads directly to adjacent areas and by metastasis (by way of the bloodstream or lymph system).

    osteogenic s. (ahs-tee-oh-JEN-ik): sarcoma of bone.

    periosteal s. (pehr-ee-AHS-tee-ul): sarcoma of the periosteum (thin tissue that surrounds and supports the bone).

    parosteal s. (pehr-AHS-tee-ul): begins along the periosteum, usually behind the knee. Slowly progressive, with eventual metastasis; prognosis better than for osteogenic sarcoma.

    synovial s. (sin-OH-vee-ul): involves the synovium of a joint, whose cell characteristerics are similar to those of the synovial membrane.

sartorius (sahr-TOR-ee-us). *Anatomy*. Long, thin muscle on the front of the thigh that flexes and externally rotates the leg. Attaches from the anterior superior iliac spine to below the knee into the tibia (shinbone).

saucerization (sah-sur-ih-ZAY-shun). *Surgical procedure*. Opening a cavity to the surface.

scab, crust. *Pathologic lesion*. Hardened dried secretions (e.g., blood, plasma, pus) that form over a wound.

scalenotomy (skay-luh-NAH-tuh-mee). *Surgical procedure*. Cutting the scalene muscle at its attachment to the clavicle (collarbone).

scalenus anterior (skuh-LEE-nus). See SCALENUS ANTICUS.

scalenus anticus (skuh-LEE-nus AN-tih-kus), **scalenus anterior**. *Anatomy*. Muscle that elevates the clavicle (collarbone) and bends the neck. Attaches from the transverse processes of the cervical vertebrae to the clavicle.

    s. syndrome, Naffziger syndrome. *Pathologic condition*. Compression of the brachial plexus and the artery between an enlarged scalenus anticus muscle and the 1st thoracic rib. Holding the arms upright may result in pain and cramping. Treatment consists of cutting the scalenus muscle.

scaphoid (SKAF-oyd), **carpal navicular**. *Anatomy*. Boat-shaped bone in the wrist.

s. pads. *Orthopedic appliance*. Inserts placed in shoes to change heel alignment during walking.

scapula (SKAP-yu-luh), **wing bone**. *Anatomy*. The shoulderblade. Large bone along the back of the chest, articulating with the ribs and the humerus (upper armbone). Attachment point of many muscles.

scapulectomy (skap-yu-LEK-tuh-mee). *Surgical procedure*. Removal of the scapula (shoulderblade), usually for tumorous conditions.

scapulopexy (SKAP-yu-loh-pek-see). *Surgical procedure*. Fixing the scapula (shoulderblade) to the chest wall.

scar, cicatrix. *Abnormal condition*. Fibrous tissue that forms over a wound during healing, replacing normal tissue.

Schanz osteotomy. *Surgical procedure*. Displacing the upper part of the shaft of the femur (thighbone) medially and giving a buttress effect to the lower side of the pelvis, to lessen hip pain.

Schanz screw. *Surgical implant*. Used in fixation devices to hold bones to an external frame, giving rigidity to a fracture or osteotomy.

Schatzker's classification. *Fracture classification*. 1. Identifies types of proximal tibial fractures. 2. Identifies fracture patterns involving the olecranon.

Scheie's syndrome (shayz). *Pathologic condition*. Hereditary disorder of carbo-hydrate metabolism (mucopolysaccharidosis) resulting in multiple organ pathology, such as enlargement of spleen and liver, scoliosis and joint contractures, possibly with bony abnormalities of the hand. Normal IQ. Less severe than Hurler's. Patient can survive into adulthood.

Scheuermann's disease, juvenile kyphosis. *Pathologic condition*. Abnormality of the vertebrae in the thoracic or thoracolumbar area; characterized by wedg-ing of at least three consecutive vertebrae and irregularities of the growth plate, resulting in a round back appearance (kyphosis). Can be painful.

Schlyme frame (shlime). *Orthopedic appliance*. Structure that holds a patient reclining on his/her back against a backrest,with the knees slight-ly bent (Fowler's position). Similar to a McConnel frame.

Schmorl's nodes. *Pathologic condition*. Herniations (protrusions) of the intervertebral disc into the vertebral body; visible on x-ray and MRI.

Schneider nail /or/ **rod**. *Surgical implant*. Self-cutting nail (tip has cutting edge to insert without pre-drilling); for intermedullary fixation of the femur (thighbone).

Schrock procedure. *Surgical procedure*. Lowering the scapula (shoulderblade) to correct Sprengel's deformity (congenital elevation of the scapula).

Schuller-Christian disease. Abbreviated name for HANS SCHULLER-CHRISTIAN DISEASE.

sciatica (si-AT-ih-kuh). *Pathologic condition*. Pain that radiates down the back of thigh and leg; caused by a herniated disc or pressure on the sciatic nerve.

sciatic nerve (si-AT-ik). *Anatomy*. Nerve exiting the pelvis that gives inner-vation to the muscles and sensation to the feet, ankles and lower legs. Comprised of the 4th and 5th lumbar and the 1st, 2nd and 3rd sacral roots.

sciatic notch (si-AT-ik). *Anatomy*. Area on pelvis formed by the inferior surface of the ilium, posterior portion of the ischium, and lateral portion of the sacrum, where the sciatic nerve and psoas minor and piriformis muscles transverse.

sciatic phenomenon, contralateral straight leg raising test, Fajersztajn test, prostrate leg raising test, well leg raising test of Fajersztajn (si-AT-ik). *Clinical test*. With patient lying on his/her back, a leg is raised with the knee in extension. Pain in the opposite leg indicates irritation of the nerve as it exits the spine. Sign of herniated disk disease.

scissors dissection. *Surgical technique*. Separating soft tissues with a scissors.

scleroderma (sklehr-oh-DUR-muh). *Pathologic condition*. Condition resulting in scar-like changes about multiple organ systems; includes pathologic changes in the alimentary tract, Raynaud's phenomenon (excessive blood vessel constriction about the fingers and hands), kidney disease, lung disease. May result in limb contractures. Forms are:

diffuse cutaneous s.: generalized skin changes; associated with Raynaud's phenomenon within one year of onset, with the appearance of skin lesions, lung disease, kidney and heart disease.

limited cutaneous s.: skin involvement limited to face and feet, chronic Raynaud's phenomenon, trigeminal neuralgia and calcifications in the skin.

systemic sclerosis: classic form, which is more likely to be called scleroderma. Significant organ involvement; affects skin to a lesser extent.

sclerosing hemangioma (skluh-RO-sing), **dermatofibroma, fibroxanthoma**. *Pathologic condition*. Type of slow-growing, benign, fibrous skin nodule; usually affects lower extremities.

sclerosing osteitis, Garre disease. *Pathologic condition*. Areas of bone become thickened and distended, but do not form abcesses. Cause unknown; thought to represent a low-grade, chronic osteomyelitis (bone infection).

sclerosis (skluh-ROH-sus). *Pathologic condition*. Chronic swelling or inflammation resulting in scarring. May occur in various organs, such as blood vessels (arteriosclerosis) or in bone (bony sclerosis). In bone, the primary change is thickening of the bony substance.

scoliosis (skoh-lee-OH-sus). *Pathologic condition*. S-shaped side curvature of the spine. May be paralytic (from polio), myopathic (associated with muscular dystrophy or muscle abnormality), traumatic (from injury to the muscle and soft tissue), congenital (failure to form properly during development), juvenile (appearing in childhood), adolescent (appearing during teen years and associated with adolescent growth spourt), or idiopathic (unknown cause).

congenital s.: generally associated with abnormal vertebrae; the spine grows on one side and is prevented from growing on opposite side, either by partial formation of a vertebra or a fusion on concave side. Present at birth.

dextrorotatory s.: direction of the curve is to the right.

levorotary s.: direction of the curve is to the left.

lumbar s.: lateral (side-to-side) curvature in the frontal plane, occurring in the area between the rib cage and pelvis.

Scotchcast. *Orthopedic supply*. Trade name for fiberglass material used in some casts.

Scottish Rite orthosis. *Orthopedic appliance*. Brace used in the treatment of Legg-Perthes disease or dysplastic hips. A pelvic band with thigh cups and a bar between the legs maintains the hip in abduction but allows flexion and extension of the hip.

scrum. *Biologic material*. Fluid produced by the body after all the cells and cellular material are removed. Usually light yellow in color.

scurvy. *Pathologic condition*. Disease caused by lack of vitamin C. Characterized by the weakening of the soft tissues and bones along with weakness, bleeding gums, edema, and skin ulcerations. In children, it affects bone development and is called Barlow's disease.

Seabright Bantam syndrome, Albright's hereditary osteodystrophy, pseudohypoparathyroidism. *Pathologic condition*. Syndrome characterized by resistance to the effects of parathyroid hormone; includes small stature, obesity, mental deficiency, delayed teeth, short metacarpal bones with a relatively long index finger, short metatarsal bones, and a tendency to develop cataracts. Calcification of the basal ganglia of the brain, hypocalcemia, and hyperphosphatemia may occur. May be hereditary.

sedimentation rate (sed rate), erythrocyte sedimentation rate (ESR). *Lab test.* Rate (in mm per hour) at which red blood cells settle to the bottom of a tube of unclotted blood. Nonspecific test used for measuring presence and intensity of various systemic inflammatory diseases.

sed rate. See SEDIMENTATION RATE.

segmental fracture. *Pathologic condition.* Break in a long bone in which an isolated central piece is not connected to either the proximal or distal fragments.

semimembranous (sem-i-MEM-bruh-nus). *Anatomy.* Large thigh muscle that bends the knee; attaches to the posterior femur (thighbone), ischium and proximal tibia (shinbone). One of the hamstring muscles.

semispinalis (sem-i-spih-NAHL-us). *Anatomy.* Large muscle along the back of the spine that gives extension and lateral bend to the spine.

semitendinosis (sem-i-ten-dih-NOH-sus). *Anatomy.* Thigh muscle that bends the knee and extends the pelvis. Attaches from the ischium to the inner side of the proximal tibia (shinbone). One of the hamstring muscles.

sensory evoked potential (SEP). 1. *Test.* Technique for determining the continuity of sensory neurons (nerves that carry tactile information) from a distal extremity to the brain. Used in scoliosis surgery to monitor for spinal cord injury. 2. *Physiology.* Impulses sent to the central nervous system by peripheral sensory nerves.

sepsis (SEP-siss). Blood poisoning. An infection involving the whole body; carried from a primary area to rest of the body through the bloodstream.

septic arthritis (SA). *Pathologic condition.* Joint infection caused by bacteria.

septum (SEP-tum). *Anatomy.* A division; thin wall of tissue (including bone) separating two areas of the body or a structure.

sequestration (see-kwes-TRAY-shun). *Physiologic process.* Containment of a type of tissue or process to one walled-off area of a body.

sequestrectomy (see-kwes-TREK-tuh-mee). *Surgical procedure.* Removal of dead tissue.

sequestrum (see-KWES-trum). *Pathologic lesion.* Dead bone tissue within the involucrum (surrounding living bone). Seen in osteomyelitis (bone infections).

serial casts. *Treatment.* Regularly (e.g., weekly) applied casts, to stretch ligaments and joints; used in treatment of clubfoot and other deformities.

seropurulent (seer-oh-PYUR-yu-lent). *Description.* Refers to both purulent and serous fluid within tissues following surgery or an infection.

serosanguineous (seer-oh-SAN-gwin-us). *Description.* Refers to fluid that is tinged with blood.

serous (SEER-us). *Description.* Refers to serum produced in the soft tissues of a wound.

serratus anterior (suh-RAY-tus). *Anatomy.* Muscle on the front of the chest wall that pulls the scapula (shoulderblade) forward into the chest to prevent winging of the scapula. Attaches to the upper ribs in front and to the anterior medial aspect of the scapula in back.

sesamoid (SES-uh-moyd). *Anatomy.* Type of small, round or oblong bone that usually acts as a fulcrum for a tendon (e.g., patella) or as protection against direct pressure on a tendon (e.g., under ball of 1st metatarsal bone in the foot).

sesamoiditis (ses-uh-moy-DI-tus). *Pathologic condition.* Inflammation of the sesamoid bone of the foot, at the ball of the 1st metatarsal bone.

sessile (SES-il). *Anatomic description.* Having a flat base of attachment.

    s. osteochondroma (ahs-tee-oh-kahn-DROH-muh). *Pathologic condition.* An osteochondroma (benign tumor of long bones) that has a broad base that attaches to bone.

Sever's disease (SEE-vurz). *Pathologic condition.* Inflammation of the apophysis (growth area) of the calcaneus (heelbone); leads to pain with walking.

shank bone. *Anatomy.* Popular term for the tibia, the larger of the two bones in the lower leg.

sharp dissection. *Surgical procedure.* Separating soft tissues with a knife or other sharp instrument. See also BLUNT DISSECTION.

Sharpey fibers. *Anatomy.* Collagenous fibers attaching a tendon to the outer part of a bone.

Sharrard iliopsoas transfer (il-ee-oh-SOH-us). *Surgical procedure.* Moving the iliopsoas tendon and iliacus muscle back from an intrapelvic position, through the iliac wing, to a lateral position on the greater trochanter, to act as an abductor instead of a flexor of the hip. Used in paralytic patients lacking hip subluxation. Similar to Mustard procedure.

sheath. *Anatomy.* Connective tissue sleeve through which anatomical structures pass. Glistening surface allows smooth motion of the encased structure against the surrounding tissue.

shelf procedure. *Surgical procedure.* Cutting the pelvic bone and fashioning a segment to form a shelf to help cover a larger portion of the femoral head.

Shenton's line, arcuate line of Shenton. *Radiographic finding.* On a frontal x-ray view of the pelvis or hip, an imaginary arch formed by the underside of the femoral neck and the lower edge of the pubic bone. May be disrupted in hip dislocation or subluxation of the hip. Used to identify subtle cases of development dysplasia of the hip.

Shepherd fracture. *Pathologic condition.* Break in the posterior process (projection) of the talus (top foot bone).

Sherman plate. *Orthopedic implant.* Thin slotted plate used for fixation of fractures. Forerunner of the plate developed by the AO.

shin, shinbone. *Anatomy.* Popular terms for the tibia, larger of the two bones in the lower leg.

    s. splints. *Pathologic condition.* Pain over the front of the lower legs; associated with a sudden increase in activity level. Felt to be due to sudden inflammation of the periosteum (soft tissue covering) of the tibia (shinbone).

shirt-stud abscess, collar button abscess. *Pathologic conditon.* Collection of pus in the web space between the fingers. Begins on the palmar side and continues to the other, making two abscess cavities with a thin portion in between, giving the appearance of a collar button.

shoe. *Orthopedic appliance.* Protective covering for the foot; also may be used in therapeutic management of abnormalies of the lower extremities.

    s. cookie: type of shoe insert; used for treating flatfoot or toeing (in or out); especially in children, to realign the weightbearing portion of the foot.

    s. lift: lift added to a shoe to equalize leg lengths.

    straight last s.: shoe in which a line from the heel through the foot is in direct line with the 3rd metatarsal bone.

    tarsal pronator s. (TAHR-sul PROH-nay-tur): made from a pattern in which left and right lasts (patterns) are reversed, i.e., right shoe on left foot.

    s. wedge: segment of leather or rubber applied to the inner or outer side of a shoe to change the weightbearing position of the foot.

Shogren's. *Incorrect spelling of SJÖGREN'S.*

short-arm cast (SAC). *Orthopedic appliance.* Cast that extends from below the elbow to the hand, not including the fingers.

short-arm splint. *Orthopedic appliance.* Plaster or fiberglass material that extends from the hand to the elbow, held in place by an elastic bandage.

short bones, os breve. *Anatomy.* Cubical bones whose sides are roughly equal. Example: lunate. See also FLAT BONES, IRREGULAR BONES, LONG BONES.

short-leg cast (SLC). *Orthopedic appliance.* Cast that extends from the foot (not including the toes) to the knee, allowing for knee flexion.

> **s. walking cast (SLWC):** cast extending from the knee to and including the foot, reinforced so as to enable walking.

short-leg splint. *Orthopedic appliance.* Plaster or fiberglass material that extends from the foot to the knee, held in place by an elastic bandage.

short wave diathermy. *Treatment.* Ultrasonic wave used in physical therapy to elevate temperatures in a small area of tissue, to relieve pain.

shoulder. *Anatomy.* Joint formed from the junction of the humerus (upper armbone) and the glenoid part of the scapula (shoulderblade).

> **s. disarticulation.** *Surgical procedure.* Amputation of the humerus (upper armbone) at the shoulder joint.

> **s. girdle, pectoral girdle.** *Anatomy.* Bony arch supporting the arms; consists of the scapula, coracoid process, and clavicle; corresponds to the pelvic girdle of the legs.

> **s. impingement syndrome, impingement syndrome.** *Pathologic condition.* Pressure of the humerus (upper armbone) against the acromium (projection of the scapula) when the arm is elevated, leading to painful irritation of the tissues between the humerus or its head and the acromium.

> **s. spica cast.** *Orthopedic appliance.* Cast that encompasses the arm and chest, immobilizing the shoulder.

shoulderblade. Popular term for the scapula, large bone along back of chest.

side pinch. *Function.* A pinch using the side of the finger against the thumb pad. See also PULP PINCH.

silastic (si-LAS-tik). *Surgical implant.* Silicone material used in interpositional arthroplasties as a spacer between two bones. Permits movement without pain.

Silfverskiöld procedure. *Surgical procedure.* Transposition of the heads of the gastrocnemius from their attachment at distal end of the femur (thighbone) to the tibia (shinbone), effectively lengthening the tendon of the gastrocnemius.

silver-fork deformity. *Pathologic condition.* Describes appearance of the distal end of the radius (larger forearm bone) after fracture: a fork lying flat with the tines facing down.

simple fracture, closed fracture. *Pathologic conditon.* Broken bone in which the bone ends do not exit the skin or damage the surrounding tissue.

sin-. Incorrect spelling of many words beginning with syn-.

single column fracture. *Pathologic condition.* 1. Break in lower part of humerus (upper armbone) involving the medial or lateral column (area that ends in the condyles). 2. Break in the vertebra involving only one of the three columns described by Denis. See DENIS CLASSIFICATION OF VERTEBRAL FRACTURES.

sinus tarsi (SI-nus), **tarsal sinus.** *Anatomy.* Opening formed by the recesses at the bottom surface of the talus (top foot bone) and the upper surface of the calcaneus (heelbone); contains blood vessels, nerves and ligaments. Continuous with the narrower tarsal canal and opens toward the outside of the joint. Lies between the posterior and anterior facets of the talocalcaneal (subtalor) joint. See also TARSAL CANAL

> **syndrome.** *Pathologic condition.* Pain in the sinus tarsi persisting many months after an ankle sprain.

sistic. Incorrect spelling of CYSTIC.

Sjögren's syndrome (SHOH-grinz). *Pathologic condition.* Chronic connective tissue disease characterized by drying of the mucus membranes, peculiar spots on the face, and enlargement of glands near the ear or carotid glands. May be associated with rheumatoid arthritis and Raynaud's phenomenon.

skelecast. *Orthopedic appliance.* Lightweight cast consisting of a series of thin, circumferential rings surrounding the affected area, connected by fortified struts. Allows for wide access to the immobilized segment.

skeleton. *Anatomy*. The rigid framework of bones that gives form to the body, protects and supports the soft organs and tissues, and provides attachments for muscles.

> **appendicular s.**: the bones of the upper and lower extremities, including those of the pelvic and shoulder girdles; forms the framework for the arms and legs.

> **axial s.**: the bones of the vertebral column, thorax and skull; forms the framework for the trunk and head.

skew foot. *Pathologic condition*. Forefoot that bends inward with the heel bending outward. On x-ray, forefoot is markedly in varus and hindfoot is in valgus.

Skillern's fracture. *Pathologic conditon*. Break in lower end of the radius (larger forearm bone) with greenstick fracture of the ulna (smaller forearm bone).

skin flap. Tongue-shaped segment of skin that has been cut (surgically or traumatically) so its blood supply remains intact; often used in surgery to cover or fill a skin defect, such as after removal of a tumor or scar.

skin graft. *Biological implant, surgical procedure*. Skin removed from an individual to be transferred from one location to another; may be taken from the same individual or from another.

> **full-thickness (FTSG)**: transplanted skin that takes the full thickness of the dermis without extending into the subcutaneous tissue.

> **split-thickness (STSG)**: transplanted skin encompassing only the most superficial layers of the dermis, used to cover an open wound.

skin traction. *Treatment*. Traction on an extremity from devices applied to the skin.

sliding arthrodesis, sliding inlay graft. *Surgical procedure*. Joint fusion in which a segment of bone is removed from half the joint and replaced by a bone segment slid down from the adjacent bone. Prevents motion at the joint.

slightly moveable articulations, amphiarthrosis, juncturae cartilaginae. *Anatomy*. Type of synarthrosis (nonmobile joint). Called a symphysis if the bones are connected by flattened disks of fibrocartilage (e.g., symphysis pubis connecting the two pubic bones at the front of the pelvis), or a syndesmosis (if connected by an interosseous ligament). See also ARTICULATION.

sling. *Orthopedic appliance*. Cloth or leather device for holding an extremity in an elevated position, to relieve pressure or weight

slipped capital femoral epiphysis (SCFE). *Pathologic condition*. In a child's femur (thighbone), a separation of the head from the neck at the growth plate; occurs between ages 10 –14. Associated with overweight individuals.

slipped disc. *Pathologic condition*. Popular term for herniated disc. Extrusion of the cartilaginous tissue in the nucleus pulposus (center of disc), which can place pressure on a nerve and result in leg or arm pain, numbness, tingling or weakness (neuropraxia).

slipper cast. *Orthopedic appliance*. Small foot cast that encompasses the heel.

Slocum procedure for patellar tendon transfer. *Surgical procedure*. Use of the inner half of the patellar tendon as a rotational flap, to help reconstruct the inner ligaments of the knee.

Slocum procedure for pes anserinus transfer. *Surgical procedure*. Transfer of the insertion of the pes anserinus (hamstring muscles) medially to help reinforce the inner ligaments of the knee.

Slocum procedure for reconstruction of the medial side of the knee. *Surgical procedure*. Method for repairing the ligaments about the inner side of the knee.

Slocum technique for arthrodesis of the posterior and posterolateral as-

pects of the spine. *Surgical procedure.* Method for fusing the back of a spinal segment; spans the spinous processes (midline protrusions at the back of a vertebra), their lamina and transverse processes.

slough (sluff). 1. *Pathologic process.* Loose tissue from infection or loss of circulation. 2. *Pathologic lesion.* Necrotic or diseased tissue that separates from the underlying, healthier bed.

sluff. Incorrect spelling of SLOUGH.

small wire external fixator. *Surgical implant.* Device used in the stabilization of fracture; holds the bone fragments from outside the body using a series of thin wires attached to a group of circular frames. See also IIZAROV EXTERNAL FIXATOR.

Smillie nail /or/ **pin**. *Surgical implant.* Small nail used to hold loose bone segments in place in areas of osteochondritis dissecans.

Smith fracture, reverse Colles' fracture. *Pathologic condition.* Break in the distal end of the radius (larger forearm bone) near its lower joint surface, with a displacement toward the palm.

Smith-Petersen approach. *Surgical technique.* Anterolateral approach to the hip joint. Used for drainage of the hip joint, in replacement of the femoral head, and for innominate osteotomy.

Smith-Petersen arthrodesis. *Surgical procedure.* Technique for fusion of the hip using a Smith-Petersen nail.

Smith-Petersen arthroplasty /or/ **mold** /or/ **mould arthroplasty**. *Surgical procedure.* Creation of a new joint by interposing inert material (plastic, metal, etc.) between the reshaped ends of bones.

Smith-Petersen cup. *Surgical implant.* Artificial hip joint using a glass cup as replacement for the acetabulum (hip socket). No longer used.

Smith-Petersen nail. *Surgical implant.* Triflanged nail used in fixation of the femoral neck.

snapping tendon syndrome. *Pathologic condition.* Symptoms of painful snapping caused by a tendon that moves abnormally across a bony prominence. Most commonly encountered by ballerinas at the iliopsoas insertion across the upper femur (hip).

snuffbox. *Anatomy.* Small space at the wrist between the extensor pollicis and abductor pollicis tendons of the thumb. If painful, may indicate a fracture of the navicular bone.

soas. Incorrect spelling of psoas (muscle).

socket. *Anatomy.* The hollow portion of a joint (female portion) or cup, into which the opposite segment fits.

Sofield osteotomy, Sofield technique for osteogenesis imperfecta. *Surgical procedure.* Cutting a severely deformed bony segment of an extremity into at least three to four small segments and threading them over a metal rod, to realign the extremity. Used in osteogenesis imperfecta to correct marked bowing of the legs or arms.

soft corn, heloma molle. *Abnormal condition.* Pressure area between the toes that results in the formation of a painful callosity. Usually macerated and softened from moistness between the toes.

sole. *Anatomy.* The bottom, or plantar aspect, of the foot.

soleus. *Anatomy.* Large calf muscle that bends the foot downward (plantar flexion). Extends from top of tibia (shinbone) to the calcaneus (heelbone).

sonogram, ultrasounography. Picture of internal structures derived from transmission of high frequency sound waves into an area, which are reflected by the tissues. Frequently used in diagnosis of hip dysplasia and evaluation of a fetus in the womb.

Southwick osteotomy. *Surgical procedure.* Cutting the proximal femur (thighbone), to realign the femoral head in the acetabulum (hip socket) in severe slipped capital femoral epiphysis. Precise cut will result in correction of alignment in three places.

Soutter procedure. *Surgical procedure.* Cutting the anterior superior iliac spine (with attached muscles and fascia) at its attachment to bone and allowing the muscles to slide distally. For relieving contractures.

spasm (SPAZ-um). *Pathologic condition.* Involuntary muscle contracture.

spasmodic torticollis, **cervical dystonia**. *Pathologic condition.* Condition characterized by abnormal tension and activity across muscles of the neck; can lead to abnormal posture and repetitive twisting movements. Can begin at any age but usually starts in 30s or 40s. No known cause or cure.

spastic (SPAZ-tik). *Clinical finding.* Having jerky, uncoordinated movements from muscle hyperactivity, usually resulting from central nervous system disease.

> **s. cerebral palsy**. *Pathologic condition.* Type of cerebral palsy (central nervous system disease); hyperactive muscle activity leads to jerky, unco-ordinated movements.

spasticity. *Pathologic condition.* Condition characterized by state of hyperac-tivity and increased muscle tone leading to uncoordinated movements and, potentially, contractures.

sphingomyelin (sfing-oh-MY-oh-lin). *Biologic substance.* Phospholipid found in the brain and spinal cord, crucial to its function. See also TAY SACKS DISEASE.

sphingomyelolipidosis (sfing-oh-my-loh-lip-ih-DOH-sus), **Niemann-Pick dis-ease**. *Pathologic condition.* Severe form of lipid storage disease. There is growth impairment with progressive neurological deterioration, enlargement of the liver and spleen, and cherry red spots or grayish haze in the reti-na. Death by age 3. A more benign form occurs rarely in adults.

spica bandage (SPI-kuh). *Orthopedic supply.* Soft dressing that uses tech-nique of overlapping bandages, applied to the body and the first part of a limb, or to the hand and a finger.

spica cast (SPI-kuh). *Orthopedic appliance.* Cast applied to a section of the body and the adjoining portion of a limb, or to the hand and an adjoining finger, in order to effectively immobilize the encased appendage. Takes its name from its resemblance to an ear of wheat.

spicule (SPIK-yul). *Pathologic finding.* Sharp piece of bone or pointed object, e.g., a piece of glass or tin.

spina bifida (SPI-nuh BIF-uh-duh). *Congenital abnormality.* Spinal column defect in which the posterior elements of the spine do not completely meet or fuse. Variable in degree.

> **cystica** (SIS-tuh-kuh): absence of the posterior bony elements of the spine allowing protrusion (in form of a sac) of the lining of the brain or spinal cord under the skin. Four types: meningocele, myelodysplasia, meningo-mylocele, myelomeningocele, which all have neurological involvement.

> **occulta**: separation of the arch of the spine, with no neurological involve-ment and no cyst or protrusion.

spinal accessory nerve. *Anatomy.* Cranial nerve that supplies the trapezius, sternocleidomastoid and levator scapulae. Exits the skull between the inter-nal jugular vein and internal carotid artery, extending into the posterior triangle of the neck.

spinal ataxia (ay-TAK-see-uh). *Pathologic condition.* Loss of muscular coor-dination due to injury or disease of the spinal cord; may be associated with syphilis or diabetes.

spinal block. *Anesthesia.* Injection of local anesthetic into the spine, to eliminate pain at a specific nerve area.

spinal canal. *Anatomy.* Bony and connective tissue channel through which the spinal cord and its membranes pass.

spinal column. See SPINE.

spinal cord. *Anatomy.* The part of the central nervous system that rests within the spinal canal; neurological structure that connects the brain to the lower extremities by multiple fibers through which electrical impulses travel.

spinal fusion. *Surgical procedure.* Fusion of the bones between two or more vertebrae, to prevent movement. Usually used for treating degenerative disorders in segments of the spine, after complex fractures of the spine, or in an effort to treat an unstable portion of the spine.

spinalis muscle (spi-NAL-us). *Anatomy.* Muscle (one of a series) that attaches to the back of a vertebra; seen in various groupings from skull to lumbar area.

spinal muscular atrophy. *Pathologic condition.* Symmetrical muscle weakness characterized by degeneration of anterior horn cells of the spine; affects lower limbs more than upper limbs. Hereditary. Three types, according to severity:

> **type I (Werdnig-Hoffman disease)**: severe form; acute, with onset at birth, usually leading to death from pneumonia in 1st or 2nd year due to weakness of chest muscles.

> **type II (Werdnig-Hoffman disease)**: intermediate form; chronic, onset at 6-12 months. Patient able to sit but not walk. Survival into adulthood. Death from pneumonia.

> **type III (Kugelberg-Welander disease)** (VO-lan-dur): least severe form; variable onset. Patient is able to walk, but gait is abnormal. Can have normal life span but with risk of pulmonary complications.

spinal stenosis (SS) (stuh-NOH-sus). *Pathologic condition.* Narrowing of the spinal canal (bony tunnel through which spinal cord passes) causing irritation and compression of the spinal cord. Other types listed under STENOSIS.

spine, spinal column, vertebral column. *Anatomy.* The backbone, extending the full length of the back. Consists of 30 vertebrae: 7 cervical (in the neck), 12 thoracic (in the back), 5 lumbar (between the ribs and pelvis), and the pelvic vertebrae (5 sacral, 1 coccygeal).

> **bamboo s**. *Pathologic condition.* On x-ray has the appearance of a bamboo stick; occurs in advanced stage of ankylosing spondylitis.

spine (tibial). *Anatomy.* The two bony projections into the knee joint from the proximal tibia (shinbone). Attaches to the posterior horn of the lateral semilunar cartilage.

spinous process (SPI-nus). *Anatomy.* The midline of a vertebra where the lamina fuse. Forms the bumps running up and down the center of a person's back.

spiral fracture. *Pathologic condition.* Break that twists as it extends along a bone, assuming a spiral configuration.

spiral groove of the humerus. *Anatomy.* Furrow in the humerus (armbone) in which the radial nerve travels down the arm toward the elbow.

splayfoot, fallen arch, flatfoot, pes planus, talipes planus. *Abnormal condition.* Foot that lacks an arch; foot whose metatarsal arch, which runs from the heel to ball of foot, is collapsed. May be congenital or developed over time.

splenius muscles (SPLEEN-ee-us). *Anatomy.* Group of muscles that pulls the head back and to the side; attaches from behind the mastoid region of the skull to the cervical and upper thoracic spine.

splint. *Orthopedic appliance.* Cylindrical device used for immobilization of an extremity; part of its circumference is rigid and the remainder is soft, to help accommodate swelling.

> **air s.**: made of inflatable material, usually for transporting a patient.

> **coaptation s.** (koh-ap-TAY-shun): placed on both sides of a fracture, maintaining pressure against a fragment.

cock-up s.: plaster or metal splint that holds the wrist in a slightly dorsiflexed (extended) position, to protect it.

dorsal s.: the rigid portion lies in the back (dorsal aspect) of the extremity.

fiberglass s.: the rigid portion is made of fiberglass.

inflatable s.: same as AIR.

long-leg s. (LLS): extends from foot to thigh; extends above the knee.

plaster/plaster of paris s.: the rigid portion is made of plaster of paris.

posterior s.: the rigid portion lies in the back of the extremity.

radial gutter s.: for holding the ring and small finger. The rigid portion is shaped like a gutter and runs along the ulnar border of the hand and wrist, from the finger to the forearm.

short-arm s.: extends from hand to elbow, held by an elastic bandage.

short-leg s.: extends from foot to knee, held in place by an elastic bandage.

sugar tong s.: forearm splint that maintains fracture alignment by stretching on the dorsal and ventral surface and around the proximal joint. Resembles sugar tongs.

Thomas s.: V-shaped metal frame running from the hip to beyond the toes; allows for traction to be applied to the leg. Usually used for patient's transport.

thumb spica s.: extends from the forearm to the hand and past the interphalangeal joint of the thumb.

traction s.: allows for traction to be applied to a limb or digit.

ulnar plus s.: crosses the finger, hand and wrist, holding the hand in an ulnar-plus position (wrist slightly extended, the metacarpophalangeal joint flexed to 90° and the interphalangeal joints extended).

volar s.: applied to the wrist and forearm; rigid portion lies in the front (volar aspect) of the extremity.

wire ladder s.: rectangular splint with crossbars, resembling a ladder. Used for temporarily immobilizing an extremity during application of first aid or in preparation for patient transport.

splints (shin). *Pathologic condition.* Pain over the front of the lower legs; associated with a sudden increase in activity level. Felt to be due to inflammation of the periosteum (soft tissue covering) of the tibia (shinbone).

split hand, lobster hand /or/ **claw, cleft hand, main fourchee**. *Congenital anomaly.* Hand separated into two parts (like a lobster's claw); associated with missing fingers and metacarpal bones.

split-thickness skin graft (STSG). *Surgical procedure, biological implant.* Skin removed from an individual to be transferred from one location to another; emcompasses only the most superficial layers of the dermis and does not extend into the subcutaneous tissue. Used for covering an open wound. See also FULL-THICKNESS SKIN GRAFT.

spondylitis (spahn-duh-LI-tus). *Pathologic condition.* Inflammation of the spine; may be infectious in origin.

ankylosing s., Bechterew's disease, Marie-Strumpell disease: autoimmune connective tissue disorder resulting in gradual fusion of the joints between vertebrae and severe limitation of spinal motion, with back and hip pain.

s. deformans (dee-FOR-muns): spinal condition characterized by the creation of large spurs and calcification of the intervertebral ligaments. Associated with back pain and stiffness. Hallmark of the condition is its prominent radiographic changes.

rheumatoid s: same as ANKYLOSING (above).

spondyloarthritis (spahn-duh-loh-ahr-THRI-tus). See SPONDYLOARTHROPATHY.

spondyloarthropathy (spahn-duh-loh-ahr-THRAH-puh-thee), **spondyloarthritis.** *Pathologic condition.* Arthritis of the vertebral joints.

> **juvenile s.**: inflammation and degeneration of the spine; may result in spinal deformity and various joint abnormalities. Affects children and adolescents. Many types.

spondylodesis (spahn-duh-loh-DEE-sus). *Pathologic condition.* Fusion of the spine.

spondyloepiphyseal dysplasia (spahn-dul-oh-eh-pif-uh-SEE-ul dis-PLAY-zjuh). *Congenital abnormality.* Syndrome characterized by short trunk dwarfism, delayed deposition of bone in the vertebrae and proximal femur, and coxa vara. Hereditary.

spondylolisthesis (spahn-duh-loh-liss-THEE-sus). *Pathologic condition.* A falling or slipping forward of one vertebra on another. See also SPONDYLOPTOSIS.

> **degenerative s.**: results from degeneration of the joints of the lower spine.
> **dysplastic s.**: caused by congenital abnormalities in the upper sacrum.
> **isthmic s.** (ISS-mik): caused by lesion (lytic, fatigue fracture or acute fracture) of the pars interarticularis (back of spine between vertebral facets).
> **pathologic s.**: occurs with bone disease (e.g., osteogenesis imperfecta, arthrogryposis), or as a result of tumor or surgery.
> **traumatic s.**: secondary to fracture in areas in the lumbar/sacral spine other than the pars interarticularis (back of spine between vertebral facets).

spondylolysis (spahn-duh-loh-LI-sus). *Pathologic condition.* Defect in the pars interarticularis (back of spine between vertebral facets).

spondylopathy (spahn-duh-LAH-puh-thee). *Pathologic condition.* Any abnormality or disease of the vertebrae.

spondyloptosis (spahn-duh-lahp-TOH-sus). Most severe form of spondylolisthesis, where one vertebrae slides off (completely displaces) another.

spondylosis (spahn-duh-LOH-sus). *Pathologic condition.* Any degenerative disease of the spine.

> **ankylosing s., Marie Strumpell disease, spondylitis deformans**: gradual fusion of the joints between vertebrae; results in severe limitation of spinal motion, round back appearance, and back and hip pain.

sprain. *Pathologic condition.* A tearing of, or an injury to, a ligament. 1st degree: ligament is stretched; generally produces pain and swelling. 2nd degree: some fibers are torn; often accompanied by weakness and bluish discoloration due to bleeding. 3rd degree: most or all of the fibers are torn; produces severe weakness and decreased mobility.

Sprengel's deformity, congenital elevation of the scapula. *Congenital abnormality.* Elevation and medial rotation of the scapula (shoulderblade). Motion is limited.

spring ligament. *Anatomy.* Very thick, strong ligament between the calcaneus (heelbone) and navicular of the foot, which supports the head of the talus (top foot bone).

spur, osteophyte. *Pathologic condition.* Outgrowth of bone usually at the edge of a joint or a vertebra; indicates an arthritic or inflammatory process. See also CALCAR.

squinting patellae. *Pathologic condition.* Knees that point toward each other; result of femoral anteversion, which causes the patella to move abnormally across the knee. Causes knee pain.

standing frame orthosis. *Orthopedic appliance.* Orthotic device that holds a small child lacking strength or muscle control in the upright position.

Staphylococcus aureus (staf-uh-loh-KAH-kus OR-ee-us). *Bacteria.* Organism normally residing in the skin; frequently associated with infections.

stasis (STAY-sus). *Function.* State of having no active flow of a bodily fluid.

Steele osteotomy. *Surgical procedure.* Cutting through the innominate bone above the acetabulum (hip socket) to allow rotation of the acetabulum. For treatment of acetabular dysplasia.

Steida fracture. *Pathologic condition.* An avulsion type of break (sudden muscle contraction that pulls its attachment from the bone) around the knee, with small pieces of bone along the side of the knee joint. Associated with a tear in the anterior cruciate ligament.

Steindler arthrodesis of the elbow (ahr-throh-DEE-sus). *Surgical procedure.* Technique for fusing the elbow: an onlay graft from the pelvis is placed along the back of the humerus (armbone) and attached onto the olecranon process (tip of elbow). Held in place by a screw placed through the upper half of the graft and into the humerus.

Steindler arthrodesis of the shoulder (ahr-throh-DEE-sus) *Surgical procedure.* Technique for fusing the shoulder: the humerus (upper armbone) is sutured to the scapula (wingbone). Obsolete.

Steindler flexorplasty. *Surgical procedure.* Transfer of the flexor muscles of the forearm to a more proximal site on the humerus (upper armbone); enables flexion by changing leverage of the muscles. Used in individuals who have flexor paralysis of the arm.

Steindler stripping. *Surgical procedure.* Releasing the plantar fascia and muscles to treat a high arch.

Steinert's disease, **dystrophic myotonia**, **myotonic dystrophy**. *Pathologic condition.* Hereditary weakness of the muscles of the face, neck and distal extremities. Patients usually present with weakness of the hands, difficulty walking, or tendency to fall. May die young from pulmonary-cardiac failure; they are especially at risk during anesthesia.

Steinmann pin. *Surgical implant.* Long, pointed pin used for fixation of fractures or as a method of bone stabilization. May be threaded or smooth.

stellate fracture (STEL-ayt). *Pathologic condition.* Star-shaped break caused by direct trauma.

stenosing tenosynovitis of the finger /or/ **thumb** (sten-OH-sing ten-oh-sin-oh-VI-tus), **trigger finger** /or/ **thumb**. *Pathologic condition.* Finger that snaps as it is brought from flexion into extension. Caused by a small nodule on the tendon that prevents normal gliding movement.

stenosis (sten-OH-sus). *Pathologic condition.* Narrowing or tightness of a structure or canal.

    cervical s.: degenerative narrowing of the cervical spinal canal, causing irritation and compression of the nerve roots and/or spinal cord.

    foraminal s.: narrowing of the neural foramen (bony opening in spine through which nerve roots exit to the body) causing compression and irritation of the affected nerve root(s).

    lumbar s.: degenerative change in the lumbar area of the spinal canal; causes irritation and compression of the nerve roots. Most common of the spinal stenoses.

    spinal s.: narrowing of the spinal canal (bony tunnel through which the spinal cord passes) causing irritation and compression of the spinal cord.

sterile. *Condition.* Free from living organisms.

sterilization. *Procedure.* Method used to render a material free from living organisms; includes steam under pressure, gas, and ionizing radiation.

sternoclavicular joint (stur-noh-kluh-VIK-yu-lur). *Anatomy.* Joint at the shoulder composed of the sternum (breastbone) and the clavicle (collarbone).

sternocleidomastoid muscle (stur-noh-kli-doh-MAS-toyd). *Anatomy.* Long muscle that tilts the skull to the side and rotates it to the opposite direction. Attached at the front of the chest at the level of the clavicle (collarbone), and at the skull at the mastoid process.

sternum (STUR-num), **breast bone**. *Anatomy*. Large bone on the front of the chest, where ribs attach.

steroid, corticosteroid. *Drug classification*. Cortisone derivative; for treating inflammatory and allergic diseases. Examples: cortisone, hydrocortisone, prednisone.

Stickler syndrome, **progressive arthroophthalmopathy**. *Pathologic condition*. Syndrome characterized by joint abnormalities (seen at birth), severe hip and knee problems, with bony enlargements of the knees, ankles and wrists; significant nearsightedness and astigmatism, possible retinal detachment. Patients generally have a normal life span and intelligence. Some systemic effects, e.g., high fever, high sed rate, splenic enlargement. Hereditary.

Still's disease, **systemic onset juvenile rheumatoid arthritis**. *Pathologic condition*. Type of juvenile rheumatoid arthritis; characterized by the onset of fever, chills, joint pain, enlarged lymph nodes and spleen.

stiloid. Incorrect spelling of STYLOID.

Stimson maneuver. *Treatment*. Technique for reduction of a traumatic hip dislocation. With patient prone and affected hip hanging over the edge of a table, the femoral head is forced back into the acetabulum (hip socket) by gravity and direct pressure.

stinger, burner. *Pathologic condition*. Sudden jolt of pain across the arm after a blunt injury to the head and neck, most commonly in football players. Usually resolves spontaneously.

stippled, stippling. *Pathologic condition*. Appearance of small, punctate calcifications in the uncalcified areas of bone in infants and children, and in some cartilaginous tissue such as the voice box. Occurs in many conditions, but may also be indicative of chondrodysplasia punctata.

stitch, suture. 1. *Surgical implant*. String- or threadlike material used to sew wounds together. Types listed under SUTURE. 2. *Surgical procedure*. To repair a wound using sutures.

stockinette. *Orthopedic supply*. Tubular cotton material applied over the skin underneath padding and plaster when casting or splinting.

Stone staple. *Surgical implant*. Four-pronged staple used for holding ligaments or tendon to bone.

straight last shoe. *Orthopedic appliance*. Refers to a shoe in which a line from the heel through the foot is in direct line with the 3rd metatarsal bone.

straight leg raising (SLR). *Test*. With the patient lying face-up, the leg is elevated, stretching the sciatic nerve; pain down the leg or in the opposite leg may indicate a herniated disc. Patients with cerebral palsy or other muscle abnormalities may exhibit tightness of the hamstrings.

strain. *Pathologic condition*. Abnormal stretch on a muscle or tendon, with injury.

Strayer procedure. *Surgical procedure*. Relieving tension on the heel cord by cutting the Achilles tendon, stretching the heel and suturing the loose and retracted upper portion of the tendon to the soleus (one of the calf muscles), allowing the foot to be dorsiflexed in neutral. Used for treatment of equinus deformity in children and adolescents.

Streeter's dysplasia (dis-PLAY-zjuh). *Congenital abnormality*. Syndrome of numerous constricting rings produced by thin bands of amniotic membrane that may encircle an arm, leg or digit in utero; may be so deep as to touch the bone and sever blood vessels and nerves. See also AMNIOTIC BAND.

195

stress fracture, **fatigue fracture**. *Pathologic condition.* Break in a bone caused by prolonged repetitive activity, such as running or marching.

stroke. *Pathologic condition.* Sudden loss of specific brain functions (e.g., speech, specific movement), from interrupted blood supply, as by an embolism, thrombosis or hemorrhage; usually results from cerebral blood vessel disease (atherosclerosis).

strut graft. *Surgical technique.* Bone graft used as a strut between two areas of bone; most frequently between two ends of a spinal curve in a kyphotic or scoliotic deformity.

Stryker frame. *Orthopedic appliance.* Has an upper and lower shell; for turning patients with paraplegia or quadriplegia, who are unable to turn themselves.

stump shrinker. *Orthopedic appliance.* Elastic sock used on the end of an amputated extremity to squeeze out the fluid and compress tissues in preparation for fitting a prosthesis.

stump sock. *Orthopedic appliance.* Stocking placed over an extremity between the skin and a prosthesis.

sturnum. Incorrect spelling of STERNUM.

St. Vitus' dance, **Sydenham's chorea**. *Pathologic condition.* An acute disease of the central nervous system: patient has involuntary irregular movements of muscles of the face, neck, and limbs, which disappear in sleep. Associated with rheumatic fever; may be infectious or toxic.

styloid process (STI-loyd). *Anatomy.* Short bony prominence at the end of a bone (e.g., ulnar styloid and radial styloid, both at the wrist).

subacromial bursitis, **Duplay disease**. *Pathologic condition.* Inflammation of the bursa of the shoulder causing pain with arm elevation.

subastralagar (sub-as-TRAG-uh-lur). See SUBTALAR.

> **s. arthrodesis** (ahr-throh-DEE-sus). *Surgical procedure.* Fusion of the subtalar joint, to correct alignment and/or to treat arthritis of the subtalar joint.

> **s. dislocation**. *Pathologic condition.* Dislocation of the foot at the subtalar joint, between the talus (top foot bone) and calcaneus (heelbone).

> **s. joint**. *Anatomy.* Joint between the talus (top foot bone) and the calcaneus (heelbone).

subchondral bone. *Anatomy.* Very hard bone underneath the articular cartilage.

subclavian vein. *Anatomy.* Blood vessel feeding into the superior vena cava; returns blood from the arm to central circulation.

subcoracoid dislocation (sub-KOHR-uh-koyd). *Pathologic condition.* Dislocated shoulder resulting in the humeral head sliding beneath the coracoid in the front.

subcutaneous. *Anatomic location.* Layer of fatty tissue underneath the skin.

subcuticular (sub-kyu-TIK-yu-lur). *Anatomic location.* Under the cuticle.

> **s. suture**. *Surgical technique.* Stitch that travels through the deep layers of the skin.

subglenoid dislocation (sub-GLEN-oyd). *Pathologic condition.* Dislocated shoulder resulting in the humeral head sliding underneath the glenoid of the scapula (shoulderblade).

subluxation (sub-luks-AY-shun). *Pathologic condition.* Refers to a bone that incompletely translates out of anatomic alignment within a joint. Once it leaves the joint, it is considered dislocated.

subluxing patella. *Pathologic condition.* A patella (kneecap) that moves to the side and slides in and out of its normal groove in the distal femoral condyle.

subsartorial canal, **Hunter's canal**. *Anatomy.* Channel in the lower leg through which the femoral artery travels; the sartorius muscle forms its roof.

subscapular. *Anatomic description.* Refers to the area deep under the scapula (shoulderblade) between the scapula and the underlying chest wall.

subscapularis muscle (sub-skap-yu-LEHR-us). *Anatomy.* Large muscle covering the front surface of the scapula (shoulderblade) that internally rotates the humerus (upper armbone). Attaches to the proximal humerus.

subtalar (sub-TAY-lur), **subastragalar**. *Anatomic description.* Refers to the area below the anklebone (talus).

> **s. arthrodesis** (ahr-throh-DEE-sus). *Surgical procedure.* Fusion of the subtalar joint, to correct alignment and/or to treat arthritis of that joint.

> **s. dislocation**. *Pathologic condition.* Dislocation of the foot at the subtalar joint, between the talus (top foot bone) and calcaneus (heelbone).

> **s. joint**. *Anatomy.* Joint between the talus (top foot bone) and calcaneus (heelbone).

subtrochanteric fracture (sub-troh-kan-TEHR-ik). *Pathologic condition.* Type of hip fracture; break below the lesser trochanter of the femur (thighbone).

subungual (sub-UN-gwul). *Anatomic description.* Beneath the nail.

> **s. abscess**. *Pathologic condition.* An abscess beneath a toe- or fingernail.

> **s. exostosis** (eks-ahs-TOH-sus). *Pathologic condition.* Bony growth at the distal phalanx, causing elevation of the nail; may be painful.

suction. *Treatment.* Application of negative air or water pressure onto a system (as in a vacuum).

Sudeck atrophy, **reflex sympathetic dystrophy**. *Pathologic condition.* Nonfunctioning extremity caused by exquisite tenderness or pain from the inappropriate firing of pain and sympathetic nerve fibers; usually triggered by an injury. Leads to scarring, loss of hair around the injured part and thinning of the skin. Treatment may require psychotherapy, physical therapy, and sympathetic blocks. In general, the longer the injured body part is not used, the more difficult it is to achieve a successful recovery.

sudo-. *Incorrect spelling of many words beginning with PSEUDO-.*

sugar tong splint. *Orthopedic appliance.* Forearm splint that maintains fracture alignment by stretching on the dorsal and ventral surface and around the proximal joint. Resembles sugar tongs.

sulcus (SUHL-kus). *Anatomic description.* A groove or fissure.

> **s. angle**. *Measurement.* On a tangential view of the knee (merchant's view), the angle created by the intersection of a line parallel to the anterior border of the medial femoral condyle and one parallel to the lateral femoral condyle. This angle should normally measure about 137°.

sulfatide lipidosis, **sulfatidosis**, **metachromatic leukodystrophy.** *Pathologic condition.* Lipid storage disease characterized by abnormal accumulation of fat molecules (sulphatide lipids) with a sulphur chain. Progressive deterioration of central nervous system, with loss of ability to walk, speech difficulty usually about age 1, death by age 10. Autosomal recessive. Most common leukodystrophy in childhood.

sulindac (suhl-IN-dak). *Drug.* An acetic acid, NSAID for treating pain and inflammation. Trade name: Clinoril.

sunrise/sunset view. X-ray of a slightly flexed knee, so the patella can be seen in outline riding in the femoral sulcus (groove) at the distal femur (thighbone).

superficial peroneal nerve (pehr-uh-NEE-ul). *Anatomy.* Branch of the common peroneal nerve supplies the anterior compartment of the leg.

superficial vein thrombosis (SVT) (thrahm-BOH-sus). *Pathologic condition.* Blood clot in a superficial vein within the leg or arm, often after intravenous infusion. Pain and induration (hardening) about the vein may resolve slowly. See also DEEP VEIN THROMBOSIS.

superior. *Location*. Refers to a structure that situates higher (closer to the head) than another. See also INFERIOR.

    s. gemellus (guh-MEL-us). *Anatomy*. Small muscle in back of hip (above inferior gemellus) that rotates the hip externally. See also INFERIOR GEMELLUS.

    s. gluteal vessels (GLU-tee-ul). *Anatomy*. Large blood vessels that supply the buttocks muscles and exit the pelvis through the sciatic notch. See also INFERIOR GLUTEAL VESSELS.

    s. mesenteric artery syndrome (mes-en-TEHR-ik). *Pathologic condition*. Contriction of first part of the intestine, from the superior mesenteric artery being pulled tightly across the intestine in spinal correction (spinal surgery or body cast) so that food cannot past through the intestine; causes vomiting.

    s. pubic ramus (PYU-bik RAY-mus). *Anatomy*. Part of pubis joining in front at the center of the pelvis. See also INFERIOR PUBIC RAMUS.

supernumery digits. *Congenital anomaly*. Extra fingers or toes.

supinate (SU-pin-ayt). *Function*. Turning the hand in the palm-up position or the foot in the sole-up position. See also PRONATE.

supination (su-pin-AY-shun). *Function*. Forearm rotated so that the palm points forward, or foot whose sole points upward. See also PRONATION.

supinator (SU-pin-ay-tur). *Anatomy*. Muscle that turns the palm upward. Attached to the two forearm bones (radius and ulna); originates from the lateral epicondyle of the humerus and upper portion of the ulna, attaches to the midportion of the radius.

supine (su-PINE). *Anatomic description*. Lying on the back in face-up position.

suppurate (SUP-yur-ate). *Abnormal process*. To form or discharge pus.

suppuration (sup-yuh-RAY-shun). *Abnormal process*. Formation of, conversion into, or act of discharging pus.

suppurative (SUHP-ur-uh-tiv). *Description*. Refers to infection associated with purulent material (pus).

    s. osteomyelitis (ahs-tee-oh-mi-uh-LI-tus). P*athologic condition*. Bone infection with pus that is usually bacterial.

supraclavicular nerve (su-pruh-kluh-VIK-yu-lur). *Anatomy*. Branch of the brachial plexus that supplies sensation to the area above the shoulder.

supracondylar fracture (su-pruh-KAHN-duh-lur). *Pathologic condition*. A break above the condyles of the distal femur (thighbone) or distal humerus (upper armbone).

suprapatellar plica (su-pruh-puh-TEL-ur PLI-kuh). *Anatomy*. Band or fold of synovial tissue in the area above the patella (knee). If inflamed or excessively hypertrophied (large), may result in chronic irritation or scarring of the fold, which may become thickened and cause symptoms that indicate a problem within the knee joint. Occasionally associated with popping and catching of the knee.

suprapatellar pouch (su-pruh-puh-TEL-ur). *Anatomy*. Large synovial-lined cavity in direct continuity with the knee joint.

suprascapular nerve (su-pruh-SKAP-yu-lur). *Anatomy*. Nerve comprised of branches from the 5th and 6th cervical (neck) nerve roots; innervates the supraspinatus (above spine of scapula) and infraspinatus (below spine of scapula) muscles.

supraspinatus muscle (su-pruh-spi-NAY-tus). *Anatomy*. Shoulder muscle that abducts (raises) the humerus (upper armbone). Originates from the scapula (shoulderblade) above the spine of the scapula and attaches to the superior facet of the greater tuberosity of the humerus.

surgical approach. *Surgical technique.* Method of accessing deep structures in ways that minimize damage to neurovascular structures and muscles.

    Avila: entry to the sacroiliac joint from the front of the pelvis.

    Codman: approach to the shoulder; begins over the deltoid muscle at the front, crosses over the clavicle (collarbone), to the back of the shoulder.

    deltoid splitting: cutting the upper part of the deltoid muscle along the length of its fibers (up and down) to expose the shoulder joint.

    Gibson: approach to the hip from back and side, for exposure of the femoral head and trochanteric area.

    Smith-Petersen: anterolateral approach to hip joint; used for drainage of hip joint, in replacement of femoral head, and for innominate osteotomy.

    transacromial (tranz-ay-KROH-mee-ul): approach to top of the shoulder through a cut across the acromioclavicular joint. See also SABER-CUT INCISION.

surgical neck fracture. *Pathologic condition.* Break in the proximal humerus (upper armbone) below the physeal plate.

sustentaculum tali (sus-ten-TAK-yu-lum TAY-li). *Anatomy.* Ridge of bone on the inner side of the heel (calcaneus) that supports the talus (first foot bone).

Sutherland osteotomy. *Surgical procedure.* Double innominate osteotomy of the pelvis; a cut is made above the acetabulum (hip socket) and another lateral to the symphysis pubis; the acetabulum is rotated to cover the femoral head. Useful in dysplasia of the hip.

suture. *Anatomy.* Joint where the opposing articulating surfaces of adjacent bones are connected by a thin layer of fibrous connective tissue; found between bones of the skull and face. One of three types of fibrous joints. See also SYMPHYSIS, GOMPHOSIS.

suture, stitch. 1. *Surgical implant.* Stringlike or threadlike material used to sew wounds together. 2. *Surgical procedure.* To repair a wound using sutures. 3. *Surgical technique.* Method for sewing or repairing wounds with sutures.

    baseball: type of locking stitch; used to repair a shredded tendon or ligament.

    braided: made of multiple fibers wrapped around each other.

    Bunnell: wire stitch inserted into a tendon with the end protruding from the wound; enables its withdrawal after the tendon has healed.

    buried: the knots have been buried within the tissue being repaired.

    cat-gut: absorbable suture made of cat-gut material.

    Ethi-bond: trade name for a nonabsorbable, braided suture made of synthetic material.

    fiber wire: nonabsorbable, braided suture made of synthetic material.

    horizontal mattress: placed across the wound in two passes, or throws, at the same depth.

    interrupted: placed individually across a wound; not connected to each other.

    Kessler: passing of two separate sutures through a torn tendon, with both tied down simultaneously to finely control the tension across the stitch.

        modified: uses only one stitch; slightly less control of the tension across the suture, but requires fewer knots and less extraneous bulk.

    Krackow: same as BASEBALL (above).

    locking: running stitch where each row is locked so it will not slide.

    monocryl: absorbable monofilament suture made of synthetic material.

    monofilament: made of only one fiber.

    nonabsorbable: same as PERMANENT (below).

    nylon: made of nylon.

    permanent: material that will not be absorbed or dissolved by the body.

prolene: nonabsorbable synthetic suture.

running: uses one long thread with numerous passes across a wound.

smooth: same as MONOFILAMENT.

subcutaneous: placed within the deep layers of the skin.

subcuticular: travels through the deep layers of the skin.

Tevdek: trade name of nonabsorbable suture material.

tie: done without a needle; to tie and close off the ends of vessels.

transosseous: passed through the bone to tie a ligament or tendon to the bone.

Tycron: trade name for a nonabsorbable, braided suture made of synthetic material.

vertical mattress: placed across a wound in two passes, or throws, one pass deeper than the other.

Vicryl: trade name for an absorbable braided suture.

suture anchor. *Surgical implant.* Screw-like device with an eyelet at the head allowing for suture material to be passed through it. Used in reattaching a tendon or ligament to a bone.

swan neck deformity. *Pathologic condition.* Finger deformity caused by uneven pull of the tendons about a finger. Characterized by flexion of the distal interphalangeal joint (last finger joint) and hyperextension of the proximal interphalangeal joint (joint past the knuckle). In the thumb, there may be partial dislocation of the metacarpophalangeal joint. Occurs most often in patients with rheumatoid arthritis or osteoarthritis of the thumb joints.

swayback. *Abnormal condition.* Popular term for lordosis, a curvature of the spine in which the concave surface of the curve faces backward.

Swedish knee cage. *Orthopedic appliance.* Brace that prevents hyperextension of the knee.

swing phase. *Function.* One stage in ambulation; leg is swung forward in preparation for initiation of the next step; occurs between toe-off and heel strike.

Sydenham's chorea, St. Vitus' dance. *Pathologic condition.* Acute disease of the central nervous system: patient has involuntary irregular movements of muscles of the face, neck and limbs, which disappear in sleep. Associated with rheumatic fever; may be infectious or toxic.

Syme amputation. *Surgical procedure.* Removal of heelbone and forefoot; the heel pad is brought up to lie under the articular surface of the tibia (shinbone).

sympathetic block. *Treatment.* Anesthetization of a body part by injecting an anesthetic drug into the sympathetic nerve trunk. For treating pain conditions and autonomic disorders such as reflex sympathetic dystrophy.

sympathetic nervous system. *Anatomy.* Part of the autonomic system; provides quick energy and response. See also AUTONOMIC NERVOUS SYSTEM, PARASYMPATHETIC NERVOUS SYSTEM.

sympathetic trunk. *Anatomy.* Chain of sympathetic nerves running along the sides of the spine carrying impulses for bodily functions.

symphalangism (sim-FAL-un-jis-um). *Pathologic condition.* Fusion of the finger joints or toe joints.

symphysis (SIM-fuh-sus). *Anatomy.* Type of articulation in which the ends of the bones are connected by a cartilage plate; do not ordinarily move or flex. One of two types of cartilaginous joints. See also SYNCHONDROSIS.

s. pubis (PYU-bus): joint between the two anterior portions of the pelvis where they join at the midline.

synchondrosis (sin-kahn-DROH-sus). *Anatomy.* Temporary joint between two bones that gets fused into solid bone by adulthood. Examples: between bones of the quadrangular space in the pelvis between the ischium, pubis and ilium. One of the two types of cartilaginous joints. See also SYMPHYSIS.

syndactyly (sin-DAK-tuh-lee). *Congenital abnormality.* Fusion or webbing of two or more digits.

syndesmosis (sin-dez-MO-sus). *Anatomy.* Joint comprised of bones joined by interosseous ligaments. Example: area at end of the tibia (shinbone), between the tibia and the fibula. One of the three types of fibrous joints. See also GOMPHOSIS, SUTURES.

synergy (SIN-ur-jee). *Function.* Activity of muscles working in coordination.

synostosis (sin-ahs-TOH-sus). *Pathologic condition.* Fusion between two bones.

synovectomy (sin-oh-VEK-tuh-mee). *Surgical procedure.* Removal of part or all of the synovial membrane of a joint.

synovia (sin-OH-vee-uh), **synovial fluid**. *Anatomy.* Transparent fluid within a joint that lubricates the joint.

synovial joint (sin-OH-vee-ul), **diarthrosis**. *Anatomy.* Freely movable joint with a synovial lining (fluid secreting membrane), e.g., knee, wrist.

synovial membrane (sin-OH-vee-ul), **synovium**. *Anatomy.* Fine membrane within a synovial joint that secretes synovial fluid, to lubricate the joint.

synovial osteochondromatosis (sin-OH-vee-ul ahs-tee-oh-kahn-droh-muh-TOH-sus), **synovial chondromatosis, osteochondromastis**. *Pathologic condition.* Multiple small cartilaginous formations in the synovial membrane that may become detached and fall into the joint as loose bodies (joint mice). Causes pain, swelling and stiffness.

synovial sarcoma (sin-OH-vee-ul). *Pathologic condition.* Malignant tumor in the proximity of a joint whose cell characteristerics are similar to those of the synovial membrane.

synovitis (sin-oh-VI-tus). *Pathologic condition.* Inflammation of the synovial membrane.

synovium (sin-OH-vee-um). See SYNOVIAL MEMBRANE.

syringomyelia (suh-RIN-go-mi-EE-lee-uh). *Pathologic condition.* A cyst within the substance of the spinal cord, leading to destruction of neural elements and resulting in loss of sensation, paralysis, charcot joints, etc.

syst. Incorrect spelling of CYST.

systemic (sis-TEH-mik). *Description.* Affecting the body generally, rather than a specific (local) area.

    s. lupus erythematosus (LU-pus). *Pathologic condition.* Inflammatory disease that commonly affects joints, especially in the hands, wrists and knees. Involves connective and vascular tissues of many organs; may be associated with severe arthritis, kidney involvement, abnormalities of the retina, and rash on the face. Usually occurs in the 3rd or 4th decade.

    s. onset juvenile rheumatoid arthritis (SOJRA), Still's disease. *Pathologic condition.* Type of juvenile rheumatoid arthritis; characterized by the onset of fever, chills, joint pain, enlarged lymph nodes and spleen.

    s. sclerosis. *Pathologic condition.* Nonspecific term used to describe a collection of conditions (scleroderma is one); results in scarlike changes in the skin and/or an organ. See also SCLERODERMA.

T

T. Abbreviation for THORACIC VERTEBRA; used with specific number (T1–T12).

tabes dorsalis (TAY-bees dor-SAL-us), **posterior spinal sclerosis**. *Pathologic condition*. Loss of sensation and positioning sense in the legs; effect of syphilis on the spinal cord.

table. Firm, often adjustable table used for patient examination or procedure.

> **fracture**: allows x-rays to pass through it (radiolucent); has multiple attachments for variability in patient's positioning and for applying traction.
>
> **Chick**: type of fracture table.
>
> **OSI**: trade name of fracture table.
>
> **radiolucent**: operating room table that allows x-rays to pass through.
>
> **Jackson**: type of radiolucent table.

tailbone. *Anatomy*. Popular term for the coccyx, the fused rudimentary coccygeal vertebrae at the tip of the sacrum that represent the bony remnants of a tail.

tailor's bunion, bunionette. *Pathologic condition*. Inflammation and enlargement of the 5th metatarsophalangeal joint at outer side of the foot (little toe).

talar dome fracture. (TAY-luhr). *Pathologic condition*. Break in the rounded surface (top) of the talus (top foot bone).

talar tilt test (TAY-luhr), **inversion ankle stress test**. *Clinical test*. Examiner applies maximum inversion to the ankle; excess inversion indicates instability of the ankle's lateral ligaments.

talectomy (tay-LEK-toh-mee). *Surgical procedure*. Removal of talus (top foot bone).

talipes (TAL-uh-peez). *Anatomy*. The foot, including the ankle.

> **t. calcaneocavus** (kal-kay-nee-oh-KAY-vus). *Abnormal condition*. Foot with a dorsiflexed heel (pointed up) and plantarflexed forefoot and midfoot (pointed down). Arch is abnormally high; seen with some forms of cerebral palsy.
>
> **t. calcaneous** (kal-KAY-nee-us). *Congenital abnormality*. Dorsiflexed (pointed up) forefoot such that the top is positioned against the tibia (shinbone).
>
> **t. calcaneovalgus** (kal-KAY-nee-oh-VAL-gus). *Congenital abnormality*. Plantarflexed (bends down) foot that turns out.
>
> **t. cavovarus** (kay-voh-VEHR-us). *Congenital abnormality*. Plantarflexed (bends downward) foot that points down with heel and toes turned inward.
>
> **t. cavus** (KAY-vus). *Congenital abnormality*. Foot that has an abnormally high arch.
>
> **t. equinovalgus** (ee-kwi-noh-VAL-gus), **equinovalgus deformity**. *Congenital abnormality*. Plantarflexed (bends down) foot that turns out.
>
> **t. equinovarus** (ee-kwi-noh-VEHR-us), **clubfoot, equinovarus deformity, pes equinovarus**. *Congenital abnormality*. Rigid, inwardly rotated foot that bends down and in; if untreated, rests on outer edge and cannot be placed flat on the walking surface.
>
> **t. equinus** (ee-KWI-nus), equinus deformity. *Congenital abnormality*. Plantarflexed foot (hindfoot points down as if on tiptoes); can lead to a toe walking deformity or be part of a rocker-bottom foot.
>
> **t. planovalgus** (plan-oh-VAL-gus), **pes planovalgus, planovalgus deformity**. *Congenital abnormality*. Flat foot that is deviated to the inner side.
>
> **t. planus, fallen arch, flatfoot, pes planus, splayfoot**. *Abnormal condition*. Foot that lacks an arch; foot whose metatarsal arch is collapsed. May be congenital or developed over time.

talipomanus, clubhand, radial clubhand. *Congenital anomaly*. Absence of the radius (larger forearm bone) and thumb, with the wrist deviated toward the thumb side.

talocalcaneal bar /or/ **bridge** (tay-loh-kal-KAY-nee-ul). *Congenital abnormality.* Bridge of bone between the talus (top foot bone) and calcaneus (heel), preventing motion of the joint.

talocalcaneal joint (tay-loh-kal-KAY-nee-ul). *Anatomy.* Joint between the talus (top foot bone) and the calcaneus (heel).

talocalcaneal ligament (tay-loh-kal-KAY-nee-ul). *Anatomy.* Ligament between the talus (top foot bone) and calcaneus (heel), located within the tarsal sinus.

talocalcaneonavicular joint (tay-loh-kal-KAY-nee-ul-nuh-VIK-kyu-lur). *Anatomy.* Joint between the talus (top foot bone), calcaneus (heelbone), and navicular; allows rotation of the foot.

talofibular joint (tay-loh-FIB-yu-lur). *Anatomy.* Joint between the talus (top foot bone) and the fibula (smaller bone of lower leg).

talofibular ligament (tay-loh-FIB-yu-lur). *Anatomy.* Ligament holding the talus (top foot bone) and fibula (smaller bone of lower leg) in position on the outer side of the foot.

talonavicular ligament (tay-loh-nuh-VIK-yu-lur). *Anatomy.* Ligament joining the talus (top foot bone) to the navicular in the front of the foot.

talus (TAY-lus), **astragalus.** *Anatomy.* Top foot bone. Bone in the ankle between the end of the tibia (shinbone) and the calcaneus (heelbone).

> **vertical t.** *Pathologic condition.* A talus that is plantarflexed (points down); usually associated with paralytic abnormalities such as cerebral palsy.

tamponade (tam-puh-NAHD). *Treatment, biologic process.* Prevention of blood or fluid into an area, by pressure.

Tanner-Whitehouse system (TW2). *Measurement.* Standard for assessment of a child's skeletal development based on wrist and hand x-rays.

tarsal (TAHR-sul). *Anatomic description.* Relating to the tarsus (hindfoot).

> **t. bars.** *Congenital abnormality.* Abnormal connections between various parts of the bones of the hindfoot.

> **t. bones.** *Anatomy.* The seven bones of the hindfoot: talus, calcaneus, navicular, three cuneiforms and cuboid. Corresponds with the eight carpal bones in the wrist.

> **t. canal.** *Anatomy.* Canal between the talus (top foot bone) and calcaneus (heel); continuous with the wider tarsal sinus. Holds blood vessels, nerves and ligaments. Separates the front from the back facets of the talocalcaneal (subtalar) joint. See also SINUS TARSI SYNDROME.

> **t. coalition.** *Congenital abnormality.* Fusion of two or more adjacent tarsal bones that are normally unconnected; may be painful. Cause of one type of rigid flatfoot. See also PERONEAL SPASTIC FLATFOOT, TARSAL BARS.

> **t. navicular.** *Anatomy.* Bone in the foot between the cuneiforms and the talus (top foot bone).

> **t. pronator shoes** (PROH-nay-tur). *Orthopedic appliance.* Shoes made from a pattern in which the left and right lasts (patterns) are reversed, i.e., right shoe on left foot.

> **t. sinus** (SI-nus), **sinus tarsi.** *Anatomy.* Opening formed by the recesses at the bottom of the talus (top foot bone) and upper surface of the calcaneus (heelbone); contains blood vessels, nerves and ligaments. Continuous with the narrower tarsal canal; opens toward the outside of the joint. Lies between the front and back facets of the talocalcaneal (subtalar) joint. See also SINUS TARSI SYNDROME.

> **t. tunnel.** *Anatomy.* Anatomic tunnel in the medial (inner) aspect of the

ankle through which pass the tibial nerve, tendons of the posterior tibialis, flexor digitorum longus and flexor hallucis longus muscles (in order, from front to back), tibial nerve and posterior tibial artery and vein.

    syndrome. *Pathologic condition*. Entrapment of tibial nerve at the level of the tarsal tunnel. Analogous to carpal tunnel syndrome in wrist.

tarsalmetatarsal. Alternate spelling of TARSOMETATARSAL.

Tarso abduction bar, **abduction bar**, **abduction bar splint**, **Denis Browne bar** /or/ **brace** /or/ **splint**, **Fillauer bar** /or/ **abduction bar**. *Orthopedic appliance*. Metal bar that holds a pair of shoes together, positioning the feet. Used for controlling leg rotation in infants.

tarsoepiphyseal aclasia, dysplasia epiphysealis hemimelica, epiphyseal osteochondroma, Trevor disease. *Congenital abnormality*. Abnormal development of osteochondromas, usually involving multiple bones in one limb. Three variations: localized (involves one epiphysis); classic (involves more than one bone in a single limb); and generalized (involves multiple bones in more than one limb).

tarsometatarsal (TMT) (tahr-so-met-uh-TAR-sul). *Anatomic description*. Pertaining to the tarsus and the metatarsus.

    t. dislocation, t. fracture-dislocation, Lisfranc dislocation. *Pathologic condition*. Traumatic dislocation of the foot at the tarsometatarsal joint. Frequently involves fractures of the bones in the immediate area.

    t. joint, Lisfranc joint, midtarsal joint. *Anatomy*. Joint complex between the metatarsal and tarsal bones (the cuneiforms and the cuboid).

tarsus (TAHR-sus). *Anatomy*. The hindfoot and midfoot. The area between the lower end of the tibia and the beginning of the metatarsal bones. Comprised of the 7 bones of the ankle known as the tarsal bones. See TARSAL BONES.

Tay Sachs disease. *Pathologic condition*. Juvenile form of cerebral sphingolipidosis; characterized by progressive spastic paralysis, blindness and mental deterioration. Underlying pathology: abnormality in storage of sphingomyelin.

T-condylar fracture. *Pathologic condition*. Fracture that extends between the two condyles and splits medially and laterally; looks like a letter T on x-ray.

technetium-99 (tek-NEE-shee-um), **technetium pyrophosphate**. Radioactive material injected to obtain a bone scan.

T.E.D. stockings. *Orthopedic supply*. Trade name of stockings designed to prevent blood clots.

Telfa dressing. *Orthopedic supply*. Trade name of thin plastic material that does not stick to wounds.

tendinitis (ten-din-I-tus). *Pathologic condition*. Inflammation of a tendon, frequently at its insertion onto the bone.

tendoachilles (ten-doh-uh-KIL-eez), **Achilles tendon, heelcord**. *Anatomy*. Strong connective tissue band that joins the triceps surae (calf muscles) to the calcaneus (heelbone); comprised of the tendons of the gastrocnemius and soleus muscles.

    t. lengthening (TAL). *Surgical procedure*. Elongation of the Achilles tendon. Used in tight heel cord conditions to eliminate toe walking.

tendon. *Anatomy*. Strong band of tissue that attaches a muscle to a bone; each named after the muscle to which it attaches, e.g., abductor hallucis tendon.

    conjoined t. *Anatomy*. Represents union of two or more muscles connecting to the same location on a bone, e.g., the iliopsoas tendon.

    t. sheath. *Anatomy*. Connective tissue sleeve through which tendons pass; glistening surface allows smooth motion of the tendon from its muscle to its distal point of attachment.

t. transfer. *Surgical procedure*. Transfer of a tendon's position at its attachment to a different position on a bone or tendon. See also TENODESIS.

tendonitis. Alternate spelling of TENDINITIS.

tennis elbow, **lateral epicondolytis** *Pathologic condition*. Inflammation of the extensor tendons where they attach to the capitellum and lateral condyle of the humerus (upper armbone), from repetitive motion in dorsiflexion of the wrist (as when hitting a backhand while playing tennis).

tenodesis (ten-oh-DEE-sus). *Surgical procedure*. Attaching a portion of a tendon to a bone or to the end or side of another tendon. Most commonly used in the treatment of nerve palsies and joint instabilities. See also TENDON TRANSFER.

tenolysis (ten-oh-LI-sus). *Surgical procedure*. Freeing a tendon from adhesions after injury or repair.

tenorrhaphy (ten-OHR-uh-fee). *Surgical procedure*. Repair of a tendon after rupture or transection.

tenosynovectomy (ten-oh-sin-oh-VEK-toh-mee). *Surgical procedure*. Removal of the inflamed lining of a tendon. Used in treatment of inflammatory disorders affecting tendons and their sheaths, such as rheumatoid arthritis.

tenosynovitis (ten-oh-sln-oh-VI-tis). *Pathologic condition*. Inflammation of a tendon and its lining.

tenotomy (ten-AH-toh-mee). *Surgical procedure*. Cutting of a tendon.

tensor fascia lata (FASH-uh LAH-tuh). *Anatomy*. Muscle that flexes and abducts the thigh; originates from the lateral aspect on the ilium (pelvis) and attaches to the proximal anterolateral tibia (shinbone) via the iliotibial band.

teres major (TEHR-eez). *Anatomy*. Muscle that adducts the arm and helps to extend and internally rotate the humerus (upper armbone); originates from the inferior lateral border of the scapula (shoulderblade) and attaches onto the proximal humerus.

teres minor (TEHR-eez). *Anatomy*. Muscle that draws the humerus (upper armbone) toward the glenoid fossa (maintains humerus against its cup in the shoulder) and externally rotates it; originates from the inferior lateral border of the scapula (shoulderblade) and attaches to the proximal humerus.

terrible triad of O'Donoghue, O'Donoghue's terrible /or/ **unhappy triad**. *Pathologic condition*. Knee injury: a tear of the medial collateral ligament, anterior cruciate ligament (ACL) and medial meniscus. O'Donoghue described as resulting from tackle injury; since discovered that most ACL tears in football players result from twisting injuries (sudden change in direction).

tethered cord syndrome, cord traction syndrome, filum terminale syndrome. *Congenital anomaly*. In patients with certain spinal defects (e.g., spina bifida), the conus medullaris (terminal end of spinal cord) becomes attached to the bone or scar tissue, preventing its upward migration with growth. Causes cord tension and can result in progressive paralysis of the bladder, bowel, and lower extremities.

Tevdek suture. *Orthopedic supply*. Non-absorbable suture material used in repair of wounds.

thenar eminence (THEE-nahr). *Anatomy*. Muscular prominence on the thumb side of the palm: comprised of the abductor policis brevis, opponens policis, and the oblique head of the adductor policis.

thenar muscles (THEE-nahr). *Anatomy*. The intrinsic muscles of the thumb:

abductor policis brevis, opponens policis, adductor policis, flexor policis brevis.

thenar space (THEE-nahr). *Anatomy*. Potential space on the palm and radial sides of the hand; can be filled with pus during certain infections.

thigh. *Anatomy*. The part of the leg between the hip and the knee.

thighbone. *Anatomy*. Popular term for the femur, the largest bone in the body; joins the hip to the knee.

Thomas ring. *Orthopedic appliance*. The part of a Thomas splint that fits around the thigh; used in the treatment of fracture of the femur (thighbone) or lower leg. The ring is held in place with a sling underneath the leg.

Thomas splint. *Orthopedic appliance*. A splint consisting of a V-shaped metal frame running from the hip to beyond the toes. Allows for traction to be applied to the leg. Usually employed during patient's transport.

Thomas test. *Clinical test*. With patient supine, one leg is brought upward to the chest, flattening the lower lumbar spine. If the opposite thigh flexes forward, it indicates a hip flexion contracture.

Thompson and Epstein classification. *Injury classification*. Identifies different types of posterior hip dislocations.

thoracic (thor-ASS-ik). *Anatomic description*. Refers to the chest thorax (chest).

    t. orthosis (ohr-THOH-sus). *Orthopedic appliance*. A brace supporting the chest and lower spine in the treatment of scoliosis.

    t. outlet. *Anatomy*. Space through which pass the major neurovascular structures of the arms.

        syndrome. *Pathologic condition*. Pain, weakness, atrophy and/or arm swelling caused by neural, arterial or venous compression of the thoracic outlet. May be due to trauma, exostoses or malformations.

    T-spine. *Anatomy*. The part of the spine comprised of the twelve vertebrae that support the ribs.

    t. vertebra. *Anatomy*. Any one of the twelve bones that make up the thoracic spine.

thoracoacromial artery (THOR-uh-koh-uh-KROH-mee-ul). *Anatomy*. Branch of subclavian artery; supplies front of the chest wall and portions of the shoulder.

thoracodorsal nerve (thor-uh-koh-DOR-sul). *Anatomy*. Nerve that supplies the muscles of the lateral chest wall and the latissimus dorsi. Branches from the posterior cord of the brachial plexus.

thoracolumbar (thor-uh-koh-LUM-bahr). *Anatomic description*. Refers to the thoracic and lumbar areas of the spine.

    t. juncture: area between T-12 (last thoracic vertebra) and L-1 (first lumbar vertebra), where the thoracic and lumbar spines meet.

thoracolumbosacral orthosis (thor-uh-koh-lum-boh-SAY-krul). *Orthopedic appliance*. Brace that encompasses the thoracic area, lumbar area and the sacrum.

thoracoscapular arthrodesis (thor-uh-koh-KAP-suh-lur). *Surgical procedure*. Fusion of the scapula (shoulderblade) to the thoracic wall to hold the scapula in correct position; for treating paralysis of the scapular muscles.

thorax (THOR-aks). *Anatomy*. The chest; the upper part of the trunk between the neck and abdomen, formed by the twelve thoracic vertebrae, the twelve pairs of ribs and the sternum.

thromboangitis obliterans (thrahm-boh-an-JI-tus), **Buerger's disease**. *Pathologic condition*. Inflammation of the inner wall of a blood vessel, leading to thrombosis (clot) in the vessel. Can result in gangrene.

thrombocyte (THRAHM-boh-site). *Anatomy*. Blood platelet; part of blood that normally initiates the clotting response.

thrombocytopenia with absent radius syndrome (TAR) (thrahm-boh-sko-PEEN-yuh). *Congenital abnormality.* Syndrome characterized by an abnormally small number of platelets and absent or underdeveloped radii of forearms. Patient may also have bleeding tendencies, mental retardation, congenital heart disease, kidney abnormalities. Hereditary; autosomal recessive. Varying degrees of severity.

thrombophlebitis (thrahm-boh-fluh-BI-tus). *Pathologic condition.* Clotting and inflammation of a vein. See also THROMBOSIS.

thrombosis (thrahm-BOH-sus). *Pathologic condition.* Blood clot in a vein or artery.

thrombus (THRAHM-bus). *Pathologic condition.* Blood clot in the vascular system; may be in the heart or in a blood vessel. See also EMBOLUS.

thumb. *Anatomy.* The first finger of the hand.

thumb in palm deformity. *Pathologic condition.* Deformity that results in the thumb being clasped within the palm. Frequent in neurological disease, such as cerebral palsy.

TIA. Abbreviation for TRANSCIENT ISCHEMIC ATTACK.

tibia (TIB-ee-uh), **shank bone**, **shinbone**. *Anatomy.* The larger of the two bones in the lower leg articulating with the femur (thighbone) proximally and the talus (top foot bone) distally.

 t. valga, genu valgum, genu valgus. *Abnormal condition.* Knock-knees; ankles remain widely separated while standing with knees touching.

 t. vara, bandylegs, genu varum, genu varus. *Abnormal condition.* Bowlegs; legs whose knees point outward, remaining separated when standing with ankles together; results in a bowlike appearance.

tibial (TIB-ee-ul). *Anatomic description.* Refers to the tibia (shinbone), the bone between the knee and ankle.

 t. artery. *Anatomy.* Branch of the popliteal artery; supplies portions of the lower leg. Divides into anterior and posterior branches.

 t. collateral ligament. *Anatomy.* Connective tissue band (1) along the inner side of the knee, connecting femur (thighbone) to tibia (shinbone); acts as a stabilizer of the knee, keeping the tibia from rotating outward; (2) along the inner sides of the interphalangeal and metatarsophalangeal joints of the toes.

 t. eminence fracture. *Pathologic condition.* Avulsion fracture (sudden muscle contraction that pulls its attachment from the bone) of the proximal tibia (shinbone) at the insertion of the anterior cruciate ligament.

 t. nerve. *Anatomy.* Branch of the popliteal nerve; supplies portions of the lower leg. Divides into anterior and posterior branches.

 t. osteotomy (ahs-tee-AH-tuh-mee). *Surgical procedure.* Cutting through the tibia to realign it, usually to correct deformities about the knee.

 t. plateau. *Anatomy.* Weightbearing surface of the tibia where the femoral condyles articulate (the knee).

 t. spine. *Anatomy.* The two bony projections into the knee joint from the proximal tibia (shinbone). Attaches to the posterior horn of the lateral semilunar cartilage.

 t. torsion. *Pathologic condition.* Inward twisting of the shin bones (between knee and ankle), which can cause a child's feet to turn inward ("pigeon-toed"). Typically seen among toddlers.

 t. tubercle. *Anatomy.* Small bump on front of shin bone, just below the knee. Serves as place of attachment for the patellar tendon.

tibialis anterior muscle (tib-ee-AL-us), **tibialis anticus**. *Anatomy.* Muscle that causes dorsiflexion and supination of the foot. Arises on the tibia (shinbone) and inserts on the 1st metatarsal and navicular on the inner side of the foot.

tibialis posterior muscle (tib-ee-AL-us). *Anatomy.* Muscle that adducts and plantarflexes the foot. Arises from the back of the tibia (shinbone) and interosseus membrane, and inserts distally on the lower surface of the foot along the inner side.

Tietze's syndrome (TEET-seez), **costochondritis, costosternal syndrome, peristernal perichondritis**. *Pathologic condition.* Inflammation, pain and tenderness of the cartilage connecting the ribs to the sternum (breastbone). The pain is exacerbated with deep breathing.

Tillaux fracture (til-OH). *Pathologic condition.* Break in the anterior, lateral articular surface of the distal tibia (shinbone) in an adolescent when the growth plate is closing.

Tinel sign (tin-EL). *Clinical sign.* Shocking sensation experienced in response to tapping the area overlying a nerve injury, regeneration or entrapment.

toenail (ingrown). *Pathologic condition.* Toenail that becomes covered by soft tissue, resulting in inflammation, infection and pain. Causes include wearing tight shoes, improper nail trimming, injuries, fungal infections, abnormalities in foot structure, or recurrent trauma to the area.

   O'Donoghue procedure for (oh-DAHN-uh-hyu). *Surgical procedure.* Removal of the lateral (outer) fourth of the nail plate and underlying matrix.

Tolectin. *Drug.* Trade name of tolmetin, NSAID for treating pain and inflammation.

tolmetin (TOHL-met-in). *Drug.* NSAID for treating pain and inflammation. Trade name: Tolectin.

-tome. *Suffix.* A cutting instrument (osteotome: tool for cutting bone).

tomogram (TOH-muh-gram). *Radiologic test.* X-ray that allows visualization of multiple sections of an area. See also TOMOGRAPHY.

tomography (tuh-MAH-gruh-fee). *Radiologic test.* X-ray process for showing multiple sections of an area (tomogram); involves moving a photographic plate in the opposite direction of the beam, both of which are rotating about a point of interest in the body.

tophus (TOH-fus). *Pathologic condition.* Deposit of uric acid crystals; seen in gout.

Toradol. *Drug.* Trade name of ketorolac, NSAID for treating pain and inflammation.

Torode and Zieg classification (ZEEG). *Fracture classification.* Identifies pediatric pelvic fractures.

Toronto orthosis /or/ **brace**. *Orthopedic appliance.* Maintains legs in abduction, allowing movement of the hips. Used in the treatment of Perthes disease in the 1970s and early 1980s.

torque (tork). *Measurement.* Rotational force.

   t. heel. *Orthopedic appliance.* Orthotic device attached to the heel of a child's shoe that rotates the foot (internally or externally) with each step.

torsion (TOR-shun). *Physical stress.* Twisting movement around an axis.

   t. fracture. *Pathologic condition.* Spiral-shaped break associated with a twisting type of injury.

torsional rigidity (TOR-shun-ul). *Physical property.* Amount of resistance a structure will mount against a rotational force.

torticollis (tor-tuh-KAH-lus), **wryneck.** *Pathologic condition.* A head that is turned and cocked to one side, with restricted rotation toward the other side; response to contraction of the neck muscles. In severe cases, can be associated with subluxation of the vertebrae. Cause may be psychogenic, ocular, spastic, or traumatic. Sometimes present at birth.

   congenital t.: present at birth; may not be apparent until age 1 or 2.

   spasmodic t., cervical dystonia: characterized by abnormal tension and activity across the muscles of the neck that can lead to abnormal posture and repetitive twisting movements. Can begin at any age but usually starts in 30s or 40s. No known cause or cure.

torus fracture (TOR-us). *Pathologic condition.* Nondisplaced break, generally at the distal end of the radius (larger forearm bone) or tibia (shinbone) in a small child. Appears as a rounded bump on the bone.

total condylar knee prosthesis (KAHN-duh-lur, prahs-THEE-sus). *Orthopedic appliance.* Artificial knee that completely covers the condyles of the femur (thighbone) and tibia (shinbone).

total contact orthosis. *Orthopedic appliance.* Describes a prosthesis used for amputations, that surrounds and touches the remaining limb on all sides.

total elbow arthroplasty (AHR-throh-plas-tee). *Surgical procedure.* Resurfacing the joint surfaces of the lower end of the humerus and upper end of the olecranon with plastic and metal so as to restore painless joint motion.

total hip arthroplasty (THA) (AHR-throh-plas-tee), **total hip replacement**. *Surgical procedure.* Hip replacement substituting the natural ball and socket of both hips with man-made parts.

> **cemented**: uses artificial parts designed to be cemented into position.

> **cementless**: uses prostheses (artificial parts) with a porous rough surface, which allows the bone to heal directly to it without cement.

> **Charnley**: cemented THA; components designed by Sir John Charnley.

> **hybrid**: the stem (proximal femur prosthesis) is cemented into position and the acetabulum is press-fit into position (inserted without cement).

> **press-fit**: same as CEMENTLESS (above).

total hip replacement (THR). Same as TOTAL HIP ARTHROPLASTY.

total joint arthroplasty (AHR-throh-plas-tee), **total joint replacement**. *Surgical procedure.* Surgical replacement of a joint.

total knee arthroplasty (AHR-throh-plas-tee), **total knee replacement**. *Surgical procedure.* Replacing the joint surfaces of the lower end of the femur and upper end of the tibia, with or without resurfacing of the patella (kneecap).

> **cemented**: uses artificial parts designed to be cemented into position.

> **cementless**: uses prostheses (artificial parts) with a porous rough surface, which allows the bone to heal directly to it without cement.

> **hybrid**: the tibia is cemented into position and the femur is press-fit into position (inserted without cement).

> **press-fit**: same as CEMENTLESS (above).

total parenteral nutrition (TPN) (puh-RENT-uh-rul). *Treatment.* Feeding a patient through major veins so as to support all his/her nutritional needs without requiring any oral input.

total shoulder arthroplasty (AHR-throh-plas-tee), **total shoulder replacement**. *Surgical procedure.* Resurfacing the upper end of humerus and the glenoid (the cup of the shoulder), to restore painless function and motion of the joint. If only the humerus is resurfaced it is called a shoulder hemiarthroplasty.

tourniquet (TUR-nuh-kut). *Orthopedic supply.* Band or inflatable balloon for applying pressure to an artery, for decreasing or stopping blood flow to an extremity.

> **elastic**: tight elastic band placed about an extremity to cut its circulation. Advantage over inflatable tourniquet: ease of application and absence of expensive instrumentation.

> **inflatable**: air-filled band placed about an extremity to cut its circula-

tion. Advantage over elastic tourniquet: ability to set the exact pressure of the band, which serves as a safeguard from excessively tight application.

trabecular bone (truh-BEK-yu-lur), **cancellous bone**. *Anatomy*. Type of porous bone having large latticework and a spongy, honeycomb appearance; filled with marrow. Example: the interior of a vertebra. See also CORTICAL BONE.

trabecular pattern (truh-BEK-yu-lur). *Anatomic description*. Refers to a honeycomb appearance; can refer to either fibrous tissue or bone.

tract. *Anatomy*. An elongated path.

 nerve t: a bundle of nerve fibers that travel together along the brain or spinal cord. In general, those along the front of the spinal cord are responsible for motor activity, and those at the back are responsible for sensation.

traction (txn). *Treatment*. Pulling on an extremity or the spine to realign it after injury (fracture, dislocation, etc.) or degeneration.

 balanced t.: pulley system that allows traction to be applied while the limb is elevated; helps to diminish swelling.

 Buck's t.: traction of a leg applied through a soft boot.

 floating t.: same as BALANCED (above).

 skin t.: traction on an extremity from devices applied to the skin.

 skeletal t.: traction on an extremity applied through a direct attachment to a bone (usually through a pin inserted into the bone).

 well-leg t: traction placed on a normal leg to exert countertraction on the abnormal leg.

traction bed. *Orthopedic appliance*. Bed equipped with an overhead attachment for allowing traction to be applied to the patient.

traction bow. *Orthopedic appliance*. Bow-shaped device for applying traction; placed on the ends of thin wire embedded in a long bone of an extremity.

transacromial approach (tranz-ay-KROH-mee-ul). *Surgical technique*. An approach to the top of the shoulder through a cut across the acromioclavicular joint. See also SABER-CUT INCISION.

transcaphoid perilunate dislocation (tranz-SKAF-oyd pehr-ih-LU-nayt). *Pathologic condition*. Dislocation of the bones surrounding the lunate (bone in wrist); associated with a fracture of the scaphoid (another bone in the wrist).

transcervical fracture. *Pathologic condition*. Break through the midportion of the femoral neck. Type of hip fracture.

transcolumn fracture. *Pathologic condition*. Break in distal portion of the humerus (upper armbone) crossing transversely across the supracondylar region.

transcondylar fracture (tranz-KAHN-duh-lur). *Pathologic condition*. Break in the distal humerus (upper armbone) or distal femur (thighbone) extending through the condyles.

transcutaneous electrical nerve stimulation (TENS) (trans-kyu-TAY-nee-us). *Treatment*. Electrical stimulation causing an irritation to the skin; decreases pain by confusing the pain fibers of the central nervous system. Person wears a device that provides minor stimulation sufficient to irritate and displace the major source of pain.

transection. *Surgical procedure*. Cutting across a structure.

transient ischemic attack (TIA) (is-KEE-mik), **"ministroke."** *Pathologic condition*. Temporary interruption in the circulation to a portion of the brain, causing dysfunction of the affected section of the brain. Resolves spontaneously.

transitional vertebra. *Abnormal condition*. Vertebra that assumes appearance of the section next to it (e.g., a 5th lumbar vertebra that takes on appearance of a sacral vertebra or 1st sacral vertebra that takes on appearance of a lumbar vertebra). See also LUMBARIZATION, SACRALIZATION.

transmetatarsal amputation (trans-met-uh-TAHR-sul). *Surgical procedure.* Removal of the foot at the metatarsal level.

transplant. *Surgical procedure.* Moving a part from one area to another (e.g., skin graft) or an organ from one person to another (e.g., kidney transplant).

   bone marrow t.: implanting marrow from a donor in an attempt to induce formation of blood cells.

transverse. *Anatomy.* Across; perpendicular to the long axis of the body or a limb.

   t. fracture. *Pathologic condition.* Break that crosses the cortices perpendicular to the long axis of the bone.

   t. plane, axial plane. *Anatomic description.* Imaginary reference plane perpendicular to the length of the body or a body part.

trapeze bed. See TRAPEZE FRAME.

trapeze frame, trapeze bed, Balkan frame. *Orthopedic appliance.* Metal struts attached to a bed frame to hold a splinted limb; provides handles the patient can grasp to move about the bed easier.

trapezium (truh-PEE-zee-um), **greater multangular**. *Anatomy.* Four-sided bone in the wrist at the base of the thumb.

trapezius (truh-PEE-zee-us). *Anatomy.* Large muscle in the back and neck that elevates the shoulder. Extends from the base of the skull to the thoracic level of the spine, attaching to the spinous processes of the cervical/thoracic vertebrae and the spine of the scapula (shoulderblade).

trapezoid (TRAP-uh-zoyd), **lesser multangular**. *Anatomy.* Small bone in the wrist, between the trapezium and the capitate; opposite the 2nd metacarpal.

trauma. *Pathologic process.* Injury.

traumatic spondylolisthesis of the axis (spahn-duh-lo-liss-THEE-sus), **hangman's fracture**. *Pathologic condition.* Break in the 2nd cervical (neck) vertebra involving the neural ring of the vertebra and separating the back of the vertebra from the body.

Trendelenburg gait. *Pathologic condition.* Waddling-like gait that occurs when weight is placed on a leg, causing the hip on the opposite side to drop. Secondary to weakness of the hip muscles or hip pain on the weight-bearing side.

Trendelenburg position. *Anatomic description.* Patient lies on his/her back (supine) with the head of the bed tilted down 45° so that the patient's head is lower than the pelvis. See also REVERSE TRENDELENBURG.

Trendelenburg sign/test. *Clinical test/sign.* Patient balances on one leg; if the hip on the non-weightbearing side drops down (from pain or weakness in the weightbearing hip), it indicates a weakness or poor mechanics of the hip abductor muscles.

Trevor disease, dysplasia epiphysealis, epiphyseal osteochondroma, hemimelica, tarsoepiphyseal aclasia. *Congenital abnormality.* Abnormal development of osteochondromas, usually involving multiple bones in one limb. Three variations: localized (involves one epiphysis); classic (involves more than one bone in a single limb); and generalized (involves multiple bones in more than one limb).

triamcinolone. *Drug.* Cortisone derivative. For treating inflammatory and allergic diseases.

triangular. *Anatomy.* Small bone in the wrist in the proximal row; articulates with the radius (larger forearm bone).

triceps (TRI-seps). *Anatomy.* Refers to a muscle that has three heads.

    t. brachii muscle (BRAKE-ee-i). *Anatomy*. Large extensor muscle on the back of the upper arm that extends the forearm at the elbow joint; originates from the glenoid on the scapula (shoulderblade), the upper part of the humerus (upper armbone), and the mid-portion of the humerus. Attaches to the back of the elbow at the olecranon.

    t. reflex. *Clinical test*. Sudden involuntary contraction of the triceps muscle in response to a tap on the triceps tendon. Tests for normal function of the muscle and the nerves controlling that muscle.

    t. surae (SEHR-ay), **gastrocsoleus**. *Anatomy*. Muscle grouping of the gastrocnemius and soleus.

trigger finger, **stenosing tenosynovitis**, **trigger thumb**. *Pathologic condition*. Finger that snaps as it is brought from flexion into extension. Caused by a small nodule on the tendon that prevents normal gliding movement.

trigger points. *Pathologic condition*. Specific areas of the body that when touched elicit pain.

Trilisate. *Drug*. A trade name of choline magnesium trisalicylate, NSAID for treating pain and inflammation.

trimalleolar (tri-muh-LEE-oh-lur). *Anatomic description*. Refers to the ankle: medial and lateral and posterior mallioli (tips of lower leg bones).

    t. fracture. *Pathologic condition*. Break in the ankle that involves the medial, lateral and posterior malleoli (tips of lower leg bones).

triplane fracture. *Pathologic condition*. Break in the tibia (shinbone) occurring about the lower growth plate; occurs exclusively in the adolescent.

triple arthrodesis (ahr-throh-DEE-sis). *Surgical procedure*. Fusion of the talus (top foot bone) to the calcaneus (heelbone), navicular to the talus, and cuboid to the calcaneus, eliminating three joints. Used to stabilize and/or correct deformity of the foot.

triquetral bone (tri-KWEE-truhl). See TRIQUETRUM.

triquetrum (tri-KWEE-trum), **cubital bone**, **triquetral bone**. *Anatomy*. Wrist bone in the second row of carpal bones, on outer side of wrist between the pisiform and the lunate.

triradiate cartilage (tri-RAY-dee-ut KAHR-tuh-lidj). *Anatomy*. The cartilaginous area in the acetabulum (hip socket) where the iliac, ischium and pubis meet. Comprises the depth of the acetabular cavity.

trisomy 21 (TRI-soh-mee), **Down syndrome**, **mongolism**. *Congenital abnormality*. Presence of three #21 chromosomes; associated with mental retardation, hyperelasticity, heart disease, oblique eyelids, flat skull and flattened facial features.

trocar (TRO-kahr). *Surgical instrument*. Pointed pin designed to fit within a sleeve or cannula; the pin penetrates tissue so that the more blunt sleeve or cannula can be delivered to its proper location.

trochanter (TROH-kan-tur). *Anatomy*. One of the two prominences on the proximal part of the femur (thighbone).

    greater t.: large prominence on the proximal femur; attachment for the gluteus medius and gluteus minimus muscles.

    lesser t.: small protrusion of bone on the proximal femur; insertion of the ilio-psoas tendon.

trochlea (of the femur) (TROH-klee-uh). *Anatomy*. Grooved area at the end of the femur (thighbone) along which the patella (kneecap) tracks.

trochlea (of the humerus) (TROH-klee-uh). *Anatomy*. Grooved area at the end of the humerus (upper armbone) where the notch of the ulna (smaller forearm bone) articulates.

Tronzo classification. *Fracture classification*. Identifies types of trochanteric or intertrochanteric hip fractures.

Tscherne classification. *Fracture classification*. Describes the severity of soft tissue damage in association with closed long bone fractures.

T-spine. *Anatomy*. See THORACIC SPINE.

tubercle (TU-bur-kul), **tuberosity**. *Anatomy*. A prominence or rounded elevation on a bone's surface.

tuberosity (tu-bur-AHS-it-ee). See TUBERCULE.

tuft. *Anatomy*. Widened end of the distal part of the distal phalanx (final bone) of a finger or toe.

> **t. fracture**. *Pathologic condition*. Break in the tuft portion of the distal phalanx of a finger or toe.

tumefaction (tu-muh-FAK-shun). *Pathologic condition*. Swelling and stiffness of a body part.

tumor, **neoplasm**. *Pathologic condition*. New, abnormal growth; may be benign or malignant.

tunnel view. *Radiographic test*. Radiologic view of the wrist or knee with the joint extended, showing the area of the carpal tunnel.

Turco incision. *Surgical technique*. Incision used in the correction of clubfoot.

turgid (TUR-jid). *Anatomic description*. Swollen.

turnbuckle cast. *Orthopedic appliance*. Body cast with a turnbuckle that may be turned to stretch or compress the body part under the cast.

Turner syndrome. *Pathologic condition*. Chromosome abnormality in females; there is only one X chromosome (total of 45 instead of 46). Result is small size, increased carrying angle of the elbow, immature sexual development, no menstrual cycles, and torticollis.

twisted neck. Popular term sometimes used to mean torticollis, a head turned and cocked to one side, in response to contraction of the neck muscles.

tx. Abbreviation for 1. TREATMENT, 2. THERAPY, 3. TRACTION.

txn. Abbreviation for TRACTION.

U

UCBL orthosis. *Orthopedic appliance*. Plastic form molded to the foot and placed in a shoe to hold the heel in specific alignment, eliminating flat foot appearance. Developed by Univ. of Calif., Berkeley laboratory.

ulcer (decubitus) (duh-KYU-bih-tus), **bed sore**, **pressure sore**. *Pathologic condition*. A break in the skin caused by pressure and immobilization.

ulna (UL-nuh). *Anatomy*. Smaller of the two forearm bones. See also RADIUS.

ulnar clawhand, ulnar-minus-hand. *Pathologic condition*. Hand with clawing of the 4th and 5th fingers and decreased sensation; from injury or transection of the ulnar nerve.

ulnar collateral ligament. *Anatomy*. 1. Connective tissue band running along the inner side of the elbow connecting the humerus (armbone) and the ulna (upper forearm bone); acts as a restraining ligament of the elbow, keeping the ulna from rotating out. 2. Connective tissue bands running along the inner sides of the interphalangeal and metacarpophalangeal joints of the fingers and thumb.

ulnar-minus-hand. See ULNAR CLAWHAND.

ulnar nerve. *Anatomy*. Nerve to the upper extremity; supplies sensation to the 5th and ulnar half of the 4th finger, and motor innervation to the muscles of the hypothenar eminence and most of the intrinsic muscles of the hand.

    palsy (PAHL-zee). *Pathologic condition*. Characteristic weakness or paralysis accompanying injury to the ulnar nerve; results in ulnar clawhand.

    release, cubital tunnel release. *Surgical procedure*. Opening the cubital tunnel to alleviate constriction of the ulnar nerve within the tunnel. Usually performed along with an ulnar nerve transposition. Used in the treatment of cubital tunnel syndrome.

ultrasonography, sonogram. *Test*. Picture of internal structures derived from transmission of high frequency sound waves into an area, which are reflected by the tissues. Frequently used in diagnosis of hip dysplasia and evaluation of a fetus in the womb.

ultrasound. *Sound wave*. High frequency sound used in certain forms of therapy and imaging modalities. See also SONOGRAM.

    u. therapy. *Treatment*. Low-intensity pulses of sound applied to tissues to stimulate healing.

uncemented /or/ **cementless** /or/ **press-fit total hip replacement**. *Surgical procedure*. Technique for replacing the hip using prostheses (artificial parts) with a porous rough surface, which allows the bone to heal directly to it without cement.

undisplaced fracture. *Pathologic condition*. Break in a bone without change in position of the fragments.

unguis (UN-gwis). *Anatomy*. Fingernail or toenail. Plural: ungues (UN-gweez).

unicameral cyst (yu-nih-CAM-ur-ul). *Pathologic condition*. Benign single-cavity cyst most commonly found in the humerus (upper armbone).

unicompartmental knee replacement (UKR), unicondylar knee arthroplasty. 1. *Orthopedic appliance*. Prosthesis for one part or one side of the knee. 2. *Surgical procedure*. Replacement of only one of the three compartments of the knee.

unicondylar knee arthroplasty (UKA) (yoon-ih-KAHN-duh-lur). See UNICOMPARTMENTAL KNEE REPLACEMENT.

unilateral. *Anatomy*. Having one side. See also BILATERAL.

    u. facet subluxation (fuh-SET sub-lux-AY-shun). *Pathologic condi-*

tion. Malalignment in one of the posterior vertebral joints (between two vertebrae).

uniplanar external fixator, monoplanar external fixator. *Orthopedic implant.* Device used to stabilize fractures and osteotomies; relies on threaded pins placed onto the bone fragments and attached to a linear, external frame.

unipolar endoprosthesis. See UNIPOLAR HEMIARTHROPLASTY, definition #2.

unipolar hemiarthroplasty. 1. *Surgical procedure.* Replacement of the femoral head with a prosthesis that allows no motion between the artificial femoral head and the underlying stem. Used primarily in treatment of displaced femoral neck fractures and some cases of avascular necrosis of the hip. The advantage of this design is its lower cost and greater sturdiness. See also BIPOLAR HEMIARTHROPLASTY. 2. *Surgical implant.* Endoprosthesis used to replace a femoral head and neck that does not have a mobile articulation between the head and neck of the implant. Also called UNIPOLAR ENDOPROSTHESIS.

union. *Function.* The healing of a fracture or osteotomy.

univalve cast. *Orthopedic appliance.* Cast cut on one side to allow it to expand in case of swelling See also BIVALVE CAST.

Unna boot (OO-nuh). *Orthopedic supply.* A soft dressing made of gelatin, zinc oxide and glycerine, commonly used in the treatment of stasis ulcers (skin ulcer from venous or lymphatic insufficiency). Developed in 1885 by German dermatologist Dr. Paul Unna.

unsegmented bar. *Pathologic condition.* Usually refers to a bridge of bone between two or more vertebrae that tethers the side it is on so that growth on the opposite side leads to progressive scoliosis.

ununited fracture (un-yu-NI-ted). *Pathologic condition.* Break in a bone that has not healed.

upper motor neuron disease. *Pathologic condition.* Category of diseases that affect the neurons in the cerebral cortex and are associated with increased motor tone, spasticity and hyper-reflexia. Example: cerebral palsy, Friedrich's ataxia.

uremia, azotemia (yu-REE-mee-uh). *Pathologic condition.* Higher-than-normal levels of urea or other nitrogenous compounds in the blood; may result in bone depletion.

urinalysis (UA) (yur-in-AL-ih-sis). *Lab test.* Chemical analysis of urine, to test for abnormal contents (e.g., albumin, pus, sugar) that may indicate systemic disease.

V

VAC dressing (vacuum assisted closure). *Orthopedic appliance*. Dressing attached to suction and applied with an air-tight seal so that continuous or intermittent suction may be applied to the wound. Allows for faster healing.

valgus (VAL-gus). *Anatomic description*. Describes relationship between parts of the body: the more distal part (farther from body) is bent away from the midline. Example: genu valgum (knock-knees: knees touching, ankles separated). See also VARUS.

> **heel v**. *Clinical finding*. With patient standing and viewed from the back, the heel is angled away from the midline of the body. Mild heel valgus is normal, but when excessive, the finding can be pathologic.

Van Nes procedure, Van Nes rotationplasty. *Surgical procedure*. Rotation osteotomy (leg bones cut into two segments and flipped backwards): the foot points back and the ankle is used as a knee joint. For controlling a prosthesis (artificial part) for a patient with a congenital, severely short femur (thighbone). Originally called Borggreve operation, for the originator of the procedure.

varus (VEHR-us). *Anatomy*. Describes relationship between parts of the body: the more distal part (farther from body) is bent toward the midline. Example: bowlegs (genu varus). See also VALGUS.

> **v. derotational osteotomy** (ahs-tee-AH-tuh-mee). *Surgical procedure*. To correct a valgus deformity: cutting the distal segment of a long bone to decrease its angulation with respect to its proximal segment.

> **heel v**. *Clinical finding*. With the patient standing and being viewed from the back, the heel is angled toward the midline of the body. Mild heel varus is normal, but when excessive, the finding can be pathologic.

vascular (VAS-kyu-lur). *Anatomic description*. Refers to the circulatory system, e.g., arteries and veins.

> **v. claudication, Charcot's syndrome, intermittent claudication, myesthenia angiosclerotica**. *Pathologic condition*. Limping caused by insufficient blood supply to the leg muscles when blood vessels are constricted or obliterated, such as in diabetes or arteriosclerosis.

vastus intermedius. *Anatomy*. Deepest of the four heads of the quadriceps muscle (on front of thigh); originates on front of the femur (thighbone) and inserts distally into the patella (kneecap) and the upper part of the tibia (at tibial tuberosity) through the patellar tendon.

vastus lateralis. *Anatomy*. One of the four heads of the quadriceps muscle (on front of thigh). Arises on the outer side of the thighbone (femur) and inserts on the patella (kneecap) and the upper part of the tibia (at the tibial tuberosity) through the patellar tendon.

vastus medialis obliquus. *Anatomy*. One of the four heads of the quadriceps muscle (on front of thigh). Arises on the inner side of the thigh and femur (thighbone) and inserts onto the patella (kneecap) and the upper part of the tibia (at the tibial tuberosity) through the patellar tendon.

vein. *Anatomy*. Blood vessel that carries blood toward the heart. See also ARTERY.

Velpeau dressing. *Orthopedic supply*. Soft cloth dressing sometimes reinforced with plaster; applied to the shoulder and arm to maintain the arm against the chest with the elbow fixed at 90°.

vena basilica, basilic vein. *Anatomy*. Blood vessel that extends from the back of the hand to the armpit, where it joins the axillary vein.

venogram (VEE-noh-gram), **phlebogram**. *Radiologic test*. Visualization of the venous tree of an extremity or region of the body after injection of dye into a small vein. Often used for identifying a vein blockage, as a thrombophlebitis, or in the identification of ongoing internal bleeding after a pelvic fracture.

venous (VEE-nus). *Anatomy*. Having to do with a vein or veins.

> **v. insufficiency**. *Pathologic condition*. Backing up of blood in a vein or groups of veins. Usually due to poor function of valves inside the veins; leads to venous enlargement and varicosities in the legs. May lead to leg ulcers.

ventral, anterior. *Anatomic location*. The front of the body or body part in the anatomic position; the ventral surface of the hand is the palm. Opposite: dorsal, posterior.

venules (VEN-yulz). *Anatomy*. Small veins.

vertebra (VUR-tuh-bruh). *Anatomy*. One of the bones of the spine. Plural: vertebrae.

> **v. plana** (vur-TEE-bruh PLAN-uh), **Calvé-Kummel-Verneuil disease**. *Pathologic condition*. Collapse and flattening of the vertebral body; most frequent in children ages 2–15 years. May be associated with eosinophilic granuloma (benign bone lesions). Plural: vertebrae.

vertebrae (VUR-tuh-bray). *Anatomy*. Plural of VERTEBRA. See VERTEBRAL COLUMN.

vertebral arch, neural arch. *Anatomy*. The bony arch at the back of a vertebra that surrounds the spinal cord.

vertebral artery (vur-TEE-brul). *Anatomy*. Blood vessel branching off the subclavian artery (1st branch). Passes through foramina on the lateral masses of the cervical vertebrae and enters the skull to supply part of the brain.

vertebral body (vur-TEE-brul). *Anatomy*. Front part of a vertebra; predominant component in the weightbearing function of the spine.

vertebral column (vur-TEE-brul), **spine**. *Anatomy*. The backbone, extending the full length of the midline of the back. Consists of 30 vertebrae: 7 cervical (in the neck), 12 thoracic (in the back), 5 lumbar (between the ribs and pelvis), and the pelvic vertebrae (5 sacral, 1 coccygeal).

vertebral disc (vur-TEE-brul), **disc, intervertebral disc**. *Anatomy*. A disk of cartilage between adjacent vertebrae; absorbs shocks and permits movement. Named after the vertebrae they reside between (e.g., C4, C5 refers to the disc between the 4th and 5th cervical vertebrae).

vertebroplasty. *Surgical procedure*. The injection of bone cement or other rigid material into fractured and collapsed vertebrae. The material is administered as a doughy paste that hardens, stabilizing the fracture and relieving pain.

vertical talus (TAY-lus). *Pathologic condition*. Foot abnormality: a talus (top foot bone) that is plantarflexed (points down). Usually associated with paralytic abnormalities such as myelomeningocele and cerebral palsy.

verus. *Incorrect spelling of VARUS.*

villous synovitis (VIL-us si-noh-VI-tus). *Pathologic condition*. Inflammation of the synovium (finger-like projections of the joint lining), which can hypertrophy (enlarge) with chronic irritation, filling the joint space.

vinculum (VING-kyu-lum). *Anatomy*. Restraining ligament of connective tissue holding a tendon to bone. Plural: vincula, vinculae.

Vinke tongs. *Orthopedic appliance*. Halo-like device for exerting skeletal traction on the skull. Points on the tongs are drilled into the skull for applying traction.

Vioxx. *Drug*. A trade name of rofecoxib, a COX-2 inhibitor.

visceral efferent nervous system, autonomic nervous system. *Anatomy.* Part of the nervous system that maintains the resting function and state of readiness of the body and organ systems. Composed of two, generally antagonistic subsystems: the sympathetic and parasympathetic nervous systems.

viscosupplementation. *Treatment.* Injection of hyaluronic acid, a gel-like substance, into a joint to help lubricate it and diminish pain.

vitamin D-resistant rickets. *Pathologic condition.* Disease resulting from the body's inability to utilize vitamin D. Results in joint enlargement, short stature and poorly calcified bone, giving rise to deformities, e.g., bowing of the legs. Frequently associated with renal abnormalities.

volar (VOH-lur). *Anatomy.* The palmar surface of the hand or forearm.

   v. carpal ligament: crosses the wrist, attaching to the hamate and trapezium and incorporating the tendons in the front of the forearm and wrist.

   v. plate: tight connective tissue band attached between the phalanges; gives stability to finger joints by preventing hyperextention and dislocation.

volar capsulotomy (VOH-lur kap-su-LAH-toh-mee). *Surgical procedure.* Cutting the capsule of a joint on the palmar side of a finger or plantar side of a toe.

volar splint (VOH-lur). *Orthopedic appliance.* Splint applied to the wrist and forearm; rigid portion lies in the front (volar aspect) of the extremity.

Volkmann's canals (FOLK-manz). *Anatomy.* Small channels for blood vessels in bone.

Volkmann's contracture (FOLK-manz). *Pathologic condition.* Muscle contracture and scar tissue resulting from death of the forearm muscles from compartment syndrome. Causes extensive swelling that results in pressure of the tissue exceeding normal pressure of the blood in the small vessels. See also COMPARTMENT SYNDROME.

Voltaren. *Drug.* A trade name of diclofenac, NSAID for treating pain and inflammation.

von Recklinghausen disease, neurofibromatosis type II. *Pathologic condition.* Syndrome consisting of the appearance of multiple soft tissue tumors (neurofibromas), specific bony abnormalities, abnormally pigmented lesions of the skin (e.g., café-au-lait spots, axillary freckling) leading to gross malformations and dysfunction. Begins in early childhood or (rarely) in infancy.

von Rosen splint. *Orthopedic appliance.* Splint that maintains abduction of the hip in infancy, for congenital dislocation of the hip.

Voorhoeve's disease, osteopathia striata. *Abnormal condition.* Abnormal lines or striations seen on x-ray in the metaphysis of long bones. There are no definite clinical findings. Rare.

V-Y advancement technique. *Surgical technique.* Method of effectively lengthening a tissue by making a V-shaped incision across it, separating the two halves, sewing the apex of the V to itself until the cut ends meet and the remainder as a V. The final repair is shaped like a Y that is longer and narrower than presurgical dimensions.

Wagner external skeletal fixation device (VAHG-nur), **Wagner fixator**. *Orthopedic appliance*. External frame for holding fragments of bone in rigid alignment; pins attached to the frame are fixated to bone through the skin. May be used in lengthening a segment of bone.

Wagner fixator (VAHG-nur). See WAGNER EXTERNAL SKELETAL FIXATION DEVICE.

Wagner procedure (VAHG-nur). *Surgical procedure*. Lengthening an extremity with a Wagner external fixator device.

wagon wheel fracture, cartwheel fracture. *Pathologic condition*. Break in the distal femur (thighbone) or proximal tibia (shinbone) in children. Named when children rode in carts and caught their leg in spoked wheels.

Wagstaff fracture. *Pathologic condition*. A displaced break of the medial malleolus (inner bump of ankle).

wake-up test. *Clinical test*. Test for spinal cord injury during spinal surgery. Patient is partially awakened and asked to move the legs; movement indicates spinal cord motor function is still intact.

walker. *Orthopedic appliance*. Aid for ambulation (walking). May have wheels in front and skids (rubber ends) in back to allow individual to put weight on the walker, thereby relieving weight on the legs.

Ward's triangle. *Anatomy*. Triangular area between the femoral head and trochanteric arc; seen on x-ray. Identifies areas of stress across femoral neck.

Watanabe scope. *Instrument*. An early arthroscope model used during surgery of large joints, to see inside the joint. Presently only of historical significance.

"water on the knee." *Pathologic condition*. Effusion (collection of fluid within a joint) of the knee joint or the membrane that surrounds it.

Weaver's bottom. *Pathologic condition*. Bursitis affecting the bursa between the tuberosity of the ischium and the gluteus maximus. Seen in patients whose work is sedentary.

web space. *Anatomy*. Space at the base of two adjoining fingers or toes.

Weber classification, Denis-Weber classification. *Fracture classification*. Defines three types of ankle fractures based on their level on the distal fibula.

Weber-Marti classification. *Fracture classification*. Describes talar (top foot bone), body and neck fractures.

webril (WEB-rul). *Orthopedic supply*. Cotton material used under a cast; the padding allows for swelling and is a soft area between the bony prominences and the plaster.

Weck knife. *Surgical instrument*. Disposable, sharp blade inserted into a handle; used for obtaining split thickness skin grafts.

wedge fracture. *Pathologic condition*. Collapse of the anterior (front) side of a vertebra.

wedging. *Treatment*. Method of correcting alignment of an extremity in a cast: cutting the cast and wedging the extremity in another direction.

weightbearing. *Activity restriction*. Refers to the weight a patient may place on one or both legs; may be partial, complete, non, or as tolerated.

well-leg cast. *Orthopedic appliance*. Cast placed on a normal leg to exert traction on the opposite leg or to restrict patient movement.

well-leg raising test of Fajersztajn, sciatic phenomenon, contralateral straight leg raising test, prostrate leg raising test. *Clinical test*. With patient lying on his/her back, a leg is raised with the knee in extension.

Pain in the opposite leg indicates irritation of the nerve as it exits the spine. Sign of herniated disc disease.

well-leg traction. *Treatment*. Traction placed on a normal leg to exert countertraction on the abnormal leg.

Werdnig-Hoffmann disease. Severe form of spinal muscular atrophy. Onset at birth; death usually from respiratory failure and aspiration in infancy or early childhood or, rarely, in early adulthood. Hereditary; recessive trait.

Werdnig-Hoffmann paralysis, infantile spinal muscular atrophy. *Congenital abnormality*. Destruction of the anterior cells of the spinal cord; eventually leads to death.

White procedure. *Surgical procedure*. For elongating the Achilles tendon: two partial cuts are made across the tendon, one high up where the tendon meets the muscle fibers, and the other distally. Since the Achilles tendon spirals as it makes its way down to the heel, the elongating effects of the two cuts are additive, making them the same as a complete transection.

whitlow, felon. *Pathologic condition*. Purulent soft tissue infection at the end of a finger.

> **herpetic w.**: herpes infection of the finger, seen in healthcare workers who work around patients' mouths (such as nurses and dentists).

Whitman plate. *Orthopedic appliance*. Rigid, metal arch support used for the treatment of flatfoot.

Wiberg angle, acetabular index /or/ **angle, CE angle, center edge (angle of Wiberg)**. *Radiographic measurement*. On a front view of the pelvis, the angle formed between a vertical line passing through the center of the femoral head and a second line from the center of the femoral head to the outer edge of the acetabulum. An angle greater than 25° is normal; less than 20° is suggestive of dysplasia.

Wilkins classification. *Fracture classification*. Describes differing severities of supracondylar humerus fractures in children.

Williams orthosis. *Orthopedic appliance*. Back brace used to immobilize the lower spine after surgery or after injury.

willow fracture, greenstick fracture. *Pathologic condition*. Break involving the splintering of a long bone; occurs in young children.

Wilson (John C.) arthrodesis. *Surgical procedure*. Extra-articular fusion of the hip joint. A large segment of bone from the ilium is inserted into a segment of bone shaved off the greater trochanter.

Wilson test. *Clinical test*. With the leg flexed 90°, the foot is internally rotated and gradually extended. Pain at the medial femoral condyle at about 30° of flexion that is relieved by external rotation of the leg indicates osteochondritis dissecans.

windshield wiper sign. *Radiologic sign*. Bone changes in the tip of the stem of an artificial hip, as seen on x-ray; indicates the prosthesis has loosened.

wing bone. *Anatomy*. Popular term for SCAPULA.

Winquist-Hansen classification. *Fracture classification*. Describes fractures of the femoral shaft in relation to percentage of total cortical diameter affected.

wire ladder splint. *Orthopedic appliance*. Rectangular splint with crossbars, resembling a ladder. Used for temporarily immobilizing an extremity during application of first aid or in preparation for patient transport.

Wolf's law. *Biological property*. Tendency of living bone to change its thickness and strength in response to stress applied against it. A change in a bone's function will result in a change in its structure.

Wolf's skin graft. *Surgical procedure*. A free, full thickness skin graft.

Woodward procedure. *Surgical procedure*. Detachment of the scapula (with its trapezius and rhomboid muscles) from the spinous processes and reattachment to the spine in a more normal alignment. For Sprengel's deformity (congenital elevation of the scapula).

Wormian bone. See WOVEN BONE.

woven bone, Wormian bone. *Anatomy*. New or immature bone seen in actively growing areas of bone: in the embryonal skeleton, after a fracture in the area of healing, or in cases of attempted fusion before the bone becomes mature and strong. The bone appears disorganized and its fibers demonstrate a random orientation. As the bone matures, the fibers become organized as dictated by the stress applied across those areas.

Wrisberg ligament. *Anatomy*. Small ligament that attaches the lateral meniscus to the medial posterior femoral condyle.

wrist, wrist joint. *Anatomy*. The bones and their associated joints connecting the forearm and the hand.

  w. disarticulation. *Surgical procedure*. Amputation of the hand through the wrist bone.

wrist-driven flexor hinge orthosis. *Orthopedic appliance*. Device that enables quadriplegics (who have normal function of C5 and C6 nerve roots) to grasp an object by dorsiflexing the wrist.

wryneck, torticollis. *Pathologic condition*. A head that is turned and cocked to one side, with restricted rotation toward the other side; response to contraction of the neck muscles. In severe cases, can be associated with subluxation of the vertebrae. Cause may be psychogenic, ocular, spastic, or traumatic. Sometimes present at birth.

XYZ

xanthoma (zan-THOH-muh). *Pathologic lesion.* Accumulation of fatty debris in histiocytes within the skin and tendons, in patients with extremely high cholesterol levels. Seen as yellow nodules in the skin and in tendons.

xenograft (ZEE-noh-graft), **heterograft**. *Biological implant.* Tissue transfered from one species to another.

xeroform dressing (ZEE-roh-form). *Orthopedic supply.* Wound dressing containing petrolatum in an antiseptic solution.

x-ray, roentgenogram. *Radiologic test.* Uses invisible electromagnetic energy beams to produce images of internal tissues, bones and organs onto film.

xyphoid (ZI-foyd), **xyphisternum**. *Anatomy.* Small bone on the lower part of the sternum that projects below the ribs.

Y fracture. *Pathologic condition.* Break usually between condyles (articular surface), spreading medially and laterally; appears on x-ray as a Y.

Y ligament, **Bigelow's** /or/ **Bertin** /or/ **iliofemoral ligament**. *Anatomy.* Connective tissue band at the front of the hip connecting the iliac spine to the femur, between the neck and trochanters. Reinforces and stabilizes the hip joint. *See also* PUBOFEMORAL LIGAMENT.

Yount and Burgess classification. *Fracture classification.* Describes different pelvic fracture patterns using the appearance of the fracture on a front-to-back x-ray of the pelvis.

Yount procedure. *Surgical procedure.* For correction of a tight iliotibial band and a flexion abduction contracture of the hip. A lateral incision exposes the fascia lata and the iliotibial band is divided.

zanthoma. Incorrect spelling of XANTHOMA.

zenograft. Incorrect spelling of XENOGRAFT.

Zickel nail. *Surgical implant.* Internal fixation device used for fractures of the upper end of the femur (thighbone).

Zielke instrumentation. *Surgical implant.* Metallic implants used for stabilizing a segment of the spine or for correcting a spinal deformity. Screws placed through the vertebral bodies are attached to each other with a threaded rod; bringing them together corrects curvature of the spine.

z-plasty. *Surgical procedure.* Multiple cuts applied to the skin or a tendon in order to lengthen a tendon or reorient/reshape a scar.

zyphoid. Incorrect spelling of XYPHOID.

ORDER FORM

Please send me _____copies DICTIONARY OF ORTHOPEDIC TERMINOLOGY
@ $29.95 per copy + shipping and handling (see table).

Please check current edition and price on our website
(www.triadpublishing.com).

Ship to: Name _____

Address _____

City/State/Zip _____ Phone _____

Fax _____ Email _____

Add current sales tax for books sent to Florida addresses.

Check enclosed for $ _____

Charge to Visa, MasterCard, American Express, Discover *(circle one)*:

Cardholder's name _____

Card number _____ Expiration date _____

**Fax to 1-800-854-4947, Phone 1-800-525-6902, or mail to
Triad Publishing Co., P.O. Box 13355, Gainesville, FL 32604**

SHIPPING & HANDLING CHARGES

	CONT. US	AL, HI, US TERR.	CANADA
Up to $30	$8	$12	$15
$30 to $80	$9	$16	$20
$80 to $200	$10	$20	$25

Most shipments to continental U.S. are sent by UPS surface; to Canada by air parcel post; to Alaska, Hawaii and U.S. territories by air mail.

FOREIGN ORDERS

Payable in U.S. funds drawn on a U.S. bank, or by credit card. Inquire as to shipping charges; email: orders@triadpublishing.com. Specify air or suface mail.

Prices subject to change without notice.

- -

HELP FOR ANYONE WITH BACK PAIN OR OSTEOPOROSIS

Get full details on our website: **www.triadpublishing.com**

☐ WALK TALL: Exercise Program for Prevention & Treatment of Osteoporosis

☐ STAND TALL: Every Woman's Guide to Preventing & Treating Osteoporosis

☐ SAVE YOUR BONES: High Calcium, Low Calorie Recipes for the Family

☐ NOT JUST CHEESECAKE: A Yogurt Cheese Cookbook. 250 delicious recipes.

☐ Osteoporosis: there IS something you can do about it. Patient education. Free.

☐ 10 Tips to Lower Fat & Calories without going on a diet. Free.

☐ Mike's Famous YOGURT CHEESE FUNNEL. Clean, simple gadget for draining liquid from yogurt to produce all-natural creamy cheese that's high in calcium, & low in fat, sodium, etc. Spread on toast or make cheesecake or other recipes.